Praise for A *GOLDEN STATE OF MIND*

"Beautifully written... engaging and nostalgic...packed with tightly woven plot lines, dazzling imagery, and historical trivia"

BookReview.com
Fiction of the Month

✍

"Witty, colorful, intricately plotted, insightful commentary on California culture"

Robert K. Tanenbaum
New York Times best selling author for Simon & Schuster

✍

"Wong's sense of Berkeley barbed humor is only exceeded by his love and understanding of the California experience . . . . should be prerequisite reading for all Cal fans and alums"

Joe Kapp
Cal's last Rose Bowl quarterback and former NFL and CFL All-Pro great

✍

"Geoff Wong has done a fabulous job of melding collegiate peccadilloes, political and cultural clashes, embellished with his natural gift of wit."

Bette Vasquez, Host of Central Valley Chronicles,
KVIE - TV

✍

"A GOLDEN STATE OF MIND just drips of Californiana... handsome farm boy Jonathan Aldon's introduction to the real world in the form of a nonstop flood of California sights and early baby-boomer trivia. Every chapter or two seems to have another song from the time... detailed descriptions of just about every square inch of the Berkeley campus - all in a time far removed from today."

The Sacramento Bee

"Geoffrey Wong is a lawyer and a third-generation alumnus of the University of California - and he's a hell of a writer, depicting the flavor, the atmosphere, and the body of California in the 1950s. He writes with passion and remarkable insight about an Iowa boy who comes to UC (Berkeley, no less) with a motto floating through his head: 'Shit flies both ways!' It's the 1950s - San Francisco and environs is recalled through such fictional characters as Sam Paean (Herb Caen), the journalist who is always reaching for another cocktail while writing a daily column about San Francisco. Wong is very good with descriptions of people, writes with a delicate touch about folks from every way of life. Guess who they are. Aristocratic Dirk Krum, writer Joan Dildeaux ('Pale, skinny, and slump shouldered, Joan's plain looks were accentuated by acne.'); Congressman Muck (from HUAC); Professor Werner Von Seller (with his Germanic beliefs about losing battles but winning the war). There's the Black Panthers. The stirrings of proud gayness. This is a sprawling, affectionate loving tribute to a massively diverse California where the impossible is not only possible but also highly probable. Wong is a very good writer indeed, about people, the era, situations, and buildings. Chinatown: 'Restaurant windows were filled with tanks of live fish and freshly cooked poultry hanging from hooks.' His descriptions of gambling and Buddy Holly's glasses and girls are beautifully paced and plotted. A vivid portrait of San Francisco at the crowning height of its glory."

The Book Reader
Fall/Winter Issue, 2001 – 2002

✍

"Rich with the traditions and absurdities of college life, the advent of civil rights movement, and a smattering of '60's songs, the book provides a nostalgic look back at a time and place that has become legendary in American social history."

Cal Monthly Alumni Magazine

✍

"Berkeley of the late fifties and early sixties is a place of legend. Geoff Wong's novel, A GOLDEN STATE OF MIND, takes the reader into the chaos, fun, and myth with imagination and humor. For those who want to explore those remarkable times with one of the participants, I recommend Geoff Wong's new novel"

Steven Koblik
Former President, Reed College, UC Berkeley '63

GOLDEN DAZE

The Sequel to A Golden State of Mind

A NOVEL BY
GEOFFREY P. WONG

National Library of Canada Cataloguing in Publication Data

```
Wong, Geoffrey P.
       Golden daze / Geoffrey P. Wong.
Sequel to A golden state of mind.
ISBN 1-4120-01719-2
       I. Wong, Geoffrey P.  .  Golden state of mind.  II. Title.
PS3623 O54 G638 2003          813'.6      C2003-901719-2
```

TRAFFORD

This book was published *on-demand* in cooperation with Trafford Publishing.
On-demand publishing is a unique process and service of making a book available for retail
sale to the public taking advantage of on-demand manufacturing and Internet marketing.
On-demand publishing includes promotions, retail sales, manufacturing, order fulfilment,
accounting and collecting royalties on behalf of the author.

Suite 6E, 2333 Government St., Victoria, B.C. V8T 4P4, CANADA

Phone	250-383-6864	Toll-free	1-888-232-4444 (Canada & US)
Fax	250-383-6804	E-mail	sales@trafford.com
Web site	www.trafford.com	TRAFFORD PUBLISHING IS A DIVISION OF TRAFFORD HOLDINGS LTD.
Trafford Catalogue #03-0492		www.trafford.com/robots/03-0492.html

10   9   8   7   6   5   4   3   2

To every person who has ever bled Cal Blue and Gold,
especially the four generations of my family who have
been blessed with the University of California experience

Fiat Lux! Go Bears!

SPECIAL APPRECIATION

Grateful appreciation to the English gardeners who troweled the manuscript for grammatical weeds: Earl Wong, Lynda Welter, and Tac Craven

Thanks to Bob, Colleen, and the gang at Willow Creek Ranch who provided the sustenance and inspiration for the Lake Tahoe chapters.

GRATEFUL ACKNOWLEDGMENT IS MADE FOR THE USE OF THE FOLLOWING:

"Be My Baby" by Phil Spector-Ellie Greenwich-Jeff Barry
Phillies 116 (Mother Bertha-Trio BMI)

"Foolish Little Girl" by Miller-H. Greenfield, Scepter 1248
(Aldon BMI)

"Venus" by Ed Marshall, Chancellorr 1031 (Rambed-Jimskip
BMI)

1

PYRAMID SCHEME

From the pile of scribbled notes, he plucked the scarlet panties reeking of cheap perfume. Using an eye liner pencil, she had scrawled

*"For a REALLY good time, call HI 3-8202
- Love, Patty Ann."*

4 a.m. in The City That Knows How.

This was Sam Paean's most creative time - the hours before dawn - when this small, compact city, was at peace with herself, the quiet moments when Paean recaptured, with verve and wit, the gossipy news of his day's trek through the heart and soul of San Francisco: her saloons and restaurants.

The glare of the fluorescent lamp illuminated the day's treasure trove: crumpled cocktail napkins, tattered matchbook covers, crinkled business cards, and the autographed, red undies - all tidbits for Paean's popular gossip column, *"Sam's Paean to The City."*

Paean hunched over his manual typewriter, his sidekick he nicknamed the loyal Royal. Nearby, a smoldering Lucky Strike plopped a trail of white across a square, metal ashtray. From the hi-fi, Sinatra crooned, *"In The Wee Small Hours of the Morning."*

Paean slurped the last of the vodka martini, pausing before he began the two-fingered duet with the loyal Royal. He tapped the sides of his aquiline nose and closed his slightly, almond eyes. At age 43, his once full head of hair was retreating at an alarming rate.

A slight breeze ushered in the moonlight flooding his Russian Hill flat, caressing the still form on the cracked leather divan, his trusty assistant and new love of his life, E Lyn Chamberlin. Curled up asleep, childlike, E Lyn was still dressed in basic black, a pearl necklace, and nylons. A pair of high heels lay crisscrossed on the oriental throw rug.

Paean took a deep drag from the cigarette, retracing the events of the evening.

He and E Lyn had celebrated the one month anniversary of their budding romance at Bernie's, the posh restaurant, showcased in the recent Alfred Hitchcock movie. They had made the round of Paean's usual haunts - Jumbo's 369, Gold Street, and the Club Hungry U - searching for "eye-tems" for the column before arriving at Paean's favorite saloon, El Toreador, known to its regulars as El Toro.

El Toro's ebullient owner, Barnaby Person, emerged from a noisy huddle to greet them. A noted writer/painter and bull fight lover, Person was a ruggedly handsome man with dark-furrowed brows. He had a medium build and wore his signature silk ascot and two-toned wing tip shoes.

"Good to see you, Sam," Person bowed.

Turning to E Lyn, Person said in a smooth, low voice, "your new hair style and wardrobe are stunning."

He kissed E Lyn gently on the cheek and added, "getting rid of those awful glasses allows dirty old men - like me - the pleasure of fully appreciating your innate beauty."

Person cleared a path through the throng - past the life-size painting of the legendary Spanish bullfighter, Manolete and the sprawling mural of the Seville bullring - and seated them at a strategically located table, marked *"Reserved - Sam Paean Only,"* where Sam had an unobstructed view of the saloon entrance and the door to the Ladies Room.

"Should have been here earlier, Sam," Barnaby said, "you missed Ava, Tyrone, Tallulah, and Noel - the usual Hollywood riffraff."

Paean quickly surveyed the charged scene. The saloon was wall-to-wall with the usual spectrum of El Toro clientele: Montgomery Street business men flirting shamelessly with beautiful, cocktail waitresses and bored, martini-sipping society matrons, ogling the tight buns of El Toro's bus boys.

At the Long Bar, a sotted male patron wearing a maroon fez - probably a conventioneer from the Midwest - was enthralled by the ample charms of the celebrated beauty, Paulette Dubois, North Beach's most famous transvestite. The Shriner waved away puffs of smoke snorting from a mounted bull's head - unaware that bartender, Maui Maehara, manipulated a plastic tube hidden in the beast's nostrils. At the far end of the Long Bar, four brightly plumed macaws glowed in a glass aviary, squawking and whistling in self-defense against the din.

At the piano, George Shearing, in his dark glasses, jammed with his quintet, playing a Latin-jazz number. The bass player leaned forward and announced Paean's arrival. Turning, the blind pianist waved in the direction of Paean's table, as his left hand marched up the Steinway in his signature chords of 7ths and 9ths.

Turning to an adjoining table, Paean tapped the shoulder of the older of two males - a bearded man dressed in a safari jacket, with a tan that glowed in El Toro's peach colored lighting.

"*'Cuban Love Song'* your request, Papa?" Paean asked.

The bearded man leaned forward, taking Paean's hand in a firm grip, said, "Who else has a thing for Cuba?"

"What brings you to town, Papa?" Paean asked.

"Needed a short break from Havana," Papa said. "Been wrestling with a book based on my wild-ass youth in Paris in the 1920's."

"Got a title?" Paean asked, pulling out a small notebook from his breast pocket.

"Toying with '*A Moveable Feast.*' "

"Delicious reading, I'm sure," Paean said, making a notation.

"What's wrong with my suggestion, '*On The Road . In France*' "? the younger man said, looking up from a book that bore the title, "*Howl.*" He had dark hair, a clean shaven, handsome face and wore a tweedy sports jacket and a button-down dress shirt.

E Lyn's eyes grew wide, recognizing the pair of famous authors. It was one thing to hear Paean speak of the celebrities he drank with but another to see them in the flesh. Sitting at the next table were Ernest Hemingway and Jack Kerouac!

"May I ask them for autographs?" she whispered.

Paean shook his head "no."

"They value their privacy," he said "That's why they come to El Torro, where all inebriates - rich or poor - are treated equally."

Person appeared, toting a large, brown paper bag.

"Here you are, Sam," Person smiled. "The pile of scraps you call news. Hope there are printable nuggets buried in this pile of cow chips."

As Paean traded barbs with the two authors, E Lyn emptied the contents onto the table and began sifting, looking for printable "eye-tems." Most were marginally newsworthy. With disgust, she stuffed the red panties into the bottom of the bag.

How hard did Paean try fending off women on the make? E Lyn wondered. She quickly scolded herself. *Forget it. Don't be a pain in Paean's ass. Being a jealous female would be unhealthy to the romance.*

But there was an intriguing item she had set aside, and it was the one that now commanded Paean's attention.

The neatly printed message, on an El Toro cocktail napkin, read:

> *"Someone is buying up Chinatown property*
> *to build a 1000 foot pyramid-shaped office building."*

The teaser triggered a visceral response. For 22-years, as San Francisco's arbiter of good taste, Paean had led the fight against the incursion of high rises into the modest skyline of the city he had fondly dubbed Baghdad by the Bay. A 1000-foot office building, in the shape of a pyramid, would overwhelm the neoclassic charm of The City's tallest structure - 183-foot Hoyt Tower - sitting on Telegraph Hill and would be a monstrous incursion into Chinatown.

Since the Gold Rush, Chinese immigrants had hand-sculpted this small, romantic town onto the hills of this magical bay. In return, the Chinese had endured racial discrimination in long-suffering silence. Tourists loved the safe, alien quaintness of Chinatown, but the cruel reality was Chinatown was an exotic ghetto teeming with 40,000 immigrants eking out subsistence from sweat shop labor. The few prosperous Chinese were not permitted to buy homes among The City's fabled hills. The thought of uprooting Chinatown residents for a pyramid-shaped high rise revolted Paean.

Where would the displaced Chinese relocate?

Oakland? Gertrude Stein once said 'there was no there, there' and the East Bay city was already too crowded.

San Jose? Land was certainly cheaper, but that small city was still agricultural, with a paucity of housing to accommodate an influx of immigrants.

Sacramento? The small, hot, dusty capital city did not have suitable industry for unskilled labor.

Paean made a note to call on Chinatown's grande dame, Grant Avenue's dowager princess, Madame Lee. He had never met the reclusive Madame Lee - nor had any other Caucasian - but her influence was well documented. Her word controlled all issues affecting the welfare of Chinatown. Colorful stories abounded of how Madame Lee, a woman in a male-dominated culture, had acquired such power and prestige. Paean envisioned a beautiful mysterious woman, resembling the silent screen actress Anna May Wong attired in a full length, silk *cheong sam,* with a mandarin collar, sculptured over a regal figure.

Madame Lee had answered prior entreaties from Paean, responding in formal letters written on red parchment, in black, formal script, he assumed was written by an American-educated secretary.

Paean padded across the room to mix another martini for inspiration. Passing E Lyn, he gently spread over her dozing form, a blue and gold blanket bearing the seal of the University of California, a gift from Cal Professor Aristotle Scott.

Returning to the Royal, Paean glimpsed the first rays of morning peaking over the Big C of Berkeley's eastern rugged foothills, illuminating the majestic bell tower, the Campanile.

After dragging one last puff from the dying Lucky Strike and draining the martini in one sustained gulp, Paean began the two-finger exercise, on the loyal Royal, that produced the fount of his existence, *"Sam's Paean to The City."*

His lead "eye-tem" began with the familiar three dot-dot-dot intro:

> *". . . Who's behind the secret skyline*
> *disaster schemed for Chinatown?"*

2

C OF TROUBLES

"Whatever happened to the sacred, hallowed halls of ivy?" Ari Scott asked of his three colleagues sipping brandy before the crackling fire of the Great Hall of the Men's Faculty Club.

Aristotle Scott, Professor of Philosophy, was deeply tanned with blond hair streaked with salt and pepper. His frame was taut, befitting a gold medal winner in the metric mile who doubled as Cal's track coach. Age 44, Ari Scott still bore matinee idol looks that made coed hearts flutter. Only furrows creeping across his brow hinted at the recent trauma of his convoluted life.

"Hells bells, Scotty," Garrick Nelquist said, emptying ashes from his meerschaum. "If it isn't one form of bull shit, it's another."

Garrick Nelquist, Professor of Political Science, had slicked-back hair and a thin, manicured moustache. He wore a tweed suit, underscoring his Anglophile preferences that did little to camouflage his rough-and-tumble youth as a collegiate boxer.

Since 1902, the Men's Faculty Club had been a bastion of male collegiality perched atop a shady knoll along the banks of Strawberry Creek, guarded by oaks and coastal redwood. The Club was a mixture of Gothic and Mission design. Above exterior walls of natural-colored, sand plaster, rows of slanting red Mission tiles of the gabled roof sheltered the upper floor's redwood shingles. Below, iridescent azaleas and rhododendrons marked a footpath to the Men's Faculty Club entry.

Inside, flames from the matte-glazed fireplace flickered shadows of mythical creatures against the steeply pitched ceiling. Along the north-south walls, twelve dragon heads carved into protruding trellises guarded ten shields fashioned from leaded glass. Each shield bore the insignia of a major university: Army, Brown, California, Cornell, and Oxford on one side squared off with the symbols of Princeton, Yale, Harvard, Columbia, and Stanford.

Nelquist read aloud a headline from the *Daily Californian* newspaper:

"William Randolph *Chandler To Speak At Cal.*
WRC Will Advocate Publish Or Perish"

"When was the last time a gubernatorial candidate risked public ridicule by showing his face on campus?" Nelquist said.

"Chandler's no fool," Jacob Aural said, caressing a brandy snifter. "He may think his speech will provoke a riot that will galvanize public support for publish or perish. Right, Sandy?"

The seeing-eye dog barked at the sound of her name.

Professor of English Jacob Aural wore dark glasses and a black, three-piece suit. His long, wispy hair was ghostly white.

"Publish or perish," Nelquist said. "What if Chandler crams that death, by paper, down our throats?" His voice trailed off as an ashen log tilted, in a shower of sparks.

Publish or perish was a transparent attack on academic tenure which protected full-time professors from arbitrary dismissals. Requiring faculty members to publish an annual work of "academic merit" would force professors to spend more time researching and writing and less time teaching. If implemented, Cal would be transformed from a university renowned for its independent, diverse, liberal education to that of a government controlled research institution.

"Teaching at Cal is like running a gauntlet," Roderick Seakin, the fourth member of the group said. "As a track man, Ari is quick enough to dodge the slings and arrows of outrageous fortune," Seakin said, borrowing a phrase from Hamlet, "but we slow-footed academic types are doomed to be punching bags for politicos."

Professor of Science Roderick Seakin was tall, big-boned, and lanky, with a long, angular face and a thick mat of silver hair, Seakin was a popular professor who delivered dramatic lectures disguised as famous scientists. Today, for a lecture on the theory of evolution, Seakin attired in a white, shaggy beard and a baggy, rumpled suit was Charles Darwin.

Ari winced at Seakin's reference to slings and arrows, as he retraced, in his mind, how outrageous fortune had thrown his orderly life into chaos.

Fall had begun with the arrival of two people inextricably tied to his past. One was his previously unknown daughter, Anna, fathered out-of-wedlock by his youthful, love affair with beautiful Olympic Italian swimmer, Sofia Cappuccino. The reunion with his long lost daughter now, a Cal graduate student, had been a godsend but also politically explosive, as her stepfather, Pablo Zarzana, a Communist, was the new Prime Minister of Italy.

The other was Ari's former Olympic teammate, Clayborn Muck, a determined rival for Sofia's affection during the 1936 Olympics. Muck had sworn vengeance against Ari for winning Sofia's heart. In September, Congressman Clayborn Muck - Chairman of the powerful House Un-American Activities Committee (HUAC) - had scheduled televised hearings to "uncover subversive elements of the Cal faculty." Ari and Garrick Nelquist had been on the top of Muck's list.

The potential scandal from Anna's paternity had been defused with the help of San Francisco gossip columnist, Sam Paean's discovery of a dark secret about Muck's henchman, HUAC Chief Investigator, Seymour Graft. The public revelation of Graft's past had derailed the hearings and prompted Muck to hastily move HUAC's anti-Communist crusade to Hollywood "to uncover and expose elements of the far flung Communist conspiracy within the movie industry."

On the domestic front, Ari had not been so fortunate. After revealing Anna's paternity to his socialite wife, Cee Cee, she had spirited their two young children, Marcus and Monique, from their Piedmont home, to the protective cocoon of her father's mansion in San Francisco. The added complication was that his ex-father-in-law, William Randolph Chandler, better known as WRC, was a candidate for Governor of California.

WRC had hired a high-priced lawyer for his daughter's divorce, an aggressive young attorney, Marvin Belly, who was asking the court to deny Ari child visitation rights, on the grounds that fathering Anna out-of-wedlock was evidence of Ari's alleged moral turpitude.

Divorce was such an extreme measure, Ari thought, a rarity, even as the promised enlightenment of the 1960's lay just two months away.

"How will it feel working for your ex-father-in-law, Ari?" Seakin said, asking the question on the mind of his colleagues. "Makes teaching here a bit sticky, I suspect."

If elected Governor, WRC would also be Chairman of the Board of California Regents, the quartet's boss.

"Sticky, murky, awkward; all the above," Ari said.

The faculty had been shocked when WRC running on a platform of fervent patriotism, had easily won the party nomination, promising to "eradicate the influence of Left Wing professors on our vulnerable youth."

"WRC's sweet revenge for our beating Muck and HUAC," Nelquist said. "He and Muck are cut from the same shitty cloth, but Chancellor Haynes won't put up with that publish or perish crap."

"Haynes may not be able to stop him," Ari said. "The Chancellor serves at the will of the Regents. If Haynes bucks him, WRC will have him fired."

Smiling beneath his dark glasses, Aural said, "If we have to publish or perish, I've got an easy assignment for myself. How about '*The Ten Greatest Rumanian Soliloquies Published in Braille?*' That should take a half page with no bibliography, right, Sandy?"

The dog barked twice.

"Here's a Poli Sci project for you, Garrick," Seakin said, a rivulet of perspiration oozing from under his white toupee. How about' *The Politics of Academic Dung - Shoveling Shit and Eating It Too!*' Should boost you into the best seller list."

Ari joined the exercise in forced mirth. "With your theatrical flair, Roderick, you could publish '*The Voracious Sex Lives of Horney Amoeba.'* "

"Touche, gentlemen," Seakin said, twirling his brandy snifter in his hands. "Any chance this is a joke, a cruel hoax? Could WRC just be posturing for the campaign?"

"Fat chance," Ari said, shaking his head. He knew his ex-father-in-law all too well. "Once WRC gets a bug up his butt, he won't give up until he has his way."

"Bug up his butt?" Aural said. "For a man of philosophy, Professor Aristotle Scott, you surely have a way with rectal metaphors!"

"Count me in for another fight," Nelquist said. "They'll have to fire my ass first. I won't be forced out by 'Governor' William Randolph

Chandler."

"You know our answer,"Aural said. "Sandy and I can always panhandle pencils on Telly." He was referring to the nickname for Telegraph Avenue, the main campus thoroughfare. "I can use that pewter cup from the Fulbright people. Knew it would be good for something practical someday."

"I missed all the excitement you three generated taking on Muck and HUAC," Seakin said. "I'm getting too old to change schools, so it looks as if Cal will be my academic Alamo," Seakin winked. "If we're going to be canned, let's go out with a bang, a big one, like the atomic scientists are always mumbling about."

Aural rose purposely, "A toast to us, gentlemen." He made a sweeping gesture with his glass in a slow semi-circle.

"To us," the others echoed.

The quartet drained the last of their brandies.

"To the Four Musketeers!" Professor Roderick Seakin said, sailing his snifter into the hearth.

"To our glorious academic future and Sandy's too," Professor Jacob Aural said, pitching his glass underhanded in the direction of the fire, Sandy barked twice in concurrence.

"Let's kick ass," Professor Garrick Nelquist said, hurtling his missile side-armed into the deep recesses of the fireplace.

"Go Bears!" Professor Aristotle Scott shouted, throwing his glass at the fiery image of William Randolph Chandler, glowering in the center of the roaring conflagration.

3

FIAT LUX

The light was blinding, but Jonathan Aldon could not summon the strength to close his eyes. His eyelids were immobile, paralyzed eye sockets splayed open by invisible forceps.

"Relax, do not fight it. Let it come to you," the soothing Latin-accented voice said - the kind of voice his mother would have described as sounding like the romantic movie, leading man, Caesar Romero. "Focus on how the swinging light spins and rotates."

From the blackness beyond, a radio softly played the Nat King Cole ballad, *"It's Magic."*

In a blurry field of illumination, a brilliant sparkling sphere swung in a low arc, spinning on its axis. Swinging and spinning, spinning and swinging. The numerals 2, 7 . . . 2, 7 . . . flashed repeatedly in his mind's eye. 2, 7 – 27, the negative number of grade points, Jonathan had fallen, in his mid-term exams – 27, the number of grade points, above a C, he would have to attain to avoid flunking out of Cal.

Jonathan felt the tension in his eyes evaporate as he followed the path of the dazzling comet in its smooth arc, like the comforting tick-tock, tick-tock of the swinging pendulum of the grandfather clock guarding the front door of the Aldon home in Clear Lake, Iowa.

"Breathe deeply and let your mind slip beyond the rhythm of the light. You are adrift, not quite awake, not quite asleep," the Latin-accented voice said, "Your lids are heavy, very heavy. They want to close, but they cannot because you have begun your journey, Jonathan, one that will free your senses. As you enter your subconscious, you will encounter many feelings, many thoughts, and many memories. Do not be afraid, as they will quickly pass."

Jonathan was floating. The opaque light gave way to dim, burnished colors, as images appeared, then dissolved. There was no up or down, no front or rear, only the vague sensation of weightlessness.

Spinning pulsating light, the suspended, orbiting glass ball at the Clear Lake High Graduation Party flashing white, diamond patterns on the banner splashed across the gymnasium:

"Happy Trails, Clear Lake Class of 1959!"

Jonathan was dancing with his co-valedictorian, Dawna Plumber. For this, his last day of high school, Jonathan was wearing the dark green, shark-skin suit, button-down white shirt, and one-inch wide, olive-colored tie Mother had purchased in Minneapolis.

Dawna was tall, thin, her dark brown hair in bangs. Thick bi-focal glasses made her blue eyes bug like an insect. She wore a layered, pink, bare shouldered, chiffon dress.

Jonathan leaned against Dawna, lightheaded from the beer he had shared with his boyhood friend, Ziggy Atherton, in the boys cloak room.

From the hi-fi, actor Tab Hunter, was warbling "Young Love," the only popular song Jonathan's mother approved. With his blond, close-cropped hair and bright blue eyes, Jonathan was, in the words of his mother, "Tab Hunter handsome."

"So, you're going to Berkeley," Dawna whispered. "I'll miss competing with you." She smelled strongly of a Max Factor fragrance his mother had received, as a free sample in the mail.

Dawna pressed herself tightly against his body. Jonathan could feel her full, firm breasts.

Strange, he thought. I never knew Dawna had big boobs.

He looked, through her thick lenses and deeply into her blue eyes. Dawna would be cute, if she didn't wear those glasses, he thought.

"Maybe, we can get together, Jonathan," she said. "Stanford's not far from Berkeley, only 40 miles." Dawna was the only other member of the Clear Lake High Senior Class going away to college.

"I always thought we had so much in common," Dawna said,

pulling Jonathan's left hand down against her right breast.

Surprised, he tried to remove his hand.

"Don't, Jonathan. That feels so-o-o good," Dawna cooed, flicking her tongue against his ear lobe.

Jonathan blushed as he felt a sudden bulge in his pants.

At the end of the dance, he rejoined his carrot-topped buddy, Ziggy, who flashed his best Alfred E. Newman grin.

"I saw you cop a feel off Dawna Plumber, you snake," Ziggy said, lowering his voice. "Are her boobs as big as her IQ?"

The Latin-accented voice intruded Jonathan's reverie.

"You will soon enter the recesses of your subconsciousness. That is where your instruction will begin." The voice of Michael Hu, the Living Buddha, was comforting, like invisible warm water gently lapping over his mind.

"In two hours, I will return to escort you back from the deep," Living Buddha said. "Do not be afraid. Listen carefully to the voices of your tutors. Each will convey important knowledge for your academic survival."

The fireworks began in the near horizon, flashing, burning, dimming slowly, finally trailing off as a glowing ember. The events of the past few months exploded, then faded before him. In the distance, he heard his buddy Ziggy's voice echoing over and over their childhood motto, *"shit flies both ways."*

The sensations of memory faded into the light, as Jonathan felt himself touch down on something soft and comforting. Then a series of familiar voices: Pimply-faced Dick Phuncque spewing chemistry equations; Ollie Punch, his wandering eye spinning furiously, breaking down the precepts of rhetoric. He could feel Royal French's 6-foot-9 inch frame hunched over him, espousing theories of warfare for his ROT-C class. Waz, in his New Jersey brogue, waxing eloquent on the reading list of Professor Jacob Aural's English class. Super Sleuth outlining the important political theories of Professor Garrick Nelquist's Poli Sci course. In the distance, he heard the voice of his roommate, Butch Tanenbloom, urging his tutors on.

Michael Hu withdrew from the circle of jabbering tutors and assumed a squatting, cross-legged yoga position. Living Buddha slowly entwined the egg-shaped, clear crystal orb with the single strand of silk thread, placing the brilliant object back into its velvet pouch. This had been the first occasion, since enrolling at Cal, Living Buddha had used his powers of hypnosis.

Like riding a bicycle, Living Buddha told himself, *once you master the technique, you never forget.*

Living Buddha had a medium build and an oval face with hooded, dark brown almond eyes that made it difficult to tell whether he was awake or asleep.

These crazy Dormies, Living Buddha thought, closing his eyes in meditation. *Why won't they accept their karma, their destiny? Why must they strive for things that were not meant to be?*

Jonathan Aldon was odd, Living Buddha thought. *It was shocking that Jonathan had chosen disinheritance by his parents, the largest hog farmers in Iowa, to defy them. The misguided freshman had rejected his destiny of inheriting the family wealth and was now poorer than any of the middle-class residents of Dooch Dorm. This was illogical nonsense.*

You cannot deny your destiny, Living Buddha thought. *Jonathan, may overcome his academic problems, but he will never survive the rejection of his destiny.*

This must be something unique to the middle-class, Living Buddha concluded. *Yes, this California middle-class with its alien notion that higher education can magically change one's destiny was strange but appealing.*

Destiny.

How different Living Buddha's life would have been without destiny. Destiny blessing Grandfather Hu so long ago. Yes, without destiny, life would have no order, no stability.

It was 1912, after the fall of the Manchu Dynasty when western powers, Britain, France, and Germany, poured into the fledgling Chinese Republic dividing up regions of China for economic development. Count Von Stroheim Krupp was one of the first German capitalists into China, establishing a base along Shanghai's tree-lined Bund overlooking the Huangpu River.

The Count's contribution to Chinese society was the introduction of menthol cigarettes to poor Chinese whose only affordable vice was smoking.

For 20-years, Grandfather Hu, who learned to speak fluent German, had been Count Krupp's faithful servant, his secret confidant. When the Count died, he bequeathed the world-wide patent for converting spearmint to menthol to his loyal servant Hu.

Michael was the only male grandchild, born during the Japanese occupation of WW II, but the Hu's had fulfilled their destiny - aided by the Count's largesse - becoming one of the richest families in China

After the war, the Hu's and other Chinese capitalists sided with Generalissimo Chiang Kai-Shek in the Chinese Civil War, pitting Chiang's Nationalists against Mao Tse Tung's Communists. When the Communists triumphed, the Nationalists and most of their capitalist supporters fled to the safety of Taiwan.

But the Hu's had a different destiny. They sought haven in Brazil where they owned and farmed thousands of acres of spearmint leaves harvested and converted to menthol for cigarettes, using the patented process Count Krupp had bequeathed to Grandfather Hu.

Michael's destiny was clear: to manage the Hu empire and return to China when the populace tired of the austere rule of Chairman Mao.

In Brazil, the future Living Buddha learned to speak Portugese and English, in addition to his family's Shanghai Mandarin. He accompanied Grandfather and Father Hu to the former slave trading port of Salvador, in the Brazilian state of Bahia. There, while the elder Hu's supervised the shipping of spearmint to American tobacco companies, Michael roamed the streets of the dilapidated, 17th century neighborhood of Pelourinho, mingling with the descendants of African slaves, learning ancient skills, including hypnosis, the black art Brazilians called "the brilliant light of knowledge," the same technique he had performed on Jonathan this evening.

From Brazil, the Hu's had witnessed the rise of American economic power. Destiny decreed that the Michael should have an American college education. Harvard and Yale required generous donations as the price of admission. Spurning what seemed to be Ivy League solicitations for bribes, the Hu's sent Michael to Berkeley, the distinguished public university, Cal, the best educational bargain in the world.

Father Hu had warned Michael to mind his studies, not to be distracted by inferior American values. But, after moving into Dooch Dorm, Michael had discovered something appealing about the Dormies, a naive charm in their shared belief that a Cal education would change their lives and fortunes.

Now named Living Buddha, Michael Hu watched, with amusement, the Dormies' competition with their across-the-street rivals, the wealthy boys of the P U fraternity. It seemed so futile, a waste of time and energy. Yet, the Dormies' boundless spirit and optimism was appealing.

What if the Dormies were right? What if a Cal education could change one's destiny? he wondered.

It was a concept contrary to everything he had been taught. As much as he enjoyed his American classmates, he was saddened by the certainty they were misguided.

No, he thought, *a Cal degree could never change destiny. Dormies were doomed to second-class citizenship, always a notch below the destiny of the wealthy, like their rivals, the P U's.*

But his Cal experience had instilled in Living Buddha something new: the ability to keep an open mind. So, he would watch what destiny had in store for these sons of the middle-class, these Dormies.

If a Cal education could affect one's destiny, then this revolutionary phenomenon would be worth witnessing . . . and blessing.

GOOD NEWS, BAD NEWS

"Papa, I have exciting news for you!"

On a bright, November day, Professor Ari Scott and his daughter, Anna Cappuccino, sat at Patty B's, a popular outdoor café on Telly. Since their introduction in September, they had met once-a-week to compare notes on the progress of their respective lives: Anna, as a Cal graduate student and Ari, as the estranged husband of Cee Cee Chandler Scott.

"Yes, Anna?" Ari said, sipping a cappuccino, the drink steamed from the coffee machine Anna's grandfather had invented.

Ari studied the features of his daughter. Anna had the same jet black hair, olive complexion, large, dark eyes, and exotically beautiful face as her mother, Sofia. Despite her conservative dress, it was impossible to ignore the voluptuous figure Anna had also inherited from Sofia.

"Papa, I am so happy for you and Mama," Anna said.

"For both of us?"

"Mama is coming to visit me," Her eyes were now pleading ". . . and you."

Ari felt light-headed, almost faint.

Sofia, at Cal? What would he say? How would he avoid being a mass of amorphous Jello?

"And what of your stepfather?" Ari held his breath, hoping against hope that Sofia would be coming alone.

"Pablo will be coming too," Anna said. "He will deliver his first speech on American soil, in Sproul Plaza."

Ari was gripped by competing emotions, the flush of excitement he had not felt for years, the chance to see the love of his life, and the dread of meeting Sofia's husband, Pablo Zarzana

Tears welled up in Ari's eyes. "How does Pablo feel about your mother seeing me after all these years?"

"Pablo is wonderful, Papa. He knows all about the *toure di amore* you and Mama shared. You will like him."

"There is more exciting news," Anna said.

Ari dabbed his eyes with a hankie and smiled "I don't know if I can stand any more excitement."

Anna's eyes flashed the same way her mother had when he had proposed marriage during their *toure di amore*. She squeezed Ari's hands tightly in hers.

"Papa, I have met the most wonderful boy," she said. "I would like you to meet him before Mama and Pablo arrive."

"Who is the lucky young man?" Ari asked, wondering what ordinary Cal student worthy of his lovely daughter's heart.

"His name is Jericho Slabio," Anna said, smiling.

Ari felt a sudden stabbing sensation in his chest. "'Save-The-World' Slabio, leader of the Guerillas For Free Speech?"

"Yes, Papa, one and the same!" Anna said, giggling like a happy, school girl.

Ari closed his eyes, feeling the onset of nausea. Jericho "Save-The-World" Slabio was a campus radical who constantly attacked the Cal administration. In his public harangues, Slabio advocated overthrowing the University "to cleanse the world of the military-industrial cabal controlling student lives."

Although Ari shared some of Slabio's political views - opposition to publish or perish - Ari could not accept Slabio's strident call for violence as a means to justify the ends. Slabio's rhetoric had incited a few incidents, but the number of students involved were small which, in police parlance, constituted only "disturbances."

The crowd for Pablo Zarzana's speech will be huge, Ari thought, *drawn by the charisma of the handsome, silver-haired Italian leader. The occasion would be perfect for Slabio and his Guerillas for Free Speech to incite a riot that would undermine Pablo's appearance.*

"Yes, your young man is quite well known," Ari said. "I've heard him speak in Sproul Plaza."

"So, you understand why I find him so fascinating, Papa. Jericho is so intelligent and passionate. He reminds me of . . ." Anna caught herself in the *faux pas*. Her face turned a bright scarlet.

"He reminds you of your stepfather, Pablo," Ari said, finishing the sentence for her. "Don't be embarrassed, darling. I'm not offended."

"Oh, Papa, you will love Jericho. I have told him so much about you and how important you are in my life. Will you meet with him?"

"How about Saturday?" Ari said, half-heartedly

"I think the two of you would get to know each other better, if I weren't present," Anna said.

So traditionally Italian, Ari thought. *Anna has fallen for this guy but wants my independent approval.*

"May I invite Garrick?" Ari said. "I think he would like to meet your famous boyfriend."

"I'd love to have Uncle Garrick meet him, too," Anna said. "The two of you can show Jericho your famous Pub Crawl." She issued a deep, throaty laugh that sounded so much like her mother.

Am I being a hypocrite? Ari wondered.

Throughout his teaching career, he had advocated the right of students to free speech. Now that his daughter had become infatuated with the radical Cal firebrand, was he now compromising his values because of petty jealousy for the new man in Anna's life?

I must be careful not to hurt Anna's feelings, Ari thought. *Remain fair. Keep an open mind. Garrick will help. Garrick is hard-nosed, yet kind and thoughtful. Garrick will steer me along the fine line between overly protective father and a loving one.*

For Anna's sake, I had better, he thought.

PRETENDERS TO THE THRONE

"Roomie, you're a brand new woman!"

Kate Howell's voice was comforting, almost reassuring, amid the noxious fumes of the chemical ingredients of the hair permanent kit.

Joan Dildeaux squinted at her own reflection in the full-length mirror. Hovering behind were the blurry images of her three, Gee Dee sorority sisters who had orchestrated the transformation.

"You look super, Dil-dee," Muffy Peachwick said.

"Absolutely," Dandy Cane added.

Wielding scissors and dabbing solution, Kate had fashioned Joan a pixie hairdo. Muffy had created a new face, applying makeup, eye shadow, and the latest lipstick shade. Dandy had given Joan a manicure and a pedicure. The make-over was completed with a spiffy, new outfit the trio had purchased for Joan from Dyan Miller's House of Fashion. The goal: to transform Joan Dildeaux, the homely, Gee Dee legacy, into an Audrey Hepburn look-a-like.

"Have a closer look," Dandy said, handing Joan her glasses.

Joan pirouetted slowly, examining the image of the "new woman." Her skin was no longer pale. Her acne was now camouflaged by makeup. The new outfit disguised her skinny, slump-shouldered figure.

Eye shadow and lipstick do add an aura of sophistication, Joan thought. *And, if I don't smile, I can hide my braces.*

"Thanks for the try, gang; but it's no use," Joan sighed, staring intently at the one feature no amount of make-over could hide.

"With my buggy, crossed-eyes, I'll never be beautiful like you."

"No, you look terrific, Joanie," Kate said.

"Really, Dil-dee," Muffy said.

"Tons better," Dandy echoed.

"Do you really think so?" Joan said, in a prayer-like whisper.

"YES!" the trio shouted, embracing the legacy.

The beautification project had been prompted by Joan's nomination as candidate for Campus Snow Queen.

I really hope Joanie is elected, Kate thought. *It would do wonders for her self-confidence.*

The Gee Dee sorority was renown for beautiful girls, and Joanie was the House of Beauty's lone exception. The *Daily Californian* had dubbed Joan's best friend and roommate, Kate Howell, the Golden Goddess, after Kate had swept five campus beauty contests in her freshman year. Muffy Peachwick, with her well-endowed figure and adventuresome attitude toward sex, had a legion of male admirers. Cute freshman pledge, Dandy Cane, was never lacking for male attention.

As a legacy, Joan Dildeaux suffered the pox of plain looks. She had been asked to join only because her mother had been a member of the sorority in the 1930's. The fact that Kate was Joan's best friend had aggravated her insecurities. For three years, the two roommates had been dubbed by snickering fraternity boys, as "beauty and the beast."

The unlikely nomination of Joan had resulted from the quartet's campaign to convince the Gee Dees to show their appreciation to their down-the-street neighbors, the Dormies, for persuading Oakland, rock and roll band, Big Berry and the Blackouts, to perform at the Gee Dee's Presents Party. The band had been the first Negro group to perform at a Cal social event and had turned a traditionally staid party into a rollicking, rolling success that was still the talk of the campus.

"Remember who you are and what you represent" was the motto of the House of Beauty, and the Gee Dee seniors had opposed the hiring of Big Berry and the Blackouts and wanted nothing to do with Kate's shocking suggestion of joining non-Greek fraternity boys, disparagingly referred to as "non-orgs," in a campus event.

To discredit Kate, the seniors had withheld their support unless Joan were the Gee Dee candidate for Campus Snow Queen. The seniors reasoned that this would be a signal to other Greeks that the nomination of Joan, the legacy, and the alliance with the Dormies must surely be a joke, as homely Joan's candidacy was surely doomed, especially where her running mate was the Dormie hunchback dwarf, Hunch Hitowski!

But Kate and her band of conspirators had other ideas. If Joan and Hunch were elected Campus Snow King and Snow Queen, it would signal the beginning of something new and positive. No longer would a girl be judged merely by her looks. No longer would a coed be shackled by physical beauty, denied the opportunity to be accepted for her intelligence and talent. It was a radical idea, but it was an idea whose time had come.

"Smile for *Life* magazine, Dil-dee," Muffy said, aiming a Brownie Hawkeye camera at the new woman. "We'll make this your official, Campus Snow Queen contest portrait."

"Wait," Dandy said, "we forgot the tiara." She plucked a silver crown fashioned from cardboard and tin foil and placed it gently on Joan's new hairdo.

"Ok, Roomie," Kate urged. "Give us your best Royal smile."

As Muffy flashed an entire roll of black and white film, Kate noticed Joan fighting back tears with a pursed lips-smile that concealed the flashing metal of her braces.

Can't wait to share this moment with Casey, Kate thought. *Yes, Casey Lee is the only male who would understand what this moment means to me.*

* * * *

"So, my little, humpback bell-ringing pal, do you think you'll be less a freak by running for Campus Snow King?" Ollie Punch said. "All you'll do is give the frat rat candidates a few laughs."

Ollie Punch was short and round with a husky frame supported by spindly legs. His wandering left eye spun at a rate directly correlated to his emotional state.

"Ollie, the Campus Snow King contest will be a lot of fun," Hunch Hitowski said. "Maybe we'll meet some nice girls, too." Hunch smiled, rubbing his claw-like hands together. "Girls aren't always impressed by handsome looks."

"For average freaks like you and me," Punch said, "we'll never have a chance with the broads." His wandering, left eye accelerated.

The ceiling of Hunch and Punch's Dooch Dorm room was festooned with stalactites of bent handles, ruptured wire and tattered shards, remnants of their testing of the aerial dynamics of umbrellas. Marking their respective sides of the room, Hunch displayed a picture of Cal's 309 foot tall bell tower, the Campanile while, on the other side, Punch displayed a 6-by-4 foot photograph of his favorite blond movie star, Suzette Mew Mew.

Aerial dynamics involved Hunch and Punch jumping off the third floor balcony with an open umbrella, testing its tensile strength. If the umbrella disintegrated during the jump, the trip to the ground took two seconds. If the umbrella did not collapse, the flight lasted as long as six seconds. The four second difference in flight time between an inferior umbrella and one with superior aerial dynamics was the difference between a hard and a smooth landing.

"Hah!" Punch barked. "Casey Lee and Royal French are wetting their pants, crowing about what a great social coup it was for the Gee Dees to name one of their own, as your partner, but look who those pretties put up!"

Casey Lee was President of Dooch, leader of the Dormies. Royal French, an army veteran of a secret war in Indo-China, his chief adviser.

"That ugly Joan Dildeaux!" Punch said, his left eye now spinning furiously. "You don't see the House of Beauty nominating the Golden Goddess, that horny Muffy Peachwick, or any of their cute freshman pledges. Screw the social precedence bull shit! Pushing Dildeaux as your partner is a half-assed gesture."

"Things always work out for the best, Ollie."

"Cut the Pollyanna goodie two shoes crap," Punch snapped.

Of the 50 sets of Dormie roommates, the pairing of Ollie Punch and Hunch Hitowski was easily the oddest. Their disparate personalities made Dormies wonder how Hunch could stand sharing the same space with Punch.

What others did not know was that the pair had shared parallel childhoods. Both were born to poor, but proud families who saw a Cal degree as a way for their son to escape his physical handicap.

At age three, Ollie Punch was tottering in the backyard when an errant arrow, fired by a neighborhood teen, struck him squarely in the left eye. Emergency surgery saved Punch's life, but he lost the eye. The Punch family was second generation, Salinas Valley, lettuce-picking, row croppers who could not afford a prosthetic eye for their son.

In grammar school, while other children played "Ollie, Ollie, Oxen-

Free," Ollie suffered the taunts of "Ollie, Ollie Punch can't see!"

The young Punch squinted his missing eye socket shut, a habit that helped him become a marbles champion. At 12, while tallying the day's winnings, Punch noticed the shattered remains of a cheap marble a competitor had wagered. The imitation or "immie" had exploded when Punch struck it squarely with his favorite Taw.

Something about the shard intrigued him. He held it up to the light of a bare bulb. It was translucent plastic and blue, a close match to the hue of his good eye.

He had an idea.

Using a scouring pad, Punch carefully sanded the rough edges of the immie. He rubbed the plastic shard for hours, smoothing it down to a thin, pliant sliver he could easily insert into the milky void of his empty socket.

The color of the fake eye was a perfect match for his other eye. However, there was a complication. The presence of a foreign object convulsed his eye muscles into twitches sending the new eye into an elliptical orbit around the edges of the eye socket.

Eight years later, Ollie Punch had become fatalistic about the unwanted attention his wandering eye commanded.

Far better the distraction of a wandering eye than the horrified stare of someone repulsed by the sight of a milky, white void, he reasoned.

As a teenager, Punch developed a hostile attitude against the curious gaze of people staring at his wandering eye.

Humiliate instead of praise, he thought. *Attack before others can hurt you.*

For those who indelicately stared at his fake eye, Punch had perfected an effective retort. He popped the former immie out of the socket, handed it to the offender, and bellowed, "suck on this."

"What do you think, Ollie. Looks rather becoming, eh?" Hunch had donned a red and white velour Santa's cap at a jaunty angle.

"Look at yourself," Punch said, grasping his roommate's rounded back, and shoving his face close to the mirror. "You look ridiculous, absolutely pitiful."

"I look like one of Santa's elves," Hunch said, smiling at his image.

For Hunch Hitowski, his deformities were accidents of birth.

During the Depression, Hunch's father left Chicago's Polish

neighborhood for the promise of work in California. Uneducated and unskilled, Hugo Hitowski became a manual laborer for United Oil, a Los Angeles oil drilling company.

Hugo married Juana Martinez, the beautiful, young Mexican maid of the owners of United Oil. The Hitowskis had six children, the first five, all girls - Juanita, Ramona, Estrelita, Rosa, and Carmen - were grown and married before a son arrived. Julio was the family favorite, born with an active, inquisitive mind, but burdened with the birth defects of dwarfism: rounded, hunched shoulders and small, claw-like hands.

In grammar school, classmates shunned him, calling him "little humpback." Julio spent hours alone in the family back yard, swinging deftly on a rope hanging from an oak tree and playing tunes on a small xylophone, talents that later would help him become Cal's Campanile carillonneur.

"Everyone is freaky in his own way," Hunch said. "We've got to do a better job at helping others see through the obvious and get to the real important stuff," he said, placing a fist over his heart.

"I think you've got your head and heart up your ass, roomie,"Punch said. His tone turned somber. "I just don't want you getting harassed and hurt by running for Campus Snow King."

"Ollie, let's make a deal. If I'm elected Campus Snow King, you promise we'll find a couple of nice girls and double date."

In their two years at Cal, neither of them had been out on a date.

Punch's wandering eye slowed to a leisurely pace. "Hunch, if you're elected Campus Snow King, I'll line up the broads, even if I have to dole cash out for a couple of ladies from Yearning Arms."

"Punch, that would cost a fortune."

"Not the usual stuff," Punch said."Couple of those Yearning Arms babes would be happy to make an easy ten bucks having coffee with us on Telly. No-sweat for them, and no social pressure for Dooch's two freaks."

"Yes," Hunch said, "That would be great! Here's to our double dating with the ladies!"

Better this way, Punch thought. *No expectations. No failures. No heartbreaks.*

* * * *

Across the street, at the Pi Upsilon fraternity, others were sharing a different interpretation of the candidacy of Joan Dildeaux and Hunch Hitowski for Campus Snow King and Queen.

"Chauncey, you are a genius," Dirk Krum said, admiring the front page headline of tomorrow's *Daily Californian.*

Dirk Krum III was President of the P U fraternity and leader of the Inter Fraternity Council, a powerful association of 57 Cal fraternities, the largest Greek system in America. He was dark-haired, with the well chiseled looks of a male model. Krum wore the standard IFC campus wardrobe of a button-down white shirt, black slacks, white socks, and black penny loafers.

A smile - part sneer, part smirk - crept across his handsome face, as held up the banner headline.

"UNHOLY ALLIANCE: GEE DEES AND DORMIES!"

"A fuggin' genius, Chauncey," Chip Fist said, snapping his fingers in approval.

Chip Fist was Dirk's roommate, a 6-foot-4-inch, 250 pound football player whose belly, nurtured by a steady diet of Hamms beer, ballooned against a soiled, white T-shirt pulled tightly over jeans. His enormous feet resembling miniature whales, were encased in rubber thongs called go-aheads.

"Nothing, really," Chauncey Remington demurred, setting down a copy of the latest in the McWilson science fiction series, *"The Chelsea Chronicles."* Remington tamped a fresh wad of tobacco into his briar pipe and drew deeply.

Chauncey Remington, dressed in a tweedy sports jacket, slacks, and argyle socks, was a 23-year old law student serving as P U Graduate Advisor. He had a handsome, well-defined face, with a thatch of chestnut hair combed straight back, emphasizing dark brown eyes framed by speckled hornrim glasses. Chauncey was the only P U who wore glasses in public - a symbol of self-confidence that underscored his reputation as a suave, "ladies man."

Krum read aloud from the *Daily Californian* article:

"The Greek system was shocked to learn the girls of Gamma Delta sorority had agreed to co-sponsor, with the Dooch Dormies candidates

for the annual Campus Snow King and Snow Queen contest.

"This marks the first time a Greek sorority has partnered with a non-org living group. The ripple effect of this pairing was felt through the Inter-Fraternity Council, many of its members who have never had the opportunity to join the Gee Dees in any campus activity.

'This development will be watched closely,' Dirk Krum III, of the IFC Executive Committee said, 'the prestige and reputation of the Greeks are be on the line.'

Tom Hobknob, another member of the IFC Ex Com, disagreed.

'The IFC should reflect an inclusive, not an exclusive attitude. We have nothing to fear from the Dormies' Hobknob said.

'He (Hobknob) doesn't speak for the IFC. The Greeks made Cal what it is, and we won't tolerate any undesirable element undermining our prestige and position, Krum responded.' "

"This is fabulous," Krum chortled. "Where did you get these photos? This should put those uppity, Gee Dee bitches in their place for pulling this stupid stunt."

Beneath the headline were a close-up of Joan Dildeaux's acne-filled, cross-eyed face and a photo of Hunch Hitowski's silhouette swinging, from rope-to-rope, in the Campanile belfry.

The caption read:

"DILDEAUX AND THE DWARF

Gee Dee & Dormie Candidates for Campus Snow King and Snow Queen"

"You forget, Dirk," Remington sniffed, drawing a long puff from his briar. "Greeks still control this campus. My contact found that shot of Dildeaux in the photo morgue of the *Blue & Gold* year book. A subtle word to the copy editor of the *Daily Cal*, and *voila*, we get editorial commentary on this distressing development."

"Dildeaux and the Dwarf has a certain *je ne sais pas quoi* lilt to it," Remington said, "a wonderful rallying cry for our PU-Kappa candidates, Chip and that cute Eileen Bonestetter."

"Bitchin, Chauncey," Fist said. "Dildeaux and the Dwarf. There's no way those two uglies can beat our babe Eileen and me!"

A sneer crept across Krum's face, turning his dark eyes into smoldering pieces of coal.

After we've humiliated her ugly roommate, Joan Dildeaux, and that Dormie hunch-back friend of Casey Lee's, Krum thought. *The Golden Goddess will come to her senses and realize she is destined to be mine!*

6

MADAME LEE

A sticky, oozing fog enveloped The City in a cool, damp shroud. In the Bay, a symphony of fog horns brayed a cacophony of throaty, two-toned warnings. The faint chatter of unseen pedestrians echoed in the distance. It was a Dashiell Hammett kind of night where Sam Spade might emerge in a tan raincoat and fedora, clutching the Maltese Falcon.

An immaculately dressed couple stood arm-and-arm in the swirling mist beneath a black, iron archway with the words *"International Settlement."*

"Maybe, we're under the wrong archway, Sam," E Lyn Chamberlin said, nodding in the direction of the other *"International Settlement"* sign further up street.

"This part of Pacific's only two blocks long," Paean said, "They won't have any problems finding two oversized *lo fahn,* even in this pea soup," Paean said, using the Cantonese phrase reserved for Caucasians. Loosely translated, *lo fahn* meant *foreign devil.*

"Oversized? You are a real pain in the butt," E Lyn said, poking Paean. "I'm rather dainty, even by Chinese standards."

Their repartee was silenced by the low growl of an auto slowly entering Pacific from Montgomery.

"Turned their engine off," Paean whispered.

Somewhere in the mist, two car doors slammed shut.

"Maybe muggers," E Lyn said, gripping tightly to Paean's arm. "What respectable people would be standing in the midnight fog, unless they were asking to be robbed?"

Whomever they were, they would be here soon, Paean thought.

The search for the mysterious Madame Lee had begun with a phone call by E Lyn to her college roommate, Jani Kay Fong. As seniors, the two had shared a tiny apartment sandwiched between two rowdy fraternities on the north side of the Cal campus. E Lyn had majored in Librarianship, Jani, in English.

Jani worked for an insurance company and was a freelance writer in the evenings and weekends, hoping to attain her dream of being a journalist. It had been ten years since their graduation, but they had stayed in touch, dining regularly in Chinatown and exchanging gossip.

"Starving for a dose of MSG, roomie?" Jani barked over the phone, referring to E Lyn's favorite Chinese dish of salted fish on salt pork patties, the pungent scent of which attracted flies for a week. Jani was tiny, under 5 feet tall, but displayed a fiery, un-Chinese temperament

"How about all-you-can-eat pepperoni pizza?" E Lyn teased, alluding to the time their fraternity neighbors partied well past midnight. Angered, Jani phoned in an order for 50 giant pepperoni pizzas to be delivered to the offending fraternity houses. Two burly delivery men convinced the frat boys to pay for "their specially ordered" pizzas.

"Your parents can reclaim you as a real daughter," Jani said, in a wistful tone. "Now that you're almost betrothed to Sam Paean. When do I meet Mr. San Francisco?"

Over the past few months, Jani had witnessed the metamorphosis of E Lyn, the former plain, library major to the stylish girlfriend of Sam Paean.

"C'mon, Jani," E Lyn said, blushing. "We're only dating. Sam has a long past with too many women for me to take him seriously," she said, more to herself than to Jani. "Any new beaus in your life?"

"I should have such luck, roomie," Jani sighed. "I scare the hell out of Chinese guys, and *lo fahn* men attracted to me are looking for a quiet, exotic."

"You're a quiet exotic, all right - like a runaway truck," E Lyn said. "Still looking for a writing job?"

"What's wrong with wanting a job where I can write and not have to answer the same BS question," Jani said, lowering her voice to mimic a male, "'what kind of Chinatown business will we get if we hire you, honey?'"

Jani's voice assumed a tone of controlled fury. "Screw you!. No one knows the race or color of the writer of the written word. Why should ethnicity have any relevance in hiring?"

E Lyn wished she had the guts to tell Jani that, in 1959 San Francisco, race still mattered. The odds were stacked against women in general, and against Chinese women in particular.

"Need a very big favor from you, Jani," E Lyn said, changing the subject.

"Shoot, roomie," Jani said. "Let's see what I can do."

"Sam needs an audience with Madame Lee," E Lyn said.

There was a long pause. E Lyn could hear Jani's brain grinding into gear.

"A very tall order, roomie," Jani said. "Madame Lee doesn't like the spotlight. I know one of her counselors, but if Madame Lee agrees, there can't be any discussion about her personal life. The meeting would have to involve the welfare of Chinatown."

"About as large as it can get, Jani," E Lyn said. "Sam's asked me to do some leg work on who's buying up property in Chinatown to build a towering, pyramid-shaped skyscraper. The impact on Chinatown will be huge."

Jani whistled softly. "I'll see what I can do, roomie; but there will be a condition, a selfish one."

"Name it, Jani," E Lyn said, "Sam will personally guarantee it."

"He has to arrange a job interview for me with the Managing Editor of *The Sentinel,*" Jani said.

"A deal," E Lyn said. "Raymond Ghee is one of Sam's drinking buddies. They sneak out once-a-month for some serious tippling."

"Better yet," Jani said. "Make that a lunch at Bernie's; and I'll play liar's dice for a job interview. That poor *lo fahn* won't know what hit him. Betcha I'll see you in *The Sentinel* newsroom within a week!"

A few days later Jani had called with instructions that Madame Lee's representatives would meet Sam at midnight, along Pacific Street, in the old *International Settlement*, once a honky tonk part of The City.

"Why the cloak and dagger stuff, Jani?" E Lyn asked.

"Madame Lee has a lot of enemies, roomie," Jani said. "There are some, both *lo fahn* and Chinese, who don't appreciate her work in Chinatown. She can't be too careful."

E Lyn had heard the rumors about Madame Lee Paean had chronicled in his column. She was a charismatic Chinatown legend who inspired deep feelings of love and hate. Despite her notoriety, Paean had never met anyone who had met her. A search of *The Sentinel's* archives turned up no photographs of Madame Lee.

But colorful stories about Madame Lee abounded. One was that Madame Lee was the widow of a prominent industrialist who escaped China during the Civil War before Mao came to power, and that the Communists wanted her dead. Another was that Madame Lee was the daughter of a liaison between a Chinatown prostitute and a wealthy Chinese gambler who died without male heirs, leaving a considerable amount of cash to his illegitimate daughter A third was that Madame Lee was a surviving granddaughter of the Dowager Empress of the Manchu Dynasty who survived the 1912 Chinese Revolution spearheaded by Dr. Sun Yat Sun - a Chinese version of the legend of Anastasia, the long, lost daughter of the Czar of Russia.

Undisputed was that the poor of Chinatown held Madame Lee in the highest regard because of the educational, health, and social programs she had sponsored for past 20-years. She was one of the few in Chinatown, and the only woman, dedicated to the welfare of San Francisco's Chinatown community.

Paean had resisted E Lyn's request to attend the meeting, but his trusty assistant had been persistent, reminding him that she had uncovered salient facts about the mysterious Pyramid and should be rewarded for her efforts.

"Mr. Paean and Miss Chamberlin, I presume," a male voice with a proper British accent said.

Turning toward the speaker, the couple saw the outline of a well-muscled man, dressed in a three-piece seat and a Tyrolean hat.

Two other men materialized from the fog and quickly frisked Paean and searched E Lyn's purse. Both wore a black turtle neck sweater with a leather shoulder holster and pistol

"Just a precaution," the British voice said. He whistled twice, and an engine turned over. Within seconds, a black limousine emerged with its lights dimmed.

"Please, do have a seat, Mr. Paean, Miss Chamberlin," the British voice said, motioning them to the rear seats/

"Wow!" E Lyn whispered, sinking into kid glove leather seat. "I've never ridden in a stretch limo before."

"Not one this large," Paean said, a tone of wonder in his voice. The limo was not an American make.

Clamoring aboard, the body guards took positions in the second row. Their escort, with the British accent, pulled up a jump seat, then barked guttural commands to the driver who switched on the head lights and gunned the limo up Pacific.

In the glow of the limo's interior lights, Paean and E Lyn noted, for the first time, that the British voice emitted from a moon-shaped, male Chinese face.

"Calphung Quock," he said, shaking hands with both. "I'm Madame Lee's aide. Thank you for your patience. The ride will be a bit circuitous, but we must be careful."

E Lyn slipped her arm through Paean's, intoxicated with the thrill of danger the limo ride suggested.

"Please feel free to help yourself to refreshments," Calphung said, motioning to a side panel.

Sliding it open, Paean found a complete bar set up.

"Don't mind if I do," Paean said, reaching for a bottle of 100% proof vodka to mix a very dry martini.

This is going to be some ride, he thought.

"Madame Lee will be with you shortly," Calphung Quock said, removing their blindfolds and taking a seat on a raised dais. "I dare say, Madame Lee deeply appreciates your patience and co-operation."

Paean and E Lyn blinked, squinting to acclimate their eyes to the darkness. The limo had driven through Russian Hill, Pacific Heights, the Tenderloin, North Beach, then to Chinatown where they were dropped off near Stockton and Clay.

"You will be safer not knowing your destination," Calphung said, handing Paean and E Lyn blindfolds.

They had been squired through the distinctive smells and sounds of Chinatown, an area Paean had often walked - sometimes staggered during the wee small hours - after closing bars on nearby Broadway. He tried to visualize where they had been: the muted clicking of mah jong tiles beneath the narrow sidewalks, the rotting odor of restaurant offal stacked at curbside, the bracing breeze on turning a corner.

They had been led down hill, then through a series of alleys.

Probably Spofford to Ross, Paean thought.

Keys jingled, then a door unlocked. They were navigated through a building suffused with a clinging scent of sweetness.

Vanilla, Paean thought. *Not a common ingredient in Chinese cooking.* Then it came to him. *Vanilla, the key ingredient in the manufacture of fortune cookies! The popular fortune cookie factory in Ross Alley!*

Exiting the cookie factory, they crossed a series of courtyards, then entered and exited several buildings, making a series of turns.

Are we going in and out of several buildings or going in circles around the same courtyard? Paean wondered.

"We're almost there," Calphung said. "Hold on to this," he said placing Paean's and E Lyn's right hands on a wooden railing.

They ascended three flights of stairs and entered a room redolent with fresh chrysanthemum. Blindfolds removed, the couple was ushered into leather and teak chairs.

The large, rectangular room had dark lacquered floors illuminated by a ring of indirect lights circling the edge of the ceiling and four thin shafts of light, one from each corner of the ceiling , directed at an ornate, golden throne in the middle of a wooden dais.

Adjusting to the dimness, the two noted the walls were painted a deep red, each bearing a large black character of Chinese calligraphy framed in gold. On each side of the dais, four people sat in the shadows, faces hidden from view. The silhouettes were of four males and four females. Paean recalled the number eight was considered lucky in Chinese culture.

"Sam," E Lyn hissed, poking him in the ribs, gazing upward.

The tall cupola of an arched ceiling was all glass through which the cool, grey fog swirled.

Calphung barked a command, and the eight retainers rose, bowing. Paean and E Lyn followed, bowing deeply, hoping their gesture reflected the appropriate respect.

"Please be seated, Mr. Paean, Miss Chamberlin," a woman's voice said, in perfect English.

They could see the outline of a female form seated upright on the gold throne, her face hidden in the shadows.

"You have met my aide, Calphung Quock," Madame Lee began.

Their moon-faced guide nodded.

"These men and women at my side, are my counselors - bright, dedicated young people who share my vision for the people of Chinatown. Since they were not allowed to attend high schools of their choice, in San Francisco, I sponsored their private, British schooling in Hong Kong, where Americans of Chinese ancestry are held in higher regard than here," Madame Lee paused. "Or, at least, where the American dollar is greatly valued."

Paean and E Lyn felt her smile suffuse the darkened room.

"Now, would you tell me about the issue that brings you here." Madame Lee said.

Paean recounted the eye-tem, the note, tipping him to the secret acquisition of Chinatown properties for the purpose of erecting a pyramid skyscraper. E Lyn reported the results of her search of the San Francisco County Recorder's Office. Ten parcels of Chinatown property had been purchased by the same person who, in turn, conveyed title to a Nevada corporation, Grand Designs, Inc. with its mailing address as a post office box at Lake Tahoe. The corporation's filing with the State of California did not list the names of any officers, directors, and shareholders.

"Registering a foreign corporation without stating any of its principals is unusual," Paean said, "and shows that someone, with powerful influence, is involved with this scheme."

"E Lyn has compiled a list of the names of the sellers, if this will be of help," Paean said, handing a neatly typed list of names to Calphung who, in turn, passed it to Madame Lee's counselors. They whispered and nodded as they read the list of names.

"Thank you, Mr. Paean, Miss Chamberlin, for your efforts,"Madame Lee said. "My counselors will contact the names on the list for any information that may be helpful."

"Tell me, Mr. Paean," Madame Lee said, "why are you and Miss Chamberlin so concerned about this issue."

"You are a diplomat, Madame Lee," Paean said. "What you're really asking is why would a pair of *lo fahn* be so concerned about Chinatown? Perhaps, you wonder whether our interest is based on the *lo fahn* habit of asking for a money reward for information?"

A ripple of chuckles emitted from the counselors.

"The thought did enter my mind, Mr. Paean," Madame Lee said, " but you don't need money. You are San Francisco royalty."

"You are very kind," Paean said. "I am well aware of your tireless efforts to educate Chinatown youth, to abolish sweatshop labor, to improve the health of the elderly, to alleviate crowded living conditions, to promote the general welfare of females, to do everything necessary for the people of Chinatown."

More murmurs and nodding among the counselors.

"I also know that traditional Chinese culture is male-dominated; and there are influential Chinatown men, especially those who have made money from the tourist trade, who resent your influence in the community and would rather have you disappear."

Madame Lee leaned forward slightly to the intersection of the four shafts of light. Paean and E Lyn held their breaths, hoping for a glimpse of her. For a moment, they saw a shock of silver hair illuminated by the crossing beams of light, but her face remained in the shadows. She was obviously well practiced in anonymity; for after pausing briefly, she reclined back into the shadows.

Damn, thought Paean, glancing at E Lyn, sharing the same thought, *A few more inches; and we would have had a rare glimpse of Madame Lee!*

"Why would Mr. San Francisco, a celebrity with no enemies, risk his popularity involving himself in a Chinatown issue?" Madame Lee asked.

"I've always believed the quality of San Francisco life is based on the international flavor of our small city by the Bay," Paean began. "I would not like to see anything that would turn The City's charming skyline into another Manhattan. This pyramid would not only trespass into Chinatown, it would also destroy The City's sense of scale, opening the door for many more high rise buildings.

"Until all the people of Chinatown, especially the men, appreciate the wisdom of your programs, anything that disrupts Chinatown life would be counter-productive to your cause," Paean said.

More murmurs and nodding by the counselors.

"You have done your homework well," Madame Lee said. "The Chinese Exclusion Act of 1882 may have been repealed in 1942, but Chinese are still excluded from all but menial jobs, from buying homes outside of Chinatown, from sending children to schools of their choice.

Madame Lee was referring to the only federal law ever passed in the history of the United States, specifically barring one immigrant group, the Chinese, from bringing families to America.

Madame Lee continued, "The truth is Chinese are tolerated, so long as they stay trapped in Chinatown, as smiling, docile photographic subjects for Midwestern tourists. So long as Chinatown's sole purpose is to bring tourist dollars to the City's coffers, it will never be more than a ghetto."

"E Lyn and I share your sentiments," Paean said, "even if many *lo fahn*, including many of my associates at *The Sentinel,* do not. I would hope, by co-operating, we may better serve our respective communities."

The counselors whispered among themselves and passed their consensus to Calphung who passed their opinion to Madame Lee.

"Of course, there is the matter of consideration," Madame Lee said.

Paean was ready with a response. He knew Chinese were proud people who did not accept welfare or charity. The offer of help must be couched in a perceived exchange of consideration - something for something - to reflect the equal bargaining positions of the parties.

"I am well aware of Madame Lee's desire to avoid the glare of publicity," Paean said.

E Lyn squeezed Paean's elbow, hoping to stop him from asking the obvious.

Don't queer the deal by asking her for a personal interview, E Lyn thought.

"However, if and when, you should change your mind," Paean said, "I would be pleased to be the first journalist to interview you."

An audible gasp emitted from the counselors. Madame Lee silenced them with a dismissive snap of her fingers.

"Mr. Paean, . . . if . . . and . . . when . . . I decide to change my mind, the interview will be yours." Madame Lee said.

Shocked, Paean's mouth dropped open. "Why would . . .?"

"I would like to repay you for your kindness to my grandson."

E Lyn and Paean exchanged quizzical glances.

"My grandson, Casey Lee, told me how helpful you were to him and his college friends, the Dormies," she said. "He also explained how kind you were to his dear friend, Kate Howell."

Small world, kismet, destiny, serendipity, Paean thought, on learning Madame Lee's grandson was Casey Lee, leader of those wildly eccentric Dormies he had encountered in North Beach, at the Big C Sirkus, and at the Gee Dee Presents Party. Kate Howell was the beautiful Cal co-ed called the Golden Goddess.

What did Madame Lee mean when she referred to Kate Howell as Casey Lee's "dear friend?" Is there a campus romance blooming between Madame Lee's grandson and the Golden Goddess?

"Calphung will be in touch with you," Madame Lee said, rising, signaling the end of the audience. "We will pass along any information we develop."

Paean and E Lyn joined the counselors in rising and bowing. Their eyes were riveted to the lacquered, hard wood floors.

What a gracious, wonderful woman, E Lyn thought. *I wish I could just run up and hug her. No,* she thought. *It would only prove I am an undisciplined lo fahn.*

"Madame Lee," Paean said, his head still bowed. "I will do everything in my power to stop the construction of the giant pyramid."

Hopefully, everything in my power will be enough to derail the largest monstrosity ever conceived for San Francisco. Paean thought.

When the *lo fahn* pair straightened up from their bows, Madame Lee was gone.

7

YEARNING ARMS

The Seeburg KD200 Select-O-Matic jukebox gleaming in its modern, sparkling, silver and glass cabinet, sat snugly in the corner of the dark, wood-paneled Pi Upsilon living room, blaring the plaintiff rock and roll song:

"Be my, be my baby,"

Finger snapping began as a polite, oscillating salute, then rose in intensity, like the sound of an army of crickets, as a triumvirate entered the P U living room. Dirk Krum III, President of the P U's, assumed a leather chair, flanked by his roommate, Chip Fist, and Graduate Advisor, Chauncey Remington.

A smile, part sneer, part smirk, crept across Krum's countenance, as he surveyed the fresh young faces of the new P U pledges.

Yes, Krum thought, *another remarkable P U class.*

Krum made a slashing gesture, with his index finger, from ear to ear, indicating the music should stop. This new rock and roll music was driving him crazy, but Krum was confident that this jarring excuse for music was only a passing fad, a novelty, albeit a dangerous one.

What ever happened to real music? Krum thought.

In 1957, as P U pledge president, one of Krum's duties was insuring the Seeburg KD200's selections reflected *"Tradition, Civility, Honor,"* the motto his grandfather, Dirk Krum I, had coined 50 years ago. Krum remembered how he had lovingly handpicked the records for the Seeburg

KD200's play list, each 45 rpm single featuring music by respectable singers like Guy Mitchell, Doris Day, Pat Boone, and Patti Page, although Krum had made an exception for Johnny Mathis, a light-skinned Negro whose ballads were irresistibly romantic to even the most straight-laced sorority girl, earning Mathis the title, "the king of make-out music."

Two years later, loud rock and roll, by Negro singers, dominated the Seeburg KD 200. There was *"What'd I Say"* by that blind piano player, *"Blue Berry Hill,"* by that fat man, and that damned *"Be My Baby,"* by that black female trio echoing incessantly through the P U house.

"Be my, be my . . ."

Chip yanked the plug of the Seeburg in the middle of the last refrain.

"Men of P U," Krum said. "You pledges have been selected for membership in the most exclusive fraternity at Cal, the best of the best. Your time in the class room is only a part of your education. It is the responsibility of P U to make you a better citizen, to make each of you a better man.

"Graduate Adviser, Chauncey Remington, our expert in matters of the fair sex, will address a common, pressing social issue."

"Yeah, boners," Chip Fist added.

Snapping fingers greeted the P U Graduate Advisor. In one hand, Remington held a briar pipe, in the other, a copy of the latest in the McWilson science fiction series, *"The Chelsea Chronicles."*

"One of your most difficult problems, as a P U, will be balancing your natural sexual urges with the goal of meeting and marrying the virtuous girl of your dreams," Remington said. Fingers snapped enthusiastically.

"As a P U," Remington continued, "you will be the target of many girls looking for a good catch. So, the question is, how do we satisfy our basic urges and still marry virgins?"

"Yeah, finding a fuckin' virgin," Fist said.

"No, Chip," Remington said, in a low smooth tone. "That's the point. There are no, using Chip's expression, 'fucking virgins.' No respectable sorority girl is going to ruin her chances for marriage by having gratuitous, pre-marital sex."

"Right, no sorority nookie," Fist said, wagging an index finger.

"But how do we get any, eh . . . experience?" Jefferson Warring asked. Warring was a dark-haired, ruggedly, handsome pledge whose pink cheeks flushed with excitement.

"That's the dilemma," Remington said, biting the briar pipe. "But, through the foresight and leadership of your President, Dirk Krum, we offer you the perfect solution."

"Screw your brains out and still find a virgin," Fist said.

"Dirk has made a special arrangement with the madam of Yearning Arms," Remington said, "so anytime you need to satisfy a sexual urge, you can spend time with their talented girls."

"Isn't Yearning Arms the boarding house featured in *Playboy?*" Warring asked. The pledge was referring to a scandalous pictorial in the September issue of the magazine entitled, "Big Boobs of Berkeley."

"Yes and no," Remington said. "Yearning Arms houses female students, but these aren't sorority girls. They're girls earning their way through college the old fashioned way, on their knees and on their backs."

"Yearning Arms is a red-light house?" Warring asked.

"That would be crass a characterization," Remington sniffed. "Let's just say these are working college girls - not anyone a P U would consider marrying - but for, shall we say, carnal necessities, it is acceptable to 'date' one within the confines of Yearning Arms."

"Dirk has negotiated a special, discount price," Remington said. "When you present yourself at Yearning Arms, you must show your P U membership card and give your secret P U handshake."

"No secret handshake, no discount nookie," Fist added.

"Remember, gentlemen," Remington said, using his briar pipe to underscore his point. "With the girls of Yearning Arms, it's just sex. Don't ever confuse sex with love."

"We'll close our meeting," Dirk Krum said, "with the singing of our fraternity sweetheart song."

As the P U's sang *"My Love Is Pure As the Driven Snow,"* Krum's thoughts turned to the glowing image of Kate Howell. Dirk's face turned dark, shuddering how Casey had come between the Golden Goddess and him. Rationally, he knew Kate was saving her virginity for him, and that her infatuation with the leader of the Dormies was nothing more than a harmless flirtation. But, deep down, Dirk could not escape the gnawing thought that Casey Lee, that despicable Chinaman, was someone to fear.

* * * *

The four marched single-file along the curb of Bowditch Street, serpentining in and out of the towering coastal redwoods, scattering iridescent corpses from liquidambar trees in their wake, and averting eye contact with passing pedestrians. A faint hint of burning syrup nipped the November air. To an unsuspecting stranger, the quartet appeared to be non-orgs. They wore no makeup and dressed in fragile, burlap skirts, over tight, black pedal pushers, frumpy sweat shirts without Cal insignia, and fractured tennis shoes. Over hair severely tied back with red rubber bands, each wore frayed, knit ski caps pulled down to their eyebrows.

The well-endowed leader walked purposely, in long strides, her fully extended arms swinging front and back. The second waddled in small, flat-footed steps, with labored breaths. The third floated gracefully, as if airborne. Bringing up the rear, the fourth, skipped childlike, giggling.

"What's the hurry, Muffy-kins?" Joan Dildeaux huffed. "You're supposed to be such an expert. This should bore you to tears."

"Dil-dee, sweetie," Muffy Peachwick said, "Just move that flat ass of yours. I'll just die if we run into anyone we know. I wouldn't be caught dead or alive in these cootie clothes."

"Gee, this is so-o-o much fun," Dandy Cane squealed from the rear, "like sneaking off to the candy store."

Candy store, thought the third, Kate Howell.

Kate smiled at the irony of the comparison. How sweet would their destination be? So un-Gamma Delta, so inappropriate for Gee Dees, respectable members of the House of Beauty, who were supposed to know who they were and what they represented.

That's the reason the plan had such appeal, Kate thought. *After this caper, Gee Dee could stand for Girl Dirty or something even more salacious!* She could hardly wait to relate the details to Casey Lee.

Yes, only Casey would understand.

"Hang a right," Muffy barked, as she led the procession down a narrow path between two, wood-shingled apartment houses. The trio obeyed, turning their faces away from the church across the street. In the distance, from a hi-fi, the Shirelles sang,

"Foolish little girl,
Wicked little girl"

The quartet struggled like rookie commandoes pushing and pulling each other over a series of dilapidated fences, scurrying across verdant side yards, arriving at a dark, back yard overgrown with a bushes and shrubs. In the cool, late afternoon mist, their labored breathing puffed clouds of steam in the shadowy mist.

They surveyed a three-story, dark-brown shingled house common to the neighborhoods south of the Cal campus.

"You sure, we're at the right place, Muffy-kins?" Joan asked.

"Dil-dee, trust me," Muffy said, batting her long eye lashes. "I'm not going to embarrass you by banging on the back door of some seminary, although it might be fun talking some cute church guy out of his vows."

Dandy Cane giggled. *Her Gee Dee big sis was so-o-o outrageous!*

"Muffy's got the right place," Kate said, pointing to the letters stenciled on a shiny brass plaque nailed above a double, oaken door.

Muffy tapped the door three times.

"Are you sure she knows we're coming?" Joan whispered, no longer as confident as she had been on leaving the comfort of the Gamma Delta sorority house.

Muffy rapped the door again, this time with authority.

"Shhh. Not so loud," Dandy squealed, pulling her ski hat over her ears. "I'm so nervous I could pee in my pants."

They heard the sound of delicate footsteps, from the floor above.

"Coming," a muffled voice said.

The back door creaked opened. In the doorway stood a middle-age woman dressed in high heels, basic black, and pearls.

Flashing a matronly smile, the woman said, "Come in, ladies. Tea is ready."

It was too late to turn back.

Each Gee Dee stepped lightly across the entryway, removing her ski cap, shaking the hand of their smiling hostess, and passing under the brass plaque - its bold letters proclaiming,

"YEARNING ARMS"

8

STAR POWER

The rhythmic snap, crackle, and pop of burning logs suffused the wood-paneled P U living room. From the patio, the soothing hiss of the P U waterfall, underscored the comforting gentleness of Perry Como crooning *"Catch A Falling Star"* from the Seeburg KD200 Select-O-Matic jukebox.

Dirk Krum III sat in the well-worn, leather P U president's chair, deep in thought. It had been a day of disturbing news. At the monthly Inter-Fraternity Council meeting, Dirk had announced, with pride, the selection of his roommate, Chip Fist, as IFC's candidate for the annual Campus Snow King contest, along with his running mate, Kappa sorority girl, Eileen Bonestetter. The IFC's custom had been to defer to the choice of its President. Thus, Dirk assumed Chip's nomination would be *pro forma.*

The Campus Snow King and Snow Queen was a penny-a-vote contest with proceeds donated to needy children for the holiday season. Imaginative fund raising activities sprouted throughout the campus, and the competition had taken on the aura of a popularity contest. The event attracted a large number of candidates, mostly non-orgs, Dirk dismissed as nobodies who enjoyed seeing their names in the *Daily Californian.* The reality was that the IFC candidate and his female running mate always raised the most money and were crowned Campus Snow King and Queen.

This year had been different. When Dirk announced Chip's selection, IFC Ex Com member, Tom Hobknob, announced the Ep Sigs would be nominating their own fraternity brother, Stefan Tillich, arguing more candidates would create greater campus interest and more money for needy children. Hobknob's announcement had been endorsed by a half dozen smaller houses and all the Jewish fraternities. In Krum's view, Hobknob was a radical disguised as a fraternity man. Previously, Hobknob had called for more emphasis on scholarship and advocated expanding fraternity membership to include non-orgs and persons of diverse faiths. Under Hobknob's approach, Christian and Jewish fraternities would no longer be segregated, and un-traditional students, non-orgs, could be accepted as fraternity brothers.

"A penny for your thoughts," Chauncey Remington said, sliding into the divan next to Dirk. Remington dropped a copy of the latest McWilson's science fiction series, *"The Chelsea Chronicles,"* on the coffee table and lit his briar pipe.

The Graduate Advisor was soon joined by Chip Fist and frosh pledge president, Jefferson Warring.

"Make that a buck for your thoughts," Fist said. "I need every penny to be elected Campus Snow King."

"Can't believe Hobknob's disloyal grandstanding before the IFC," Dirk said, taking a long swig from a bottle of Hamms beer. "I'll crush him like a bug."

"My thoughts exactly," Remington said. "Hobknob's testing the waters by pushing his Ep Sig brother. If Tillich comes in a respectable second behind Chip, Hobknob might be emboldened to run against you for IFC president."

"I need Chip to win convincingly," Krum said, slamming the bottle of Hamms on the end table.

". . . for you and the reputation of the P U house," Remington added. "The problem is Chip's really running against two candidates: that Sig Ep, Tillich, and that Dormie dwarf, Hitowski. Both could siphon off votes from Chip and either could sneak in."

"What do you suggest?" Krum said. "We'll have to raise over two thousand bucks to win."

"Difficult, but not impossible," Remington said, relighting the briar. "You could announce the appearance of a famous, Hollywood movie star who would sign autographs for a buck."

"Who?" Krum sighed. "We don't have any P U alums in the movie business, do we?"

"How about Rock Hudson?" Remington said.

"Rock Hudson?" Warring said, his eyes growing wide. "After '*Pillow Talk*,' he's the most popular actor in Hollywood! Rock would guarantee every girl on campus asking for his autograph."

"Rock! What a stud!" Fist said, snapping his fingers in approval.

"How would we get him?" Dirk asked.

"Easy," Remington said. "My dad is his Hollywood attorney. Met Rock a few times myself. He spends a lot of time with friends in The City. He'd be glad to make a campus appearance for a worthy cause, like helping Chip be elected Campus Snow King."

"Wow," Krum said, envisioning the adoring throngs of females drawn to Hollywood's masculine sex symbol.

And if Kate Howell is sweet to me, Dirk thought, *I'll arrange a private meeting with Rock Hudson.*

"Chauncey," Krum said, excited by the idea. "You've got the green light to tap into your dad's connection to get us the Rock!"

* * * *

Suzette Mew-Mew sat on the edge of a chaise lounge made of white, polar bear fur, facing the black and white portrait camera of Helmut Lange. The sexy starlet, the latest Hollywood blond bombshell, was dressed in a white silk evening dress that clung to her voluptuous body like a plaster of Paris mold. Beneath the dress, her legs were discreetly crossed, her delicate feet encased in white, spiked heels. Her left eye was hidden behind her platinum blond hair that fell to her smooth, bare shoulders, but her right eye, slightly almond-shaped, stared alluringly into the lens. Her pouty lips, forming a perfect "O," were slightly parted, as if she were cooing. Her long delicate fingers rested on back of a jet black cat squatting comfortably on her lap. The feline glared haughtily, oblivious to the blinding studio lights and the photo crew.

This photo, gracing the cover of November 7, 1959 issue of *Life* magazine, was referred to as "the cat's meow" shot. An enlarged version - a 4 by 6 foot poster - graced the wall on Ollie Punch's side of the room he shared with Hunch Hitowski.

"Suzette, my lovely darling," Punch moaned, his left eye spinning dizzily. "What I would give to trade places with that lucky black cat."

"She probably can't spell a certain three letter word for a feline animal beginning with 'c' and ending in 't,' Hunch Hitowski teased.

"What are these funny looking stains," Butch Tanenbloom said, standing on his tip-topes, sniffing the poster, running his fingers over her chest. "Ollie, you haven't been having one-handed sex with Suzette?"

"Suzette, please forgive these heathen barbarians, for they have no appreciation of true beauty," Punch said.

"Heathen barbarians? Were you referring to me?" Casey Lee said, feigning anger, as he entered the room with Royal French, All Pro, Ruby Lips, and Jonathan Aldon.

Casey Lee was tall for an Oriental - six feet - with a thin, wiry build, short-cropped, black hair, and slightly almond eyes. He spoke flawless English, in a smooth, mellifluous tone.

Royal French was Casey's right-hand man, a 6-foot-9 inch Army veteran. All-Pro was affectionately called Rooster Face but was blessed with a deep, booming voice that made him the popular disc jockey on campus radio station KALX. With his effeminate features, Ruby Lips worked part-time disguised as a gypsy, Gifted Florence, the Telly fortune teller. All were academic tutors of freshman, Jonathan Aldon.

"Hate to disillusion you, Punch," Ruby said, rocking side-to-side, hands on his hips. "I think the cat lady is a guy in drag!" Dodging a pillow thrown by Punch, Ruby said, "tsk, tsk, Ollie. We all have our little sexual deviations."

In the background, the All-Pro broke into his impression of Eddie Fisher singing *"If Ever I Needed You, I Need You Now."*

"Let's call this meeting to order," Royal said. "Ruby, Jonathan, the floor is yours."

Ruby recounted the incident that had prompted this strategy session.

It had been a slow day at Gifted Florence's. Ruby, in a black, female wig and a flowing peasant, gypsy dress, had been giving his new assistant, Jonathan, clad as a Rumanian serf - with a bandana and a black patch over one eye - instructions on palm reading, when the bells of the front door jangled, announcing the arrival of a client.

A towering figure filled the open doorway, blotting out the sun. The behemoth wore a T shirt, Bermuda shorts, go-a-heads, and a hunting cap pulled down tightly around his head.

"Gifted Florence?" he asked.

"My darling, handsome hunk, please come in," Ruby said, batting

his long, fake eye lashes. "Gifted Florence at your service." Ruby drew the drapes of the large bay window overlooking Telly. "This is my serf, Gorky," Ruby said, motioning Jonathan away from the light illuminating the crystal ball shimmering in the center of the small round table.

"Please, sit, sit," Ruby said. "You must not be ashamed of coming to see Gifted Florence. Take off that silly cap." With a delicate sweeping motion, Ruby plucked the hunting cap, revealing the beet-red face of Chip Fist.

"I am here to help you in your time of need," Ruby cooed. "As my sign promises, I see all, know all."

A look of panic gripped Chip Fist's face. "If my P U brothers knew I were here, I'd never hear the end of it," Fist whispered. "They think only girls and wimps come to you for help."

"You are obviously a very virile boy," Ruby said, in a soothing tone, "no one would mistake you for a girl. Although . . . " Ruby stopped, resisting the urge to finish his thought about the alternative.

"Tell Gifted Florence about your problem," Ruby said. "It will be heard in the strictest confidence. My serf, Gorky, is quite deaf."

Fist began, in halting speech.

"We were having a beer bust with our neighbors, the Gee Dees. I was drinking with Muffy Peachwick who's supposed to be a hot number."

"A woman of loose morals?" Ruby said, arching an eyebrow.

"Yeah, I guess," Fist said. "I mean she's supposed to screw like a bunny."

"In some circles, that might be a ringing endorsement," Ruby said, blinking his lashes.

"Anyway, we each drank a six pack; and I snuck her up to my room; and we took off our clothes and started to do it."

"Intercourse?" Ruby asked, plucking a hair from his eyebrow.

"Intercourse, humping, fucking, it's all the same," Fist said.

"So what was your problem, Big Boy?" Ruby asked. "Couldn't get it up?"

"Hell, no! I can always get it up," Fist said. "Muffy must be really experienced, because she wanted to be on top. So I'm laying on my back when all of a sudden she starts laughing. Not a giggle, but big 'Ha-Ha's.' "

"Is she into funny sex?" Ruby said.

"No," Fist said, in a whisper, "She points to my dick and says it's the teen-siest she's ever seen on a football player. To make things worse, she said my gut was so big, there was no way she was going to fit my peck-ette in - that's what she called it, my peck-ette - because it was too short and my gut was too big."

"Poor dear, what happened," Ruby said.

"I just lost it. I shriveled up faster than a turtle in danger," Fist said. "So, unless I can find a way to make my dick grow, I'll will be the laughing stock of the campus. I can't let this happen while I'm running for Campus Snow King."

"My poor darling," Ruby said, pinching Chip's cheek. "I have just the cure for you. It's a sex aid . . . the Bulgarian Hard-on-ski."

Ruby waved Jonathan to open a drawer of a hutch.

"Hard-on-ski?" Fist asked, a quizzical look on his face.

"Yes, it looks like that Big Rubber you fraternity boys use to fire missiles from the rooting section," Ruby said, receiving the device from Jonathan.

"How does it work?" Fist asked.

"Patience, you brute. Gifted Florence will tell you all, but you must not share this sex secret with anyone! Not even your roommate."

"I swear I won't tell a soul, not even my roommate, Dirk. Besides, news of my peck-ette would harm the P U's reputation as bandits."

Ruby began, "in the privacy of your room, wrap one end of the Bulgarian Hard-on-ski several times around the shaft of your peck-ette, . . er, I mean your organ.' "

Fist nodded enthusiastically.

"Then, loop the other end several times around a door knob." Ruby. said, giving Jonathan a sly wink.

"And then? . . . And then?" Chip asked.

"You lean back on your heels - stretching the Hard-on-ski as far as it will go - rocking your body back and forth gently, at least 100 times. It will help if you play background music on your hi-fi. Something encouraging, like 'Locomotion,' by Little Eva."

"The Hard-on-ski works?" Fist asked.

"Silly boy," Ruby said. "Gifted Florence would never prescribe something that doesn't work? Or course, it works! By having the Hard-on-ski pulling on your pud, at least 100 times a day, your pecker *will grow a quarter-inch a week, a whole inch in a month!"*

"Wow! An inch a month!" Fist said. "When should I stop?"

"You wouldn't want to hurt someone with something that's too big."
Ruby said. "Six months will be about right, even for that ravenous sex
machine, Muffy Peachwick."

"What do I owe you?" Fist said, unrolling a wad of bills.

"This will be enough," Ruby said, plucking all but a five dollar bill
from the roll.

"Thanks a mill, Gifted Florence," Fist said, rolling up the Hard-on-
ski, stuffing it into his shorts. "You too, Gorky," he said, pulling the
hunting cap over his head and exiting.

The Dormies howled until tears flowed on hearing Ruby's story of
his encounter with Chip Fist.

"What was the juicy info you got from him?" Butch asked, adjusting
his spats.

Jonathan picked up the story.

"While Chip was moaning about how Muffy Peachwick was calling
his penis, a peck-ette, he let it slip that he was especially embarrassed
about his size, because Hollywood's most studly male star was going
to be a special guest for the Campus Snow King contest. Chip could
only imagine how big Rock Hudson was and how he would pale in
comparison!"

"Rock Hudson's helping the P U's?" Punch barked. "How can
Hunch compete with Rock? We're doomed!"

The dorm room became silent.

"Unless . . . we come up with someone as big as Rock," All Pro
said, from the rear of the room. "And I don't mean the size of his
pecker."

"Who do you have in mind?" Casey said.

"My uncle is Suzette Mew Mew's hair stylist," All Pro said.

"Is he cute?" Ruby said, puckering his lips. "Would he find me
sexy?"

"Shut your mouth, Ruby," All Pro shouted. "There are a lot of
Hollywood hair stylists who aren't queer."

"That's not what I hear," Ruby said.

"You're suggesting?" Royal asked, suddenly taking a keen interest
"My uncle tells me Suzette Mew Mew has a thing about stray cats
that are put to sleep," All Pro said. "She keeps a dozen stray cats around
her house."

"So," Casey interjected. "Let's say you contact Suzette Mew Mew
through your uncle and ask for help in raising money to save stray cats
by a Berkeley activist group called . . ."

"Campus Crusade for Cats," Royal yelled, "the CCC!"

"Yes," Casey said. "If Suzette makes a celebrity appearance to sell
autographs, the Campus Crusade for Cats will donate one half of all
monies raised to saving stray, campus cats!"

"Hear, Hear!" Hunch shouted, jumping up and down. "Cheers for
Suzette Mew Mew, Ollie's cat lady."

"Darling, Suzette," Punch said, his wandering eye spinning dizzily.
"Imagine, you, LIVE, in my arms."

"Better rent a cat costume, Ollie," Butch said. "Cause there's no
other way you're gonna get close to that blond, four star general."

9

'TOMIC TEFLON

"A beautiful day for a public execution," Garrick Nelquist said, surveying the growing crowd. "Hope it's short and merciful."

"Good luck," Roderick Seakin said, "William Randolph Chandler's never been at a loss for words, not as a publisher, not as a captain of industry, certainly not now, as a political candidate. When it comes to belaboring bad news, he's tough to beat. Wouldn't you agree, Ari?"

"Don't pick on Ari," Jacob Aural said, stroking Sandy's head. "We don't have a say in who our in-laws are."

Ari Scott shared his colleagues' sense of dread. During his marriage to Cee Cee, his father-in-law, WRC, confided how he savored crushing an enemy, a joy akin to "pulling the wings off a butterfly."

The self-proclaimed "Four Musketeers" were among the 2,000 members of the Academic Senate seated in the plaza in front of Dwinelle Hall. Each wore a black gown accented with a scarf bearing the colors of the professor's discipline: Ari Scott, in the dark blue of Philosophy; Professors Garrick Nelquist and Aural Jacob, in the white of Humanities; and Professor Richard Seakin, disguised as himself, in the golden yellow of Science.

Dwinelle Hall was a jarring testament to the campus architecture hastily erected to accommodate the influx of Post War students, Cal's first concession to quantity over quality. The building was architecturally bland, a five-story, U-shaped concrete leviathan jammed into the banks of a south fork of Strawberry Creek, blocking the panorama of San Francisco Bay, its two perpendicular, outstretched wings pleading for acceptance among its classically designed, Beaux-Arts neighbors.

Despite Dwinelle's intrusion into the eco-system of Strawberry Creek, its ungainly size and shape did provide a utilitarian function. Dwinelle and its plaza provided a setting for public events too large for the Greek Theatre and too small for Memorial Football Stadium.

Thousands of students squatted on the sun-drenched uphill slope, like a giant human amoeba, swelling east past Wheeler and South Halls almost to the base of the Campanile, spilling south through Sather Gate and splaying north beyond Durant and California Halls.

ROT-C students, in military uniforms, waved placards:

"Patriot WRC For Governor,"
"A Vote For WRC = A Vote For A Sane University"
"Yes, On Publish Or Perish"

Bearded Pseudo-Beats, students dressed in the garb of San Francisco Beatniks, carried signs proclaiming:

"Publish or Perish - Perish the Thought,
"WRC = Willie's Really Crooked"
"Vote No To False Patriotism"

The University orchestra, seated in a C formation, at the entrance to Dwinelle Hall, heralded the arrival of the guest speaker by performing *"Pomp and Circumstance."*

A polite applause, mingling with scattered choruses of "boo's," rippled through the assemblage, as Chancellor Haynes, dressed in a light blue scarf of History, led a beaming William Randolph Chandler from the front door of Dwinelle Hall to the podium. Three-hundred feet above the throng, in the belfry of the Campanile, Hunch Hitowski swung effortlessly among the bells, banging out the mournful tune, *"The Hanging of Danny Deaver."*

"Ladies and gentlemen., friends of this great university," Chancellor Haynes intoned in a deep voice over the cacophony of competing catcalls. "I present a candidate for Governor of California, William Randolph Chandler."

A polite ripple of applause from the Academic Senate was lost in the jousting of competing chants. IFC and the ROT-C students roared,

> "Fire Left Wing Profs!
> Fire Left Wing Profs!"

Psuedo-Beats and non-Orgs chanted,

> "Fascists Suck!
> Fascists Suck!"

Chancellor Haynes ripped the microphone from its cradle and roared in a booming tone that echoed off the eastern foothills, silencing the crowd.

"LADIES AND GENTLEMEN, FRIENDS OF THIS GREAT UNIVERSITY."

"Cal's cherished tradition of free speech requires us to listen, with respect, to the views of others with whom we may passionately disagree. I urge you to listen to the views expressed by Candidate Chandler, whether you agree with his views or not. Our reputation, as a bastion of free and unfettered speech COMMAND it. Our sense of civility and hospitality DEMAND it."

Members of the Academic Senate resumed their polite applause, a subdued gesture, joined by the students en masse.

"Thank you, Chancellor Haynes," William Randolph Chandler said, bowing in exaggerated, mock appreciation.

William Randolph Chandler - WRC - was tall, big-boned with broad shoulders and large hands befitting a former football lineman for the USC Trojans in the 1920's. A thick shock of white hair framed a well-chiseled face with deep set eyes.

"Patriotic faculty and students of California," WRC began, "I bring a message of HOPE and PROMISE. For too many years since America defeated the forces of global tyranny in the War, those of the academic world, especially many this faculty who, under the rubric of academic freedom, would subvert the teaching mission of this university by claiming cockeyed, mushy-brained notions, like Higher Truth, that are dangerous to the very moral fiber of this great country."

Ari Scott felt the laser heat of his ex-father-in-law's steely gaze. The reference to Higher Truth was an intentional dig, as Ari had garnered international acclaim for a series of philosophical lectures and papers on the notion of Higher Truth.

"Hah," Seakin grunted.

"The ass hole is getting personal, Scotty," Nelquist muttered.

"One man's Higher Truth is another's lowest baseness," Aural said, in a measured tone.

WRC continued.

"But we can stop this pervasive, corrupting influence, NOW! If elected as your next Governor, I promise to implement a program that guarantees the patriotic dedication of EACH and EVERY Cal professor. Right thinking students and academicians KNOW what I'm advocating. It's PUBLISH OR PERISH!"

Choruses of boo's emitting from the Academic Senate swept up to the Campanile where Hunch Hitowski clanged the *Cal Fight Song*.

Chandler raised his arms in a victorious gesture.

"WHO better to implement and insure the success of publish or perish than a member of your own faculty who truly appreciates the necessity of research as the life blood of a great university, a distinguished professor who has agreed to champion the cause of publish or perish.

"I am pleased to announce that, at a meeting yesterday, the Regents tentatively approved the selection of the person to administer the publish or perish program. It is my pleasure to introduce him today.

"May I present that distinguished scientist, the defender of the Free World in the class room and at the Cyclotron who has graciously agreed to be accept this grave responsibility: Professor WERNER VON SELLER!"

WRC waved his arms back and forth like a college cheerleader, as Werner Von Seller rose from his seat, among the members of the Academic Senate, turning slowly, bowing at each quadrant of the circle, amid the shouts of competing factions.

Von Seller was portly and short-legged and walked with a side-to-side gait. The waddle and a long pointed nose had inspired the nickname, the Prussian Penguin, among his detractors. On his right eye, he wore a monocle that magnified the perfectly round eye. In his left hand, he carried his trademark sterling silver cigarette holder with a smoldering French Gaulois.

"Shit," Nelquist said, "I thought we ran that wack-o up the hill and chained him to his atomic reactor."

"Von Seller's got more political lives than a cat," Aural said.

Sandy barked twice in agreement.

At the start of the school year, the Prussian Penguin had been recruited by Congressman Clayborn Muck with the promise of more federal dollars for atomic research in exchange for his support of HUAC's hearings on the Cal campus.

When Muck had been discredited and HUAC had canceled its hearings, Von Seller had quietly retreated to the sanctuary of the Cyclotron where he supervised the atom smasher.

"To insure that students will not suffer from the lack of instruction while professors research their papers," WRC said, "I will ask the legislature for an appropriation to pay for the finest teaching assistants to provide hands-on education.

"I intend to hire a corps of Teaching Assistants, all of whom are graduates of that GREAT private university, my alma mater, the University of Southern California!"

"My God," Ari said, envisioning an army of tan, crew-cut TA's dressed in SC crimson and yellow overrunning the Cal campus.

WRC's announcement was like waving a red flag in front of a snorting bull, a slap in the face, as SC was the antithesis of Cal. SC stood for football and partying. Cal was academics and intellectualism.

There will be demonstrations and riots, Ari thought, *the damage from which the campus may never recover.*

Despite Chancellor Haynes admonition, the Academic Senate rose in choruses of boo's, joining those raining down from the eastern foothill sweeping through Sather Gate, as the ROT-C cadets and IFC members joined in jeers.

This was no longer a conservative or liberal issue. WRC was promising a calculated attack on the very soul of the campus, a frontal assault on the shared value of every Cal student and faculty member: Cal's superior academic environment. It was one thing to tolerate the annual slaughter by the Trojans on the football gridiron, it was another to be humiliated academically by SC Teaching Assistants.

From Sather Gate, a rising chorus rained down on the podium,

"Bull shit! Bull shit!"

Stupid fools are playing right into my hands, WRC thought, waving Von Seller up to join him.

Von Seller waddled to the podium where WRC raised his arm, like a winning prize fighter. A pencil-thin smile crept across the Prussian Penguin's face, as the choruses of boo's washed over Dwinelle Plaza

Never underestimate the persistence of atomic leadership, Von Seller thought.

WRC retreated from the podium, his arms outstretched in the "V" for victory salute made famous by Winston Churchill.

Ari shuddered at the thought of the impending bloody war that would be waged for the heart and soul of the Cal campus, as cascading choruses of boo's continued to envelope Dwinelle Plaza.

10

MUSIC AND ROMANCE

"Oooh, oooh, oooh, oooh.
Oooh, oooh . . . Oooh-oooh-oooh"

The falsetto voices, in a syncopated cha-cha beat, echoed through the cavernous Dooch living room, more groaning than cooing. The male chorus was attempting to sing the Frankie Avalon ballad, *"Venus."*

"Hey, Venus! Oh, Venus!
Venus, if you will,"

"GIRLS, PLEASE!" Ruby Lips rapped the music stand with the thin shaft of a quivering baton.

Leaning forward, hands on his slender hips, he said, "You tone-deaf Dormies don't have a friggin' clue!"

Ruby Lips had just completed a late shift as fortune teller at "Gifted Florence" and was still attired as a gypsy woman, in a peasant dress and a bandana. Melting mascara began to trickle down his cheeks.

Ruby tapped the music stand several more times. He rolled his eyes in disgust and puckered, "Darlings, sing! Sing as if you want to get laid, need to get laid, have to get laid. Channel those raging hormones!"

Even if you've got snow ball's chance in hell of actually getting laid, he sighed to himself. *Why do straight guys waste so much energy on unrequited sex?* he thought.

"Jeez, what I put up with to help you heter-o guys get a little vicarious nookie," Ruby sighed.

Ruby suppressed a smile at the enfolding scene before him. To his right, Butch Tanenbloom was demonstrating the rhythmic intricacies of the new dance, the chalypso - similar to the cha-cha with an extra half beat - perfect for those without any rhythm or timing.

"*One-two, CHA-CHA-CHA-CHA!*" Butch shouted.

A line of enthusiastic Eng-ineers stomped their feet and chanted in unison with Butch, but their feet had minds of their own.

Dormie Eng-iners are hopelessly spas-modic, Ruby sighed.

To Ruby's left, Casey Lee was trying to coax a melodic verse out of a half-dozen frosh who claimed choir experience. Each carried a mimeographed sheet of the lyrics to the Number One song in America, "*Venus,*" by Frankie Avalon.

It began as a brainstorming session as to what it might take for the Dormies to wangle a social exchange with a sorority. Hunch Hitowski had proposed a moonlight serenade

A notice had been posted on the ceiling of the Dooch elevator:

"Pajama Serenade Practice - 11p.m. Tonight"

"Is a nocturnal serenade like a nocturnal emission," Royal French said. "How should we dress ? Dirty raincoats from the T & D?"

Royal was referring to raincoats dispensed to patrons of the girlie movie house, the T&D, affectionately referred to as the "Tuff & Dirty."

Fifty Dormies had answered the call, including seventh floor Eng-ineers, the entire Frosh class, and others looking for a study break.

They appeared in various degrees of un-dress: pajama tops, pajama bottoms, togas fashioned from bed sheets, jockey shorts, robes, T-shirts and Bermuda shorts. In deference to modesty, Ollie Punch who slept in the nude, wore a jock strap - an athletic supporter - and nothing else.

"Be realistic, we don't have the looks, the threads, or the bucks to impress anyone," Punch said, his left eye spinning leisurely.

"True," Casey said, "but you're giving too much credit to fraternity guys. Not all sorority girls are hung up on looks and money."

Casey continued, "I believe, given the opportunity to get close , some of our Dormal types would have a chance to get somewhere, even with members of the House of Beauty."

"Easy for you to say," Punch said, a tinge of envy in his voice. "The

Golden Goddess has the hots for you." His wandering eye picked up velocity whenever he became aroused, and the image of Kate Howell in a compromising position made his eye spin like a gyroscope.

"Guys, Casey's right," All Pro said, "Looks aren't that important. Women go crazy over my deep, sexy radio voice. I get more blind dates than you can imagine."

"Better that your dates be blind, All Pro." Super Sleuth had quietly slithered into the ersatz dance studio. "When broads get a load of your rooster-like face, you never see them again. Take it from someone who studies campus beauties seriously. Punch is right. Good looking broads are always turned on by looks and dough - stuff we don't have!"

"No, listen," Casey said. "Even the most unapproachable, stuck up female appreciates the Big R . . . Romance. Not the 'Will I meet my Prince Charming?' kind of romance. I'm talking about every woman's insatiable need to be stroked spiritually and emotionally by a touch of fantasy, a hint of the sublime. They go bonkers when they receive something thoughtful, something as simple as a schmaltzy poem, a single flower, or a sentimental song, a gesture treating them special. This stuff gets your foot in the door. The rest is up to you."

"On the button," All Pro said. "Guys listen to my radio show for the music; but women tune in for my flowery dedications and gushy song intros. I'd love to believe my radio voice is that sexy; but the truth is my female listeners are turned on by what I say, not how I say it. Do you think beautiful women really get turned on by the looks of that little schmuck, Eddie Fisher? He gets babes like Debby Reynolds and Liz Taylor because of his songs, not because he's handsome."

"And singing stupid, sappy songs, like 'Venus' is going to do the trick?" Dick Phunque said. Phuncque was the balding, pimply-faced leader of the Eng-ineers. "Will music transform us poor, ugly Eng-ineer Dormies into handsome Prince Charmings?"

"Casey's got a point," Butch said. "When you've got a hot product, broads frequently forget what the package looks like. Phunque, look what happened to the Eng-ineers at the Big C Sirkus when you were serving Kerrs beer. Those sallies were all over you like a cheap suit."

Phunque began to salivate. "Yeah," he remembered. "That was the closest I've ever been to some of those stuck-up beauties. I could smell their fragrances mingling with the scent of Kerrs. I was standing so close I could have licked their bodies before they finished a beer."

"Don't horn in on my territory," Lizard said, licking the tip of his nose and flicking the bottom of his chin with his six inch tongue. "I'll take care of the licking for all you frustrated, perverted Eng-ineers."

Groans emitted from the Eng-ineers, then silence, as they awaited Phunque's response.

"Ok," Phunque said, wiping drool with his sleeve. He whipped out the slide rule Eng-ineers wore like swords on their belts. "Getting close to those untouchables again would be good enough for me. That could be the highlight of my social life! Let's do *"Venus!"*

"Venus!" echoed the seventh floor Eng-ineers, as they unsheathed their slide rules from their belts and brandished them like swords.

"Ok, girls," Ruby Lips said, tapping his baton."Let's try it from the top. Get those hormones cooking. Pretend the essence of your masculinity is oozing through your throats. Sing with passion! Pretend those gullible soror-whores are about to swoon from this 'swonderful crooning and slip their prissy little hands into your half-zipped flys!"

"Butch!" Ruby shouted, "give us those chalypso moves."

Butch shouted and swayed from side-to-side like a giant wounded snake, leading Eng-ineers in the syncopated steps of the chalypso with his spats adorned shoes.

The Dormies began in quasi three-part harmony.

"Oooh, oooh, oooh, oooh,
Oooh, oooh . . . Oooh-oooh-oooh"

"Almost orgasmic!" Ruby Lips shouted, dashing from one end of the singing, sashaying group to the other. "More falsetto, girls!"

Ruby Lips surveyed the chaotic scene, a mass confusion of sound and step. No Dormies sang the same lyric or danced the same step.

Ruby waved his baton at the 50 would-be singers and dancers, none of whom were not paying one iota of attention. Yet, somehow despite dissonant singing and out-of-synch stomping, the mob arrived at the ending to *"Venus"* at approximately the same time.

Energized, Ruby stood on his tip-toes, and waving his baton led the Dormies in the closing refrain:

"Oh, Venus! Hey, Venus!
LET MY DREAMS COME TRUE!"

11

HELPING HANDS

"The art of sex is a two-edged sword," the middle-age woman said, in precise diction. She looked at her guests seated at the small, oval teak table, inlaid with mother-of-pearl. "Are you sure you want to proceed?"

"Yes," the four said in unison.

They were on the top floor of Yearning Arms, in an airy room of glass overlooking a leafy canopy of Coastal redwoods where birds twilled contrapuntally to the Monotones groaning "The *Book of Love*" from a neighborhood stereo.

The hostess was a handsome, silver-haired woman with a finely chiseled jaw, a petite nose, and sparkling grey eyes. She was dressed in a tailored black suit accented with a strand of large pearls and single pearl earrings. She had the graceful, patrician air of a society matron. Her name was Wanda Majic, proprietor and madam of Yearning Arms.

If my parents knew why we're here, Kate Howell thought.

Kate's classic beauty had earned her the nickname she detested, the Golden Goddess. She was slender, small-boned, 5-foot-5, but carried herself taller. She was the first member of the Gee Dee house to let her blond hair grow out into the new longer hairdo, the "flip," that accentuated her sparkling blue eyes, complemented her high cheek bones, and underscored her well-defined chin. After winning a series of beauty titles as a freshman, Kate had tired of public life and refused to enter any more beauty contests.

If boys would stop treating me as if I were on a pedestal. Kate often thought. *If only they would treat me as a person and talk to me the way Casey does.*

Glancing at her sorority sisters, Joan Dildeaux, Muffy Peachwick, and Dandy Cane, Kate retraced the events that brought them to this private audience with Wanda Majic.

It had begun with a supply of The Pill Dandy Cane's stewardess sister, Candy Cane, had brought from Boston where research was being conducted on the effectiveness of a female birth control pill, Enovid. The four had made a solemn oath to take The Pill until the end of the semester, February, 1960, and to compare notes.

Kate had not experienced any side effects from The Pill, but she did notice a strange, new sensation during her secret, chaste, tete-a-tete meetings with Casey Lee in his room at the top of Dooch Dorm. Whenever she looked deeply into his exotic eyes, she felt a pleasant wetness in the most private part of her body, accompanied by a burning flush in her cheeks. Surely, Casey had noticed but was too much a gentleman to comment on it.

After Kate confided the phenomenon to her roommate, Joan Dildeaux had admitted to a sudden fixation on "tight male buns" she attributed to The Pill. Thus, it was not surprising that the quartet of Pill poppers should expand their interest, in sexual matters, by embracing Muffy's idea to consult with the Berkeley's expert on sex, Wanda Majic.

"I assume you're all virgins." Wanda. said, "You certainly look it."

Three of the four nodded, but Wanda was surprised to hear Muffy mutter, "Sometimes, looks are deceiving."

Muffy's given name was Mergetroid, a name she used until that fateful summer she went to Paris as a high school exchange student. Among her female siblings, Muffy had been the eldest and brightest Peachwick, but the plain Jane of her family - the one who wore thick glasses and had a flat chest. How she had envied the attention lavished on her younger sisters blessed with winning smiles and big boobs!

While in Paris, Muffy bought a pair of the revolutionary new contact lenses - not yet available in the States - and experimented with a breast growth pill that she swallowed with copious quantities of French wine. Initiated to sex by several experienced Parisian boys, she returned with a new nickname, a new bust line, and a new sexual attitude.

Wanda studied the faces of the young women, looking at each intently. *So innocent, so naive,* she thought. *Was I ever this young?*

She continued. "Historically, the duty of the groom, on the wedding night, is to initiate his virgin bride to things he has learned while sowing the wild oats of his bachelor life.

"There have been other college girls who wanted to learn about sex at Yearning Arms, but you're the first who would rather be observers than participants. Is this a way of saving your precious virginity while learning a few tricks of the trade?" Wanda asked.

"Ladies, let me totally frank. I can't allow lookie-looking while my girls are working. It would be bad for business if clients had to perform before a live audience. Voyeurism would violate my house motto: *'Trust, Discretion, and Privacy.'* "

"Don't you have two-way mirrors?" Joan asked. "I thought all . . . eh, . . . houses had them."

"I think you're referring to that awful issue of *Playboy*," Wanda sighed. "I should never have allowed that photographer to take photos of my girls."

Madam Majic continued, "As a visitor, you may ask questions of any of my girls, but if you're going to be here regularly, I'll have to put you to work."

Reading their minds, Wanda said, "Men are funny about female virginity. If you can satisfy them in ways - other the missionary position - you can still be a virgin for marriage purposes."

"Good point," Muffy said. "Ever wonder why guys who claim they love and respect you don't want to screw before marriage but have no problems asking you to put your hands or mouths on their dicks?"

"Gross," Joan said, her face turning a beet red. "Wash your mouth and hands out with Listerine."

She grabbed Muffy's hands and held them up close to her thick glasses. "Muffy-kins, what is that white fuzz growing on your palms? Wouldn't be handy hair, would it?"

Dandy giggled, "Muffy's right. In high school, plenty of guys asked to play with other parts of my body."

Although only a freshman, Dandy Cane was accustomed to male attention since she was ten years old. The youngest of the three Cane sisters, born a year apart, Dandy and her sisters, Sandy Cane and Candy Cane, were raised on the beaches of Orange County. They often passed as triplets, each with deep tans, bright blue eyes, tow-headed, Dutch boy hairdos, and tight, trim surfer figures. Candy was a stewardess on the CAT Airlines flight Jonathan and Butch had flown to San Francisco, and Sandy was an aspiring, B-movie starlet.

"Wanda," Kate said, "are you saying that there are things we can do at Yearning Arms without sacrificing our virginity?"

"Certainly," Wanda said, "You girls can help out in the Mardi Gras Room. One of the reasons Yearning Arms is popular is we understand some of our customers are embarrassed to be here. Yet, we appreciate they're here to deal with basic urges they can't satisfy elsewhere."

"You offer slightly naughty services?" Kate asked.

"Yes, that's why you girls would be perfect working in the Mardi Gras Room. The clients and the girls dress up in costumes and masks, so no one can be recognized. We have wonderful, ornate costumes that would be fashion statements in New Orleans or Venice."

"But, if we agree to work in the Mardi Gras Room, what will we have to do to these masked marvels?" Muffy asked.

"The only physical contact permitted in the Mardi Gras room is masturbating the client," Wanda said matter-of-factly.

"Just getting guys off?" Muffy's grinned. "I can handle that."

"Are gloves ok?" Joan asked, a look of disgust spreading across her face. "Yuck, the thought of touching those things . . ."

She looked at Kate. *If the Golden Goddess is willing to give it a tug, I guess I'm willing to give it a jerk.*

Kate nodded, a trace of apprehension on her face.

Wanda interjected. "Ladies, it isn't that disgusting. With a little practice, you may learn to enjoy 'chocking the chicken.' At least you'll be saving your virginity for marriage."

"But," Wanda paused, "under no circumstances will there be any kissing. I consider kissing the most intimate physical act. If you get emotionally involved with a client, do it outside of Yearning Arms. Are we clear on that point?"

Wanda pushed a button behind an Impressionistic painting, and a small elevator door slowly opened behind a full length mirror.

After descending one floor, as the elevator opened, Joan intoned, "Ladies lingerie, Mardi Gras costumes . . . hand jobs."

They exited into a dimly lit room with chandeliers illuminating wall-to-wall, red flocked wall paper.

"Reminds me of the interior of Bernie's restaurant," Kate said, surveying the Mardi Gras room.

"A 19th century boudoir," Joan said. "I already feel at home."

Wanda led them to a deep walk-in closet. Inside, the ten foot walls were lined with rows of exotic costumes and masks.

"It's like Halloween," Dandy said, rushing to select a mask of a child's face with a halo perched on top.

"Trick or treat," Muffy said, trying on a dragon's head mask.

Making their selections, they lined up for inspection.

"Perfect, ladies," Wanda said, drawing a silk draw cord. A young woman dressed in a sequined leotard and a glittering feline mask appeared and curtseyed.

A cat for a cat house! Kate thought.

The new arrival had a petite frame with a pair of spectacular breasts that made Muffy look like a boy.

Kate noted Muffy's stunned expression, part envy, part awe, as she checked out the cat lady from top-to-bottom.

"Ladies," Wanda said, "may I present your tutor, Sascha."

"Or, Boob-us Gigant-us," Joan whispered.

"Sascha is not her real name," Wanda said. "We don't use our true names here. When you walk out of Yearning Arms, your civilian life is your own. So what will your 'professional' names be, ladies? Choose a moniker your customers will find memorable, something that will give you distinction."

"Call me Miss Prim, as in prim and proper," Kate said, snapping a cat 'o nine tails. "I'll be naughty but nice."

"My name is Whore-tense, the intellectual hooker," Joan said, trying on spiked heels and mesh nylons.

"I'll be Tinker Bell," Dandy added, giggling behind the child's mask, waving a star-tipped scepter

Alternating her fists up and down, as if she were milking a cow , Muffy said, "I'm Harlotte, the Yearning Arms Handy Woman."

From a brown paper bag, Sascha produced a bunch of raw, green fruit and handed each a banana.

"Pretend the banana is an aroused male organ." Sascha held her banana in an upright position. "Gently massage the top end with the tips of your fingers."

Sascha's voice was perky , youthful, like any coed, Kate thought.

As Sascha turned, Kate thought she saw something unusual in the eye holes of her mask. Kate leaned forward for a closer look. Her initial assessment was true. Peering out from Sascha's ornate cat mask were an unusual pair of eyes: one green, the other orange.

"Now, grip the banana with the tips of your fingers and slide them lightly up and down along the entire length," Sascha continued. "That's right. Tantalize those bananas."

Oh, my God, Joan thought. *She's teaching us 'choking the chicken.' I swear, I'll never touch another banana as long as I live.*

From a stereo speaker mounted high in the corner of the Mardi Gras Room, Johnny Otis sang the rock and roll ditty, *"Willie and the Hand Jive."*

12

FAREWELL, HELLO

"I'm a gutless wonder, but what can I do?" Jerry Fart-ing said, fighting back tears. "I can't live without money." He slumped his dark brown, crew-cut head between his knees.

Jonathan had hastily called a meeting in the Dooch living room. Present were the other three freshmen Jonathan had shared so many memorable events: Farting's roommate, Tommy Tubbins, a tall, cherub-faced freshman; and Jonathan's roommie, Butch Tanenbloom.

Jonathan handed a letter, written in a perfect script, to Butch who read it aloud.

"Dear Gerald,

Your dad and I have reviewed your midterm grades, and we must express our displeasure with your C's. Mediocrity will not be tolerated by the Farthings. The cause of this academic disaster must be the distractions of living among those low-class boys at Dooch. During dorm registration, I told you the proper living group for you is the P U fraternity where you would be among your own kind.

You have not attended rush parties at the P U house, so we have decided that it, is in your best interests, to join the P U's <u>immediately</u>. *I have been assured by P U President, Dirk Krum III that, as a legacy, you will be accepted without question. We are pleased you will be following in the footsteps of other Farthing men.*

Young Dirk told us living at Dooch will only expose you to sordid, depraved influences from which you may never recover! You may have become superficially attached to a few Dormies, especially that nice Jonathan Aldon (who should also be living at the P U House!), but lifelong friendships can only be nurtured among the brothers of a superior fraternity, such as the P U's. In time, you will learn to appreciate the wisdom of our decision.

Sincerely,
Mom

PS If you do not join the P U's, we will have no choice but to stop your monthly allowance. We trust such drastic action will not be necessary."

"Gosh," Tommy Tubbins said. "Is joining a frat such a big deal?"

"It is for families who count on important business contacts for their success and well-being," Fart-ing said. "Mom really believes I'm wasting my time making friends with . . . poor guys . . . like you."

Jonathan recalled the look of horror on Mrs. Farthing's face during the P U's red ink, bomb attack on the Dooch dorm reg line and her prophetic words, *"I told you not to live in this God awful place!"*

Butch draped his right arm around Jerry's head in a gentle headlock and tapping him on the chin, said, "Easy, Fart-ing, baby. Getting your folks P O'd isn't the end of the world."

"But getting cut off from my allowance is," Fart-ing said, "How can I survive without money?"

"What about getting part-time jobs like me?" Jonathan said.

"You don't understand," Fart-ing sniffed. "I've never worked a day in my life. While you were paper boys or grocery baggers, I didn't have a care in the world. Everything was done for me. Work was always something only poor people did."

"It's never too late," Jonathan said. "I really like my part-time jobs."

"I just couldn't," Fart-ing said. "Dressing up like a gypsy boy with Ruby at Gifted Florence's, or getting chapped hands from chemicals counterfeiting ID's with Royal French, or dirtying my nails cleaning Hunch's playing cabin in the Campanile . . ." Fart-ing began to sob. "I'm sorry, Jonathan. I didn't mean to put you down."

Images of Jerry Fart-ing's life, as a Dormie, flashed through Jonathan's mind: Fart-ing walking on his hands backwards under Sather Gate as he changed his name from Farthing to Fart-ing; Fart-ing barfing after his initiation into Dormie "bowling;" Fart-ing, as part of the Campanile RF with Tubbins, Butch, and Jonathan; and Fart-ing, as member of Operation Red Foxtrot when delirious Dormies carried off the goal posts after Cal's historic upset of the SC football team.

After all these adventures, he's giving us up? Jonathan thought.

"We'll still be friends?" Fart-ing asked, wiping his reddening eyes.

"Buddies forever," Jonathan said, offering a handshake.

"Gosh, you can visit us anytime," Tubbins said.

"You can be our Dormie eyes inside the P U house," Butch said.

"I'll never forget you," Fart-ing said, forcing a weak smile, "and all the great RF's we had. When I'm settled, I'll have you over for a beer. When the P U's get to know you, they'll see how cool you guys are."

Jonathan bit his lip. In his mind's eye, he saw himself giving the same, hopeful, farewell speech had he been in Fart-ing's shoes. Had he made a huge mistake by taking a different path in defying his parents?

"Hey, Jerry," Butch said. "You'll always be Fart-ing to us, so get used to us calling you by your 'real' name in public, even in front of your new P U buddies."

Fart-ing hugged each, turned, and without looking back, left. The trio watched ex-Dormie, Jerry Fart-ing, head bowed, disappearing slowly into the Fall mist, as new P U pledge, Gerald Farthing.

* * * *

A thin male with skin stretched over six feet of bone, eased out of the elevator, holding a tattered suitcase in each hand. He wore a faded T-shirt, its partially torn breast pocket jammed with a phalanx of ball point pens guarding a stack of index cards. A crumpled pair of white chinos hung precariously on his waist. Sewn brown patches covered rips on the knees of his pants.

A grin rippled around the bulbous nose supporting black, hornrim glasses. Thick chestnut hair lay like a coonskin cap on his angular head.

"Holy, crap!" Butch said, peering out from his room. "Hey, Junior! Look who's here. It's our favorite cabby."

Jonathan stepped around Butch and rushed to greet the arrival.

"Rod Organ! What are you doing here?" Jonathan asked, pointing at the suitcases. "Dropping off a new Dormie?"

"You might say that," Organ said, winking.

"Like who?" Butch said, padding up the hallway.

"Like me!" Organ said, dropping the suitcases. One split open, spilling clothing on the floor.

"I've spent so much time in Berkeley helping you Dormies with your crazy RF's, I thought I'd transfer from San Francisco State," Organ said, "Besides, I'm tired of sleeping at the beach in my woodie."

Jonathan recalled how he and Butch had hired Rod Organ at the San Francisco Airport for the ride to campus. For an extra five dollars, Organ had thrown in a quick tour of Chinatown and North Beach. In front of the famous Beatnik hangout, City Lights Bookstore, Jonathan and Butch had come to the rescue of a buxom blonde in the clutches of two assailants. In the ensuing scuffle, the gallant duo learned, first-hand, the true identity of Paulette DuBois, The City's most notorious transvestite. Only quick action by Organ and his woodie had saved the pair from further embarrassment. Later, Organ had played an important role in derailing a fake Beatnik riot intended to drum up support for Congressman Clayborn Muck and HUAC.

"Heard Fart-ing became a turncoat and joined the P U's, so here I am, your brand new Dormie!" Organ said, stuffing clothes back into the frayed suitcase.

"Some trade," Butch said, slapping Organ's back with his huge hands. "Lose a Fart-ing, gain an Organ."

"Better yet," Organ said, swinging a clenched fist, side-to-side like a pendulum, "the Dormies get private transportation. My woodie is in the parking lot behind Dooch."

"Jeez," Butch said, "Whadda choice! Get a date and have no wheels, or embarrass a date in that God awful woodie."

"First thing's first, Brooklyn," Organ said. "Let's see you get a date, before you think about borrowing the woodie."

Escorting the new Dormie to the room he would share with Tommy Tubbins, Jonathan asked, "what'll you major in?"

"Not sure. My mom wants me to look into merchandising."

"Merchandising what?" Jonathan asked.

"Men's fashions," Organ said with a straight face.

Butch is right, Jonathan thought. *It was sad to see Fart-ing leave; but Organ and his woodie will fit right in with the Dormies.*

13

CAPITALISTIC PUB CRAWL

The full moon glistened on the swirling river, a mix of single malt Scotch, French red wine, cognac, Irish coffee, gushing then snaking gracefully along Montgomery Street, in the heart of San Francisco's financial district. The flow diverted into two streams as they engulfed the remnant of a broken taillight, each fork carrying flotsam of goose liver pate, escargot, Caesar salad, Chateaubriand, and baked Alaska. Glowing, green horseflies awakened from evening hibernation by the delicious offal, circled lazily above. The source of the orange-brown bile lay sprawled, head first, in the gutter heaving spasmodically to the clanging of a distant cable car.

"Aaaggghhh," moaned the cause of the oozing, putrid stench.

"There, there," the booming voice of Garrick Nelquist said. "Just barf the rest of your guts out, Jericho. You'll feel better tomorrow."

Nearby, Ari Scott paced, dreading the arrival of the Saturday night paddy wagon collecting public drunks.

I don't need this kind of publicity, Ari thought, envisioning an eye-tem in Sam Paean's gossip column:

> *"What campus radical spilled his*
> *swel-eagant dinner while chaperoned*
> *by a duo of Cal's best known profs?"*

The evening had begun inauspiciously. Keeping a promise that he would meet Anna's new boyfriend, Ari, with Garrick in tow, had driven to the intersection of Telly and Bancroft where Jericho "Save-the-World" Slabio stood on an inverted wooden crate, exhorting a crowd with a harangue against "bourgeois American capitalist values" which, according to Slabio, was "the root cause of the working man's plight."

Hoping to put the young radical at ease, Ari had dressed casually in a tweed sports jacket, tie, and slacks. Always the Anglophile, Garrick wore a dark, pin-striped double-breasted suit with a red kerchief peeking from the coat pocket.

Easing into the bus zone behind the crowd, Garrick held the door open, motioning Slabio into the backseat. Introductions were hastily made, as Ari gunned the Dodge down Bancroft.

Hope no faculty members saw us, Ari thought.

Glancing in the rearview mirror, Ari noted Slabio was dressed in worn blue jeans, torn sneakers, and a tattered T shirt with the slogan,

"The Rich Suck and Swallow the Fruits of the Poor's Labor"

Slabio's eyes were blue and beady. His hair was dark brown, thick and curly like the puffed body of a blow fish, a style, a few years later, Blacks would call an Afro.

"Never ridden a DeSoto," Slabio said, lighting up a Kools. "No capitalistic monstrosities like this where I come from."

Thank God, Cee Cee took the Caddy, Ari thought.

"And where is there?" Garrick asked dryly. "Lodi?"

"Nah," Slabio said, blowing smoke over the front seats. "Ever hear of Winnemucca?"

"Nevada?" Ari said. "How can you afford out-of-state tuition."

"I qualified as a disadvantaged student under Berkeley's new admissions policy," Slabio smiled. "Being a disadvantaged student has other benefits. Profs are easier on you. I don't have to attend class, write papers, or worry about grades. Gives me time for my speeches."

"And what do your parents do?" Garrick said, tamping fresh tobacco into his meerschaum.

"If the truth be known, I come from a capitalistic, law enforcement background," Slabio said. "My mother owns a strip joint. Dear old Dad is the county sheriff. That's the reason I know so much about the enemy."

Ari shot Garrick a look of disbelief.

Slabio smirked. "I know what you're thinking. That you're superior because I'm a poor out-of-state slob. This is what the California dream is all about. Outside people can waltz in and takeover bloated, corrupt institutions like the University of California and mold them into a new model, one dedicated to the poor and downtrodden. Soon, we out-of-staters will control everything."

Slabio leaned forward and rested his chin on the top of the front seat.

"Let's get something straight, professors. I wouldn't be riding with you bourgeois capitalists except for the promise I made my honey to get to know her loving 'papa.' This whole evening is going to be a pain in the ass. It's totally against everything I believe in; but, if it's gonna please Anna, I can pretend with the best of them." Slabio blew a large puff of smoke at Ari's frowning image in the rearview mirror.

Stay calm, Ari told himself, feeling anger welling inside. *Don't let Slabio get under your skin. You'd be playing right into his hands.*

Ari turned up the sound of the car radio playing the McGuire Sisters singing *"Something's Gotta Give,"* to drown out any further comments. In self-defense, Garrick, puffed billows of pipe smoke toward the back seat

"Would the gentleman desire a complimentary jacket?" Bernie's distinguished silver-haired, maitre d,' Terrence Nulligan said, frowning at Slabio's T-shirt.

Slabio shook his head, pointing to the slogan of his T-shirt, said, "I want the capitalist pigs here to squirm at the truth."

Ari bit his lip, while Garrick rolled his eyes.

"I believe the gentleman declines your kind offer," Ari said, "May we have the Chandler family table," Ari said, slipping Nulligan a ten.

"Certainly, Professor Scott, Nulligan said, "the Chandlers are not dining here tonight," the maitre d' winked.

"So, this is the famous hangout of 'Frisco capitalism?" Slabio said, pivoting in his chair, showing off his T-shirt. "The red, flocked wallpaper looks like the inside of a French whorehouse." Slabio slapped the table, laughing.

From a corner table, Sam Paean had noted the arrival of the odd trio. He had already received tips about Ari's beautiful daughter, Anna, dating Cal's notorious student radical.

"Dining with Jericho 'Save-the-world' Slabio has to be the ultimate act of tolerance, even for two noted liberal profs, eh?" Paean said to his girlfriend and girl Friday, E Lyn Chamberlin.

The romance must be getting serious, Paean thought. *Why would Ari Scott risk his social reputation by being seen in public with someone as inflammatory as Slabio. Lovely Anna deserves someone better than this rhetorical blow hard.*

"Garcon," Slabio said, snapping his fingers at the tuxedo'd server presenting oversized, red felt menus. "I'll have a *Glen Livet*. Make that a double."

"Immediately, sir," the waiter said.

"Great service for a bourgeois dump," Slabio said, leaning forward, whispering in a conspiratorial tone. "I've never had single malt scotch before, but those *Esquire* ads look inviting."

"You read *Esquire*?" Garrick said, emptying the meerschaum. "I didn't think radicals read capitalistic trash."

"My motto is 'know thy enemy,' " Slabio said. "Can't fight things you don't understand."

"And what about *Playboy*?" Garrick said, giving Slabio a wink.

"A flesh rag," Slabio said, emptying the scotch in one sustained slurp. "But, *Playboy* does have stimulating articles. Garcon, I'll have another," he shouted, waving the empty glass in a circle above his head.

"So you read the articles?" Garrick said.

"With all due respect, Professor Nelquist, let's cut the holier-than-thou crap. I hear there are copies of *Playboy* stashed in the reading room of the Men's Faculty Club where you old farts can get your rocks off, in private."

"Let's order," Ari said, changing the topic. "Jericho?"

Looking up from the menu, Slabio said, "Since you two are picking up the tab, I'll have every decadent dish I've heard about." He inhaled the second double *Glen Livet*.

"Know thy enemy," Garrick muttered under his breath.

Slabio licked foie gras from his butter knife and ripped pieces of french bread with his teeth. "Same texture as peanut butter," Slabio remarked, gouging another mound of foie gras.

Escargot, cooked in garlic and butter, were served in the shell. Using a tiny fork, Garrick demonstrated how they were to be eaten. Ignoring the instruction, Slabio picked up a shell and, in a loud slurp, sucked the creature from its home.

"The shells aren't edible," Ari warned, hoping to avoid the spectacle of Slabio crunching the creature's habitat.

Slabio sipped his third single malt scotch, as the waiter made Caesar salad at table side.

"I'll be damned," Slabio said. "Raw egg and my favorite fish, anchovy. I have anchovy pizza, at least twice a week."

Ari shuddered, imagining Anna kissing the anchovy inhaling radical. *They say love is blind*, he thought, *but Anna has nothing in common with this young man. Does Slabio really remind Anna of her stepfather? Pablo Zarzana has to a prince, in comparison.* Ari thought.

In graceful movements, the sommelier decanted a French Cabernet Garrick had selected.

"Let me sniff the cork," Slabio said. "I saw Cary Grant do it in *'North by Northwest.'* " He nodded approvingly. "Smells better than Thunderbird!" He flipped the cork over his shoulder."It's a joke!" he chortled."Thunderbird doesn't have a cork. It's got a twist off."

The waiter carved medium rare Chateaubriand at table side.

"Make that two large slices for me, waiter," Slabio said, snapping his fingers twice. "Mmm, this capitalistic lifestyle is not all that bad," he said, shoveling meat into his mouth.

Ari and Garrick dined in stunned silence as they watched Slabio wolf down large chunks of meat without chewing, washing them down with large gulps of Cabernet.

It's now or never, Ari thought.

"What qualities of Anna appeal to you."

Garrick braced himself for the response, cradling his forehead in the palm of his left hand

"Can I be totally honest, Prof? No bull shit? Man-to-man? Who knows? I may be calling you 'papa' in the future."

Garrick coughed, choking on an imaginary piece of beef.

"Sure," Ari said, placing his utensils on the table, now wishing he had never broached the topic.

"Anna's got a tremendous intellect," Slabio said, his speech slurring.

Ari felt his stomach begin to churn.

"And . . ." Garrick said, peering into Slabio's beady blue eyes.

"And," Slabio sighed, picking up his wine glass, "she has the best set of tits I have ever seen." He drained the wine in a gulp.

Garrick gripped Ari's elbow and kicked his friend in the shin.

"Besides the obvious, young man, what else is there about Anna that appeals to you," Garrick asked.

Filling his glass from a second bottle of French wine, Slabio swirled the Cabernet before gulping it. Slabio's head swayed from side-to-side, his slurred speech now more pronounced.

"The way I see it. I marry Anna, and my political future is insured. Imagine being the son-in-law of Pablo Zarzana." His blue eyes squinted in a smile, "and, almost a relative to the next ass hole Governor of California."

"And . . ." Garrick egged Slabio on to share more of his dream as after dinner cognacs were served.

"The world is changing. The Sixties are almost here. Time for people like me to lead the downtrodden masses in an uprising against two centuries of capitalist exploitation," Slabio burped. "I will be to California what Pablo is to Italy."

"You see Anna as part of this Utopian future?" Ari said. How he wanted to throttle Slabio with his bare hands.

"Prof, be realistic," Slabio said, taking a swig from a snifter. "I think Che Guevara said it best. 'If you can't eat your enemy's food, drink his booze, and fuck his women, you don't have any business in politics.' "

Ari twisted away from Garrick's restraint and throttled Slabio's neck with both hands, spilling half the contents of the snifter over the slogan emblazoned on his T-shirt.

"Listen, you little two-bit demagogue. You do one little thing to hurt Anna, and you'll have nothing left between your legs." Ari snarled.

"Ahem," a voice said from above. "Ari, Garrick, so good to see you again." It was Sam Paean.

Ari released his grip.

"Yes, Sam. Hi, E Lyn," Ari said, rising.

"Looking mighty fetching tonight, Miss Chamberlin," Garrick, said, standing, kissing the back of E Lyn's hand.

"Who might be this young man be?" Paean said. "Could it be, the famous campus radical, Jericho "Save-the-World" Slabio?" Extending his hand, Paean said, "I'm Sam Paean. This is my assistant, E Lyn."

"Yep, this is humble me," Slabio said, draining his cognac.

"How did you enjoy dinner?" E Lyn said.

"This is a free country," Slabio said. "And when the food and booze are free, it makes capitalistic grub palatable."

"May I quote you on that," Paean said, removing a small notebook from a breast pocket.

"Sure, what the hell," Slabio burped. "When in Rome, do as the Romans do. If I'm gonna violate my principles breaking bread with the enemy, might as well go all the way. Quote me word for word, Paean; but make sure you spell my name correctly. That's one 'A' and one 'O,' in Slabio, not two 'O's." He picked up Ari's snifter from the table.

"Where're you going from here?" Paean said, eyeing Slabio sipping from Ari's snifter.

"We're sporting gentlemen," Garrick said. "We're taking Jericho on the Pub Crawl Ari and I popularized in our youth. Care to join us?".

A sustained burp issued from Slabio, emptying Garrick's snifter.

"I would hate to bear witness to Mr. Slabio's initiation into this ritual," Paean said. "Bad for my digestion. Time for El Toro, E Lyn."

Ari, calmed by Sam and E Lyn's repartee, reseated himself, as the dessert, Baked Alaska, was ignited, sliced, and served to Slabio's applause.

Keep your cool, Ari reminded himself. *Anna is infatuated, but she is strong and smart. She'll see through this phony. As for the matter at hand, you ungrateful pipsqueak,* thought Ari. *Let's see how really tough you are.*

Ari ordered another two brandies for Slabio and nodded to Garrick who was now smiling broadly. Garrick lit the meerschaum and blew a long sustained puff at "Save-the-World" Slabio devouring the dessert.

Wobbling out of Bernie's, Slabio said, "Show me this famous Pub Crawl Anna bragged about. I'll drink your asses under the table."

Hailing a cab, the trio stopped at the Buena Vista Café where Irish coffee was invented. After two, Slabio scoffed, "Nothing but caffeine and sugar. Let's find some real booze."

A second cab took them to Broadway where Ari and Garrick, with Slabio in tow, began the Pub Crawl.

Zigzagging bar-to-bar, the trio matched drink-for-drink at Kelly O'Wong's Irish Pub, Quoth The Craven's Saloon, Tac's Tavern, Gold Street, Club Hungry U, and every pub, bar, and gin joint between.

At the end of the Pub Crawl, the trio was still standing, but Slabio's early copious consumption at Bernie's was taking its toll.

"Let's get a little fresh air and walk back to the car," Garrick said, his head pounding.

"Sure," Ari said. He had been pacing himself carefully. "Walk or crawl, we'll hoof it back to the car."

"Anything you fucking capitalists do, I can do better," Slabio said, farting in defiance.

The three were within two blocks of Bernie's, when Slabio began tottering side-to-side. Brushing away Garrick's hand, he said, "Don't need your bourgeois help."

Half a dozen paces later, Slabio listed to one side and crumpled slowly to the pavement, his head and hands dangling in the gutter.

After a few labored breaths, the flood of bile exploded from Slabio's innards, creating the stream now flowing along Montgomery Street.

"The Left Wing Paradox," Ari said, referring to Garrick's pet socio-political theory that always elicited affectionate boo's from his students. Garrick's tongue-in-cheek observation was that radicals who advocated greater rights for the downtrodden became victims of the very people they championed. History was littered with radicals who fomented unrest and revolution, only to find themselves disposable after the revolution. Garrick pointed to Robespierre's fate during the French Revolution and Trotsky and Kerensky's demises after the Russian Revolution.

"My sentiments exactly," Garrick said, holding his nose, "With his proclivity for seduction, this is a very volatile combination. Two-bit demagogue reduced to a common drunk. Kid's a real ass hole, an egregious one at that, but you'll have your hands full showing his true side to Anna. When women fall in love, there's no accounting for their lack of good taste."

Ari nodded. He had to find a way to expose Slabio's dark side. Anna's future depended on it.

Now snoring blissfully, Slabio continued to ooze the last vestiges of his capitalistic, gourmet mis-adventure.

Gazing into the night sky, Ari saw a smiling apparition, a beautiful ghost from his youthful *toure di amore*.

Yes, Ari thought. *Sofia will be here soon. Mothers always know how to deal with daughters.*

14

PRITTI DIVA

"Rogers, . . . Mr. G. Dreyers Rogers?"

A hand shot up among the students jamming the doorway of Professor Jacob Aural's English 1A class.

Sandy barked twice.

"Thank you, Sandy," Professor Aural said, patting the head of his seeing-eye dog. "Dreyers is an interesting name, Mr. Rogers. You may take any of the empty seats."

A handsome boy with flashing eyes and an athletic build muscled through the crowd and up the tiered levels of the main lecture hall of South Hall, the mid Victorian-Second Empire styled building erected in 1873, that was still used for classrooms by the English Department.

"Dockter, . . . Mr. Doctor K. Dockter?" Professor Aural called. "Another unusual name. With a name like that Mr. Dockter, I trust you are a pre-med major?"

A tall, rugged student with sun-bleached blond hair and a sly grin bounded into the classroom.

There was only one vacant seat left.

"Geez," Butch Tanenbaum grumbled. "Nothin' but frat-rats. How about a babe, Junior?" Butch said, eyeing the last empty seat, next to Jonathan that had been formerly occupied by Roz Tess.

After the Angel of Death had posted mid-term grades, 12 of the 40 students of Professor Jacob's English 1A had dropped out. Eight received C's, two, D's, and two, including Jonathan, were failing.

"Crashers," students who had patiently attended Professor Aural's lectures without credits and without assigned seats, were now awaiting the result of a random lottery printed in Braille, plucked from a beret by Roz Tess, a striking brunette with a winsome smile, who had received the only A on the midterm exam. The grade earned Roz Tess the seat of honor, in the center of the front row.

"Diva, . . . Miss Pritti Diva?" Professor Aural announced, "Pritti Diva, present?"

As Professor Aural reached for another name, a firm female voice shouted from the hallway, "Here, sir!"

As the throng parted, a chorus of appreciative whistles greeted the new arrival.

"Apparently, Miss Diva is a popular selection," Professor Aural said.

Whistles, now accompanied by good- natured hoots, followed the girl, as she walked up the steeply pitched lecture room toward the empty seat next to Jonathan.

"Whoa, Junior," Butch said. "A three star General!" Butch leaned his 6-foot-5-inch frame, in an exaggerated bow, making a sweeping gesture, directing Pritti Diva to the seat next to Jonathan.

"Stop it, Butch," Jonathan whispered, "This is embarrassing."

Through clenched teeth, Butch hissed, "The meek shall NOT inherit the earth, Junior." He stepped behind the empty seat.

Pritti Diva, didn't walk, she sashayed with a confident air, smiling broadly at her new classmates. Her clothes were not a part of the standard campus wardrobe. She wore a gold-colored dress, pearls, and low heels, something more common to a sales person in a fancy women's store than a freshman student.

Jonathan noted that she did not carry her books hugged tightly to her bosom like other coeds, but carried them in one hand, swinging her arm gracefully like a pendulum. As she approached, Jonathan saw the reason for the wolf whistles. Despite her thin, small frame and her loose-fitting dress, it was obvious Pritti Diva was well-endowed. The left side of her face was hidden behind a flowing hairstyle sculptured around a finely chiseled face, reminding Jonathan of Father's favorite actress, Gene Tierney.

"Thanks, Sir Gallant," she said to Butch, gracefully easing herself into the chair to Jonathan's right.

"Butch Tanenbloom, from Brooklyn, at your service. The charming fellow, next to you, is my buddy, the esteemed Jonathan Aldon from

Clear Lake, Iowa."

Butch clasped his giant hands on Jonathan's shoulders and forcibly rotated his body 90 degrees to the right to face the new member of the class.

"Pritti Diva," she said, looking squarely at Jonathan. "I'm new to Berkeley, too."

Jonathan felt his face flush as he looked into her dazzling emerald eye. He recalled his giddy reaction speaking to the CAT Airline stewardesses on the flight from Minneapolis, but there was something different, something mysterious, something alluring about this gorgeous female seated inches away.

"Regrets to the rest of you," Professor Aural said, bidding the disappointed throng adieu. "Better luck next semester."

"For those of you who are remaining for the rest of the semester, may I offer you a pearl of wisdom," Professor Aural said, pacing back-and-forth in front of Sandy who had taken up a spot in the warm sunlight streaming in from the window.

"When you enrolled in this class, you assumed English 1A was reading a certain number of books and writing a certain number of papers."

Several class members nodded.

"With the poor showing on the mid-term exam, you should now appreciate that neither raw intelligence nor creative fluff is a guarantee of success.

"You are among the best and brightest in the world, *la creme de la creme,* so it is not my intent to retest your IQ's. Doing well does NOT depend on memorizing lines from famous literature. It does NOT depend on flowery book reports. It does NOT require the use of fancy, multi-syllabic words. It certainly does NOT depend on sounding like me as you write exam answers.

"What I hope to accomplish is helping you use your God-given gifts to change your perspective of the world. No, I'm not talking about brain-washing, as some of the more conservative members of our faculty suggest, but rather, through the spoken and written word, to challenge you, to stimulate your imagination, to encourage clear and creative thought, with the ultimate goal of creative problem-solving, in a rapidly changing world.

"Some of you may believe I derive some sadistic enjoyment in engaging Mr. Aldon in embarrassing discourse. Some may think I pick on him because he's from Iowa."

"You're not?" Butch said, drawing laughter from the class.

"That must be Mr. Aldon's alter-ego, Mr. Tanenbloom," Professor Aural said, "No, I'm not."

"What I'm trying to do is encouraging all of you to question values ingrained from birth. I call on Mr. Aldon, because Iowa is the least diverse state in the country and its shared community values have not changed over the past century. Isn't that true, Mr. Aldon?"

"Yes," Jonathan said, wondering if Professor Jacob were a long lost son of Iowa.

"Iowans have rigid beliefs that work well in the Heartland of America but would not be successful in a society as diverse and dynamic as California. Would you agree, Mr. Aldon?"

"Yes," Jonathan said, feeling the warm gaze of Pritti Diva's green eyes suffusing him.

"I hope your vocabulary will expand beyond one word responses, like 'yes' or ' no,' Mr. Aldon."

"I do too," Jonathan said, reminding himself that he would need to work on oral responses in his nightly tutoring at Dooch.

"Good, Mr. Aldon. I see improvement already. 'I do too' is a three word response!"

Exhaling in relief, Jonathan turned toward Pritti Diva who returned his gaze with a smile that made her emerald eye iridescent. It was this precise moment when Pritti Diva brushed back the sweep of her cascading hair - like a camera shutter clicking - revealing the flashing brilliance of her other eye.

Jonathan blinked, thinking he had witnessed an illusion.

The color of Pritti Diva's other eye was orange.

15

THE POUND OF MUSIC

Freed from the shackles of a wire corset, ropes undulated up toward bronze and green-hued bells suspended from the ceiling of the Campanile. Normally, the bottom of the ropes were wired to 61 wooden batons of a golden oak console, within a roofless, rectangular, glass-enclosed playing cabin. At their upper-reaches, the ropes were tethered to individual bells weighing from 29 pounds to over 4118 pounds.

Inside the cramped playing cabin, above 29-foot pedals, the 61 wooden baton were arranged in rows like the keys of a piano. Carillonneurs were trained to play the bells by depressing the batons with their hands while dancing an agile jig on the foot pedals.

Hunch Hitowski watched the ropes serpentine gracefully up to his vision of heaven. Above, the curved arches of each of the four quadrants of the belfry had been carved from solid pieces of California granite and paneled with Italian ornamentation of coffers with rosettes like the Campanile's namesake in St. Mark's Plaza in Venice.

The 61 bells, in clusters of varying sizes, were suspended in orderly rows by an intricate network of metal braces. The original 12 English bells, installed in 1917, were covered with the green patina of oxidation. Later, 49 French bells had been added, some still glinting splotches of their original bronze hue.

Hunch hopped onto a narrow rampart circling the glass walls of the playing cabin, nimbly swinging from rope-to-rope, banging the bells in deafening, rhythmic flight, shaking the belfry in a musical temblor. Miss Betty Burdick, Campanile chime mistress, preferred her assistants playing at the console, but Hunch loved the freedom of being musically airborne. Royal French had noted that, in a certain light, the outline of the little hunchback, swinging from bell-to-bell, resembled Victor Hugo's description of Quasimodo from *"The Hunch Back of Notre Dame."* Hunch began his the noon concert with , *"Long Ago and Far Away."*

Seventy-five feet below, beneath Roman numeral VI of the Campanile's clocks, Jonathan Aldon sat in the comfortable cocoon of the chime mistress's office replete with all the comforts of home: shower, kitchenette, and library. He sat in the sitting area reserved for visiting dignitaries. Books for his afternoon classes were stacked on the floor.

Hunch had convinced Miss Burdick that the belfry playing cabin needed regular cleaning to promote the well-being of its carillonneurs. Thus, five days-a week, Jonathan hoofed up the 316 steps to the belfry and polished the glass walls of the playing cabin to a sparkle before Hunch's noon concert. This high-rise duty should have paid only the minimum wage of $1.00 per hour, but Miss Burdick liked the young man and offered Jonathan a generous $1.50 per hour.

Since meeting young Jonathan during the Campanile RF, Miss Burdick had been taken by the wholesome personality and clean-cut looks of this earnest young man. If the truth were known, Jonathan was the vision of the grandson she never had and in a way, reminded her of dashing Irish Wes O'Chita, who had broken her heart in her senior year at Cal 41 years ago. Single, she had dedicated her life to cataloging and cross-referencing the music to thousands of tunes performed by Hunch and the other Campanile carillonneurs.

There were two benefits of Jonathan's job at the Campanile. One was the delicious, home-made cookies Miss Burdick baked. The other was he could study in the bell tower office until his 2 p.m. class.

Jonathan felt the soothing vibration of the office walls, as the minute hand of the Campanile clocks advanced, a sensation that felt like the rocking he and his childhood buddy, Ziggy, had experienced inserting a nickel in a metal box, marked *"Swedish Massage,"*on beds at Clear Lake's Blue Horizon Inn.

Jonathan had finished his reading assignment for Professor Aural's English 1A Class, anticipating what areas he might be called upon to address. Professor Aural no longer intimidated him. He was beginning to understand why the professor was challenging him to think on his feet, why it was more important to be analytical and clear-thinking than to fumble for a memorized, "right" answer.

Jonathan pulled a crumpled letter from his back pocket.

"Dear Johnny-Boy,

Sorry about not writing. Busy slopping pigs for Aldon Farms.

Your parents came back from Berkeley and went nuts (especially your mom) telling everybody in town how they had disowned you because you had turned into a Crazy Beatnik. At the Methodist Church, your uncle Reverend Granger, even led a prayer for your salvation!

I was plenty worried until your Uncle Mike and Aunt Pearl told me the real facts about your split with your parents.

Your folks invited Pop and me for Thanksgiving. Damned tough not talking about you. Whadda you gonna do? Gobble, gobble!

Study real hard. I'll be rooting for you.

"When" by the Kalen Twins, Number #1 on K-HOG radio.

Your buddy (and the OTHER Amazin' Double A's),

- Ziggy

PS 1:Ever run into any of those big-titted gals living at that Yearning Arms boarding house we saw in Playboy? I think of you every time I drool over those kazoobies. You lucky dog!

PS 2: Don't ever forget, Johnny-Boy, 'Shit flies both ways!' "

Shit flies both ways, thought Jonathan. The boyhood motto he and Ziggy had coined for the Amazing Double A's now sounded naive and far removed from his life at Cal.

Shit flew only one way these days, always in his direction, he sighed.

"Everything, ok, Jonathan?" Miss Burdick said, peeking her head around the corner of the library.

"Cookies were delicious, as usual," Jonathan said with a grin that made her blush."You treat me better than my own mother." He bit his lip, thinking how true that was.

"I'll never take the place of your mom, Jonathan. Just want you to be comfortable, and I'll do my little something to help you make your grades. Hunch told me how difficult it's been."

"Everything you do makes a positive difference to me, Ma'am,"

Jonathan said, suddenly feeling a pang of sadness.

"Keep your chin up, Jonathan," Miss Burdick said.

Jonathan produced a ball point pen and tablet and began to write. His head and heart were filled with conflicting thoughts and emotions, as he reached out to his link to Clear Lake, Iowa, now an alien land.

"Ziggy:

Thanks for the pep talk. I'll need a lot of help to get my grades up to a C. The Dormies are tutoring me every night. Can you believe I get hypnotized for some of these learning sessions - like those geezers we used to laugh at when they got the old fleegle eye from Marvelous Mandrake at the Cerro Gordo County Fair - but it REALLY works!

Part-time jobs are keeping a few bucks in my pocket. Working with Ruby Lips is like dressing up for Halloween. Helping Hunch Hitowski in the Campanile is fun but turning me deaf! Making fake ID's with Royal French, makes me feel like a spy. An exotic kind of education!

Don't faint, but I DID meet a gal from Yearning Arms (sits next to me in English). She wasn't one of girls we saw in Playboy, but Pritti Diva is absolutely gorgeous. Butch calls her a three star General. Can you imagine a girl with one green eye and one orange? Swear, I'm not joshing! We talk a lot, but I'm too chicken to ask her out. With so little money, what could I offer? Butch is always suggesting something crazy, but I guess I'm doomed to admiring her in silence.

Had Thanksgiving with my Oakland relatives, Reverend Ike, his wife Doris, and their three sons. More food than you can eat in a week.

MJ's musical career has really taken off. He and Big Berry and the Blackouts have a recording contract to perform "Louie, Louie." The song has driven the campus nuts! AJ was voted Northern California high school football player of the year. We're hoping he'll come to Cal. I'm really worried about RJ. His Black Panther friends have run-ins with the Oakland Police - mostly pushing and shoving - but their leader Huey got a hold of some guns from the Che Guevara Fan Club. Reverend Ike and Doris are praying for RJ's safety.

Your Crazy Beatnik Buddy (the Other Amazin' Double A)

Jonathan

PS Bobby Darin's "Mack The Knife" #1 in the Bay Area."

Jonathan sealed the letter, licked and affixed a four-cent stamp for first-class postage.

In the belfry, Hunch Hitowski concluded his noon concert with a melancholy rendition of *"I'm Always Chasing Rainbows."*

16

BLUE LIGHT SPECIALS

On the rugged eastern foothill, above the Berkeley campus, is a triangulation of Cal's most endearing symbols. The northern point is the 10,000 seat, Greek Theater sculptured into a eucalyptus grove in 1903. Overlooking San Francisco Bay and the Golden Gate, the concrete bowl was patterned on the theater at Epidaurus.

At one corner of the triangle, rising from Strawberry Canyon, is the perfect oval of Memorial Stadium built in 1923, with a seating capacity of 75,000. Inspired by the classic design of Roman sports arenas, Memorial Stadium is often described as "the most beautiful place in America to watch a college football game."

To the east, at the apex of the triangle, squats the Big C. The 40-by 20-foot block concrete letter was built in1905 during a driving rain storm, when students forming a human chain, passed raw materials up the hill where concrete was mixed and poured.

Well above the Big C sits a circular, concrete building resembling a wheel of white cheese where a few, with security clearances, work at the atom smasher housed within its bowels. This is the Cyclotron, the domain of noted atomic scientist, Professor Werner Von Seller.

On a clear night, the view from the Cyclotron is breathtaking. The gleaming necklaces of the Bay, Golden Gate, and Richmond-San Rafael bridges float in a half circle of light above the black waters of San Francisco Bay. A blanket of lights from hundreds of thousands of Bay Area homes blink in rhythm to distant fog horns braying forlornly.

Standing before this sweeping panorama, Von Seller adjusted his monocle and savored the last puffs of a Gaulois encased in the sterling silver cigarette holder.

Von Seller had furnished his office in minimalist Danish. His one extravagance was an eight foot, ebony desk, appropriately dramatic for a scientist exploring the mysterious world of atoms. Behind the desk, a long closet, with folding accordion doors, housed a hi-fi stereo system and a bed with a firm mattress.

In the evening, as he worked alone, Von Seller turned the hi-fi stereo to full volume, immersing himself in the music of his favorite Wagner opera, *Die Walkure*. He had discovered that playing Wagner while the atom smasher did his bidding provided a contrapuntal symphony of sound and fury that could not be duplicated elsewhere.

The Cyclotron - not that childish Big C - is the true apex of the Cal triangle, Von Seller thought. *Yes, the Cyclotron was a bastion protecting the naive and gullible public from the foibles and excesses of modern life. Where else could the secrets of the atom be unlocked to serve the military and society, than here in his beloved Cyclotron?*

Von Seller was well aware of his derisive nickname, the Prussian Penguin, liberal faculty members snickered behind his back. But he had unwavering faith in himself and even more faith in the power of the atom. History would accord him a place of honor for his dedicated work.

When his family had left Germany, 25-years ago, Von Seller was already a child prodigy. His wealthy industrialist parents, fearing Hitler's war plans, fled to Austria, then to Denmark, and eventually to California.

The teenage Von Seller enrolled at Stanford, at age 15, and quickly mastered the concepts of nuclear fission, becoming the youngest member of the Manhattan Project, developing the atomic bombs dropped on Hiroshima and Nagasaki. As the Cold War set in, Von Seller was an obvious choice to head up atomic research at Cal, the most distinguished public university in the world.

Occasionally, Von Seller questioned himself about his on-going fight with the weak-minded, left-wing element of the faculty.

I am the supreme survivor, he reminded himself. WRC's patronage in asking him to administer publish or perish would be the pivotal turning point in his life.

Von Seller had sacrificed his youth for the cause of the atom. There were times when he longed for a normal social life others enjoyed.

At international conferences, he had discreetly explored the wonders of female flesh, visiting highly recommended brothels. He admitted there was a certain thrill in dallying with girls, especially very young girls, but there was no greater thrill than his hours spent at the Cyclotron's control panel.

Tonight, he had finished his first weekly newsletter to the faculty entitled "Cyclotron White Paper #1." The title had a certain understated cachet that would irritate his fuzzy-brained enemies. Von Seller reported, in detail, his efforts to recruit graduate assistants to conduct classes, while the faculty was busy satisfying its publish or perish requirement. He particularly relished describing his USC recruits as "distinguished doctoral candidates from that pre-eminent private university to the south." He knew what an angry stir this would cause, but he had considered Cal's traditional "holier than thou" attitude toward the SC Trojans infantile and nonsense.

Wasn't the western actor, John Wayne, an SC grad?

If he played his cards correctly, Von Seller was certain he would merge the resources of Cal and SC into a symbiotic colossus of atomic research facilities that he, alone, would control for the benefit of mankind. Yes, administering publish or perish was just the beginning of his ascension as a revered figure in the academic, scientific community.

He pressed the concealed button beneath his desk, admitting him into the heart of the Cyclotron, the air-conditioned room adjacent to the atom smasher. Walking purposefully to the ten foot control panel, he pushed the series of coded signals to the atom smasher, advising his mistress that her master was ready for tonight's work.

The cyclotron hummed obediently, inducing flashing red numbers on her dials. As she approached maximum speed, she emitted a blue light, deepening in intensity, until the entire Cyclotron was bathed in a luminescent blue glow, visible to airplanes flying through San Francisco Bay airspace.

At these moments, Von Seller felt a rush of exhilaration, akin to the times he spent with those very young girls; but the seductive blue light of the atom smasher aroused him like no young girl ever could.

He held tightly to the two rails of the control panel, as the atom smasher whirled to maximum speed, the velocity needed to smash a tiny atom into elemental particles. His face was now awash in her deep blue glow as the atom received the Cyclotron's full force and fury in an orgasmic explosion.

Von Seller felt emotionally lifted into orbit, falling, then fading into a sublime abyss of heavenly blue.

Yes, this was the core of his existence!

* * * *

The outline of a reclined figure laying sideways on the bed was visible against the moonlit sky. A trio of assistants squatted nearby, while a rapt audience huddled on the floor of the darkened room.

"Ready?" one assistant whispered.

"Yes," the prone figure replied.

A raspy click and a white flame leaped from a Zippo lighter held by the nearest assistant, Butch Tanenbloom. For several seconds, the flame gently flickered near the prone figure.

"Got one coming," grunted the reclined figure.

"Hurry," the second assistant urged, extending a measuring tape.

"Yes!" the prone figure shouted, as a low, "whoosh" of methane gas issued, turning the flame blue, as it blasted horizontally toward the second and third assistants, one holding a tape measure, the other a stop watch.

"Five and one-half inches!" Jonathan said.

"A full second!" Punch announced, clicking a stopwatch, as his eye spun in an excited orbit.

The crowd broke into applause and the flame blower was mobbed. by fellow freshmen.

Cherub-faced freshman Eng-ineering student, Tommy Tubbins, had set a new Dooch record for lighting flatulence!

"Any challengers to the new champ?" Living Buddha said, picking up the blackened tape measure.

"Waz can top that," Royal French said. "You should be stuck with him in the dorm elevator when he cuts the cheese. Whew!"

"We want Waz! We want Waz!" a chorus of voices chanted.

"I'll get him," Hunch, the Campanile carillonneur said.

It was a typical Friday night at Dooch Dorm. Creative competition was substitution for a dateless social life for the Dormies. Following an indigestible dinner, as flatulence bloated the rooms and hallways of Dooch, Dormies devised creative ways to pass the gaseous night away.

Lighting farts was one.

All-Pro intoned his deepest dee jay voice, announcing the arrival of Waz.

"And now, our NEW CHALLENGER - from the Garden State of New Jersey - that INTREPID, campus traffic enforcement officer, your friendly Meter Mel, THE GAS WITH CLASS. The ONE, the ONLY, WAZ-Z-Z!"

Cheers, mixed with boo's greeted Waz's arrival. He had a lanky build, with long arms dangling almost to the knees. Dark brown hair lay flat on a small head from which small, dark eyes squinted. Waz's long, pointy nose underscored the thick nasal, New Jersey accent that seemed to bypass his lips and emit directly from his nostrils.

At a young age, Homer Wazlewski acquired the name, Waz - not a short for his surname - because of his fascination for the movie, *"Wizard of Oz,"* which he pronounced "Wiz-a-Waz." Growing up in Hoboken, Waz excelled at the neighborhood sports of riding beat-up motorcycles and shooting pool.

In high school, Waz's life was transformed. Riding bikes and hustling pool bets were no longer stimulating. The vision of California, as a mystical place, as his somewhere over the rainbow, consumed him. He read about a wonderful educational opportunity offered by Cal to the new generation of middle class students.

His buddies laughed and called him high falutin' when he sold his motorcycle and placed the money, along with his pool winnings, in a college fund. Waz dutifully attended classes, diligently did his home work, and spent Sundays at the Public Library. To the surprise of the neighborhood, Waz earned an out-of-state scholarship to Cal for deserving "disadvantaged students."

His life would be changed forever.

"Hey, you guys know better than to roust an intellectual. I was about to relieve myself of Mystery Meat . . . ," Waz protested.

Royal English and Mo McCart tossed Waz onto the bed, turned him on his side, and unceremoniously yanked off his pants.

"We want gas! We want gas!" upper classmen chanted.

Lights were doused.

Punch said, "Waz, the Dooch upperclassmen are depending on you to uphold our honor. Frosh Tubbins set a new Dormie record of five-and one-half inches for a full second."

"Too much pressure," Waz protested. "Gotta relax."

Waz warmed up taking deep breaths, his body heaving into contortions.

"Never too much pressure, Waz," Mo teased. "Let 'er rip!"

"Ten second count down," Hunch warned.

"Ok, Ok, It's percolating," Waz said.

"Five, Four," the freshmen shouted.

All Pro flicked on the Zippo and moved the flame close to Waz's exposed buttocks. Living Buddha held a Brownie Hawkeye camera, poised to record the moment.

"Three, Two. . ." the upper classmen shouted.

The sound of a dull "ph-o-o-o-t" from Waz's buttocks. A giant blue flame flashed illuminating the faces of the stunned crowd

"Got it on film," Living Buddha said. "Didn't need a flash!"

"Open the door before we're asphyxiated," Butch shouted through the thick cloud of ignited methane.

"Seven inches!" Punch screamed, looking at markings of the seared measuring tape.

"Three full seconds! Hunch said, staring at the stopwatch.

"A new Dorm record, and possibly a new world record," Royal French shouted."I'm gonna submit this to Guinness for immediate consideration!"

As Waz pulled up his pants, upper classmen shouted "shower him! shower him!"

Boosting Waz on their shoulders, Dormies rushed him down to the bathroom to throw him fully clothed into a shower to celebrate the gaseous achievement.

Watching the happy throng zig-zag down the hallway, bouncing off the walls, Casey thought. *If only this heat source could be put to practical use!*

17

TEMPLE OF CAMPHOR

Blustery Pacific winds penetrate the Golden Gate, gusting and swirling into San Francisco Bay, spreading easterly over a 1000- miles of meandering inland delta waterways, traversing California's great Central Valley, eventually subsiding at the base of the Sierra Nevada mountains 100-miles away. As ocean breezes serpentine through the Cal campus, only one point of topography is impregnable, where even the strongest gust is diverted by a fortress of trees, the Eucalyptus Grove.

The seedlings of blue gum eucalyptus trees had been imported from the Australian island of Tasmania, 24-years before the colony founded by British convicts, joined the British Commonwealth. They had been planted at Cal in 1877, to provide wind shelter for a running track. Like emancipated inmates, the blue gum eucalyptus thrived in their new home, near the south fork of meandering Strawberry Creek.

By 1959, the Eucalyptus Grove, freed from its natural enemies, had flourished, mushrooming into the tallest eucalypti in the world and the tallest strand of hardwood trees in North America.

Towering over the Life Science Building, the Eucalyptus Grove consists of a series of graceful columns reaching toward the heavens with scepter-shaped leaves forming a shield against the sun's intrusion. In the late afternoon, a few shafts of light burrow through the leafy canopy, ethereal beams of brightness bathing the interior of the grove in a brilliant, golden glow, illuminating bands of swirling colors within the gray bark of the blue gum eucalyptus.

Despite the Eucalyptus Grove's mystical beauty, few venture into the Grove and fewer linger in its peaceful environs. Although appealing visually, the Grove is repellant to the olfactory senses, for the Eucalyptus emits a pungent camphor, like the stench of a popular, oily salve parents slather on the chests of coughing, wheezing children.

It was in here that Ari Scott found solace for the loss of his love. During weekly visits, Ari noted that, at a certain time of the day, a singular intense ray of sunshine formed a circular beam in the exact middle of the Grove, illuminating a small, carved wooden bench.

Like many philosophy students, Ari considered himself spiritual, not religious. Yet, once a week, Ari made the pilgrimage to the Grove bench, where, amid the medicinal smell of camphor, beneath the rustling of the leafy canopy, and the gurgling of nearby Strawberry Creek, he grieved the memory of his love lost.

Ari continued the ritual until he yielded to the persistent pursuit of beautiful coed, Cecelia "Cee Cee" Chandler, daughter of newspaper publisher William Randolph Chandler, a young woman to whom no one ever said "no." On the day of his engagement to Cee Cee, Ari returned to the Eucalyptus Grove to say goodbye to Sofia's memory.

Now, ten years after his farewell, the Eucalyptus Grove was the site of a miraculous reunion. Entering the sanctuary, Ari inhaled the scent of camphor, the salve of his years of mourning. It was the time of day when the singular beam of light bathed the bench in an incandescent circle of light. His head bowed, Ari eased himself into the familiar pew.

For the first time in a decade, he allowed himself the pleasures of memory.

It was the tumultuous summer Olympics of '36 prior to the War where Hitler planned to demonstrate the superiority of his Aryan nation. History trumpeted the exploits of Jesse Owens capturing four Olympic gold medals, but Ari had contributed to the debunking of German superiority by winning the metric mile for America. Entering the last lap of the race in third place, Ari passed teammate, Clayborn Muck, and, in a lunging finish, edged the favorite, Gunnard Lange.

Muck had been more than Ari's rival in the mile. He was one of a legion of ardent suitors for the affection of Italian breaststroke swimmer, Sofia Cappuccino, whose voluptuous figure proved to be a buoyant disability against her reed-thin rivals.

When Sofia gave her heart to the unaffected, naive Ari, Muck, the scion of Boston aristocracy, swore vengeance on Ari that was almost realized during the HUAC hearings Muck had recently scheduled.

After the Olympics, Ari and Sofia, undertook their toure di amore - romantic days and nights amid the ruins of Rome, the beaches of the Italian Riviera, the ancient canals of Venice, the magnificent art of Florence, exchanging the undying pledge of lovers.

Arriving at Sofia's hometown, Milan, Ari had asked Sofia's father, Giuseppe Cappuccino, the inventor of the machine that brewed the world famous coffee drink, for his daughter's hand in marriage. A traditionalist, Giuseppe would not grant permission to someone who was not yet gainfully employed. Ari returned to California, promising to return for Sofia after completing his graduate studies.

As the War exploded over Europe, Ari was shocked by the news that Mussolini had imprisoned "bourgeois capitalists" including Milan's renown Cappuccino family. In her last letter, Sofia described the family's plight as inmates in Palermo Prison. When America entered the War, Ari volunteered for the OSS, serving as an intelligence officer during the invasion of Italy.

As the Allies pushed up the Italian "Boot," Ari clung to the hope that he would find Sofia. At Palermo, he found only ruins. A survivor of the prison remembered a Cappuccino family but believed they had died before the Allied invasion. Ari retraced the toure di amore, seeking information about the Cappuccino's. In Milan, he walked the grounds of the family estate destroyed by artillery fire, tearfully remembering their vows of love.

Sofia was dead.

It was not until the *Look* magazine article on Italy's charismatic Communist leader, Pablo Zarzana, that Ari learned that Sofia had survived the war and married Zarzana. Then came Sofia's letter, announcing that their daughter, Anna, the offspring of their *toure di amore*, had been admitted to Cal as a graduate student.

Anna's sudden appearance brought Ari unbridled joy but signaled the end of his marriage to Cee Cee who would not accept Ari's "bastard love-child."

The Campanile's chimes interrupted Ari's reverie. Recognizing the tune, Ari smiled. Hunch Hitowski was playing the War favorite,

"Sentimental Journey."

An unseen force made Ari glance over his shoulder.

For a moment, he was stunned. Twenty paces away stood a vision, virtually unchanged by the passage of time.

Ari rose and stood silently drinking in her beauty. The face was slightly fuller, but her hair was still a jet-black mane. Sofia's eyes sparkled with the same burning intensity that captivated him 23-years ago. She was dressed in a tailored gray suit with a scarf bearing the tri-colors of the Italian flag. Despite its modest styling, the dress failed to conceal Sofia's voluptuous figure.

Ari walked purposely toward her, each step removing a year from their separation, until he stood before her. Once again, he was the naive college boy under the magical spell of the love of his life.

What was he to do? What did he want to do?

The puzzle was solved by a pair of arms swarming the two, joining them in a three-way embrace. It was Anna.

"Papa, Mama," Anna whispered. "I love you both."

The trio hugged silently, tears streaming down their faces.

Anna broke the embrace, wiping away dripping mascara. "You have a lot of catching up to do. I'll see you at Pablo's speech." She kissed each on the cheek. "See you later."

Walking backwards, blowing a kiss to each, Anna joined Jericho "Save The World" Slabio waiting in the shadows of a Eucalyptus.

Arms encircled around each other, Ari and Sofia waived at the retreating figures. The former lovers held hands, smiling from across the years.

"Scotty, you have become distinguished-looking, eh?" Sofia said, stroking Ari's salt and pepper hair.

"Darl—," Ari caught himself before uttering the old endearment. "You and Anna could pass for sisters."

"I see you are no longer my tongue-tied swain," Sofia teased.

"After our *toure di amore*, I was never the same," Ari said, drawing Sofia to him. I tried to find you during the War," he said, reliving the pain of that desperate search.

"I know, dearest Scotty. It was a terrible time. Let me share the first few years of Anna's life with you," Sofia said, leading Ari back to the wooden bench.

"I must know everything about the years of your life I lost," Ari said.

They held hands tightly, as she retraced the past.

When Anna was born, I was torn between my love for our darling baby and the shame my family faced, their only daughter, mother of an illegitimate grandchild. I stayed at the family estate, fearing the public scorn of Milan. I did not have the courage to tell you, Scotty.

Mussolini imprisoned us and seized all the family property. At Palermo, we were treated well; but Papa was a broken man. The thought of returning to ruins after the War was too much to bear. Papa lost the will to live and died of a broken heart.

When the Fascists abandoned the prison to invading Allied forces, Mama and I moved to Lucca where we lived with a cousin until Italy surrendered. Returning to Milan was disheartening. There was nothing left.

Ari nodded, recalling the devastation he had encountered.

Sofia recounted how, after the War, she, Anna, and her mother had moved in with an aunt; and all three of the women worked, struggling to make ends meet.

Ari pressed Sofia's head to his chest and stroked her luxurious hair, as she continued.

Sofia described how, as a young, unwed mother, she had met the firebrand, Pablo Zarzana, who was willing to marry her and help raise a child that was not his.

Ari fought back the tears he felt for Sofia's ordeal.

"The rest is history, Scotty. Pablo was so strong, so loyal, so devoted to us. I could not refuse his marriage proposal."

"How did you escape your . . ." Ari asked the burning practical question confronting anyone in Italian politics.

" . . . poverty?" she asked, reading his mind.

"We had been married a few years and were struggling, when a representative of Papa's old law firm found me. He said Papa had set up a trust account for me when I reached 30. The account contained royalties from his world-wide patent on Cappuccino machines."

Sofia looked at Ari with dark eyes that seared holes in his soul.

"And the trust fund changed your lives?" he asked.

"Cappuccino coffee had become world famous. The royalties made me an heiress. I became the banker for Pablo's causes."

The irony of the similarity of Pablo and Ari's brides was evident. Both men had married into wealth - Pablo unwittingly, Ari naively - but both marriages had taken different paths.

"Do you . . ." Ari could not finish the question.

"Love him?" Sofia whispered. "I have never loved another like I loved you, Scotty. Pablo and I share a different kind of love. We are joined by the adversities we shared, as outsiders and undesirables, in post-War Italy. We have a deep loyalty and affection that I cannot describe. It is not the passion you and I shared in our *toure di amore*, but it is a strong bond that has kept us together as a family. I can never repay the debt I owe Pablo for rescuing us from the streets of Milan."

Pulling her face away from Ari's chest, Sofia said, "Now that you are enjoying your lovely daughter, do you feel the pride of a Papa."

"I do. I have never experienced such joy since Anna's arrival," Ari said. "Cee Cee left me because she didn't want to share my love for Anna; but, looking back, my marriage was doomed from the start. I am close to my children, Marcus and Monique; but Cee Cee and her father are trying to prevent me from ever seeing them again."

"Scotty, nothing can deny your love for your children."

"And us?" Ari said, in a whisper.

Ari had dared to ask the question weighing on his mind.

"We had our *toure di amore*," Sofia said softly. "We will always have our *toure di amore*."

They held each other in a long, silent embrace.

She had spoken the Higher Truth he had tried desperately to ignore. The memory of their love and of their *toure di amore* would bind them for the rest of their lives; but their realities were now irreconcilable. Sofia's destiny was that of the dutiful wife of the Prime Minister of Italy. Ari was destined to champion academic freedom. Their child, Anna, would forge the gap between the former lovers. That was their shared destiny.

"Sofia, there is a matter of parental concern I must share with you." Ari said somberly.

"Papa Scotty," Sofia teased, "it would not be your feelings about a certain young man Anna is seeing, eh?"

"Am I that obvious?" Ari asked.

"Let's say Anna notices your face turn angry whenever Jericho Slabio's name is mentioned."

"Am I being an overly protective father?" Ari asked, suddenly embarrassed by the transparency of his feelings.

"No more than Pablo," Sofia said, giving Ari a knowing smile.

"Does Pablo think he's a phony too?" Ari shouted in joy.

"Let's say, since Pablo has had many enemies during his political life, he is always careful with anyone who showers him with adulation. For the most part, the young man is impressive. He says all the right things, " Sofia paused.

"But?" Ari sensed a reservation.

Sofia continued. "Pablo is uncomfortable with Slabio's belief that violence is necessary to implement social change. Pablo has advocated nonviolence all his life. He sees danger in anyone urging force to impose his will on society."

A wave of relief swept Ari.

"And what of Anna?" Ari asked.

"You must give her time to realize she has made a youthful mistake," Sofia said. "Slabio is not cut from the same mold as Pablo. Trust her to learn this in her own time. Anything you say will only hinder her eventual realization."

Sofia placed her arms around Ari's neck. "Scotty, dearest, Anna inherited the best from both of us and has been raised with Pablo's wisdom. Do you believe that an engaging, even charming young man can suddenly change a lifetime of values? Be patient."

The Campanile bells chimed 4 p.m.

"Pablo will be speaking soon," Ari said. "I would like to hear him."

Arm-in-arm, the former lovers - now loving parents - exited Ari's temple of camphor, leaving behind swirling eddies of dying leaves, as the incandescent beam of sunlight retreated into the dark canopy of blue gum eucalyptus.

18

DOG DAY AFTERNOON

Pausing, haunch-deep in water, Ludwig von Schwarenberg squinted across the tree-lined plaza at the massive granite and terra cotta structure blocking his hillside view. Where small specialty shops once flourished, the east side of Telly, next to Sather Gate, was now dominated by the massive, U-shaped five story building flanked by two, three-story wings. Without its neoclassic portico, seemingly an architectural afterthought, Sproul Hall resembled the other U-shaped building, Dwinelle Hall, squatting along Strawberry Creek, 100-yards to the northwest.

It was ironic that this banal looking building was named for retired University President, Robert Gordon Sproul, a beloved figure among students, faculty, administrators, and alumni. Nothing about Sproul, the building, captured a scintilla of the spirit and soul of the Cal quintessential renaissance man, Robert Gordon Sproul whose charisma, energy, charm, political savvy, dedication, and wit had transformed Cal from one of many, land grant universities, into "the best public university in the world."

Ludwig was accustomed to large gatherings in Sproul Plaza but there was something different about the swelling crowd. This was not the day the thin man with the large Adam's apple, wearing small spectacles perched on his hook nose, descended 30-steps and neatly pinned pieces of paper on a bulletin boards.

No, Ludwig thought. *The crowd was too noisy to be waiting for the Angel of Death.*

Ludwig stepped gingerly from the water and circled the fountain bearing his name.

This is also not a day when speakers take turns shouting at each other, he thought. *The size of the crowd was also much larger than the usual noon hour ebb and flow.*

The competing banners stretched across the Ionic columns of Sproul Hall were the largest Ludwig had ever seen. The top one read,

"Cal Welcomes Pablo Zarzana"

Below, another said,

"Go Home, Commie Creep"

An hour before, Ludwig had watched that professor, the one called the Prussian Penguin, arrive with the large contingent of soldiers with the letters *"Natl. Guard"* stenciled on their helmets How Ludwig disliked the squat, short-legged professor who visited his fountain! With great fanfare, the professor pretended to be friendly by offering an overripe apple, announcing, to anyone within listening range, that he and Ludwig were "countrymen" from the same region of Germany.

How disgusting! Despite his German name, Ludwig was proud of his all-American pedigree.

A few minutes later, that disheveled student, the one with the mushroom-shaped hair, the one called Jericho "Save-The-World" Slabio, who always spoke in Sproul, marched a parade of scruffy-looking cohorts across the length of Sproul without speaking once.

He must be ill, Ludwig thought, watching Slabio and his entourage disappear around the north end of Sproul Hall.

Today was also the rarest of days when no one had brought him anything to eat. No treats. No snacks. Despite the numbers swelling Sproul, no one was paying any attention to him.

Nothing good will come of this day. He could feel it.

Something told Ludwig he must leave his beloved fountain before something bad happened.

Tomorrow will be a better day. Normalcy will return to Sproul and Ludwig's Fountain; but for today, something in the air, told him to leave. Now.

Emerging from the Eucalyptus Grove, Ari and Sofia strolled, arm-in-arm, up hill past the neo-Babylonian architecture of the fortress-shaped LSB (Life Sciences Building) with its Art Deco medallions of lions, rams, snakes, fish, crabs, and geckos. The couple angled between California Hall's Sophomore Lawn and the Chinese lion of Durant Hall, veering right, toward the swelling throng beyond Sather Gate.

High atop the Campanile, Hunch Hitowski, clanged *"My Happiness,"* on the carillons.

"Scotty, the Cal campus is so beautiful. I see why you love it so."

Ari squeezed Sofia's hand affectionately.

If only the fates had been kinder, he thought. *Sofia and I would have lived "happily ever after" among the beauty of the campus.*

Passing through Sather Gate, they saw the throng parting to allow the campus celebrity to pass.

"Ludwig! Ludwig von Schwarenberg!" many yelled.

"Scotty, look. It's a pure-bred German short-hair pointer."

"Ludwig, here, buddy," Ari said, reaching into his jacket pocket.

It's that nice Professor Scott, Ludwig thought. *He always has a treat for me.*

"How about them bazookas?" Butch said, pointing to the curly, red-haired girl with a generous bust line, standing by the podium on the Sproul Hall steps. Few Cal coeds appeared in public without at least a blouse or sweater, but the red head wore only a tight fitting red T-shirt without a brassiere.

The Dormies huddled against a wooden fence surrounding the skeletal outline of the new Student Union Building next to Ludwig's Fountain.

"Her boobs defy the law of gravity," Punch said, his left eye spinning in orbit. Ogling the voluptuous redhead, he said, "Wonder if she'd consider helping Hunch and me in our umbrella experiments on aerial dynamics?"

"Her name is Lotta Ackshon," Royal said, "Leader of the Campus Anti-Bra Crusade that claims bras are symbols of imprisonment by men. Her nickname is "Treasure Chest.""

"She should be a tailing assignment," Super Sleuth whispered, sizing Lotta Ackshon up.

"You sneaky devil," Casey said. "Tailing that bra-less wonder would be solely in the interests of aesthetics?"

"Certainly," Super Sleuth said. "I wouldn't waste my shadowing skill on anyone who was unworthy of appreciation."

"Jeez," Butch said. "How do you tail these babes without leaving a trail of drool?"

"Elementary, my dear Tanenbloom," Super Sleuth said. "My advocation is strictly intellectual."

"Bet your dong serves as a divining rod," Royal teased.

"Shhh," Casey said. "Looks like Lotta Ackshon is going to hype the Campus Anti-Bra Crusade before Slabio introduces Pablo Zarzana."

On the edge of campus, at the intersection of Telly and Bancroft Way, Professor Werner Von Seller circled impatiently. His childhood memory of Hitler's troops was that of unwavering dedication, crisp precision and singular efficiency. Since coming to America, he had never dealt with the military; but he assumed that all militaries were more or less the same, especially one that had routed the Third Reich.

"Colonel Jones," Von Seller asked for the third time, this time deploying a calmer demeanor. "You and your troops will quash anything that appears to be a disturbance, won't you?"

"My orders are clear, Professor," Colonel McReynolds Jones said, in a patient tone. "My troops are not to engage students unless we are attacked first."

McReynolds Jones was a middle-aged veteran, with a trim physique, and clear blue eyes. He had surveyed the growing crowd that clearly outnumbered his company but felt no imminent danger. The students were no older than most of his troops and reminded him of his own college-age grandchildren.

"What if you are provoked?" Von Seller persisted.

"There must be an actual assault," Colonel Jones said dryly, "My boys will not be provoked."

The last thing the Colonel wanted was the blood of civilians on his hands, especially college students. McReynolds Jones had fought in Europe and in Korea. He had witnessed too many young lives lost in war. No matter how ugly things might get today, this was not real combat.

"But aren't those rifles loaded with real bullets?" Von Seller asked.

"No," Colonel Jones smiled. "I'm here for crowd control only."

"Unarmed!" Von Seller said in disbelief. "What kind of military do we have that cannot protect itself, much less the peaceful element of this campus, against violent radicals?"

"Crunchy, Munchy! Crunchy, Munchy!" a voice chirped.

It was the campus street vendor pushing his bicycle-wheeled ice cream cart. Crunchy Munchy wore his familiar white jumpsuit, military boots, admiral's cap, and black hornrim glasses.

"Go away," Von Seller said, waving off Crunchy Munchy.

The sight of the ancient ice cream man always unnerved Von Seller. Crunchy's wrist bore crudely carved numbers, the badge of a Nazi death camp survivor. Von Seller's family had left Germany before the War, and he had always felt an uncomfortable sense of uneasiness about Hitler's *Final Solution*.

"I'll have an Eskimo Pie, sir," Colonel Jones said, handing Crunchy Munchy a quarter. "Keep the change."

"Crunchy Munchy," the ice cream man chirped, tipping his cap.

"Why are you so sure something will happen?" Colonel Jones said, peeling the wrapper off the chocolate-dipped, vanilla ice cream bar.

Von Seller averted the Colonel's piercing gaze and inserted a fresh Gaulois into his sterling silver, cigarette holder.

This is not what he had expected when he sent a note to his patron, WRC, William Randolph Chandler.

Von Seller lit the Gaulois, inhaled deeply, and blew a stream of smoke over the Colonel's shoulder insignia.

Von Seller had suggested WRC's candidacy for governor would be enhanced if he denounced the appearance of Italian Prime Minister, Pablo Zarzana. Surely, that campus radical, Jericho Slabio, would take the opportunity to incite an anti-government riot. WRC's outspoken stand for law and order on campus would certainly boost Chandler's candidacy. Von Seller urged WRC to exercise his influence among the Regents to call out the National Guard to quell any disturbance arising from Zarzana's appearance. Secretly, Von Seller hoped the sight of armed troops, massed on campus, would be like waving a red flag before the nose of a mad bull. A riot would surely erupt, and he and WRC would reap the windfall of public outrage that would follow.

But this pacifist, Colonel McReynolds Jones could thwart my plans, Von Seller thought. *How can there be a riot if troops refuse to be baited by unruly students? Calm down. Trust Cal students to irrationally overreact to these toothless troops*, he told himself. *Yes, there would be a riot whether Colonel Jones wanted one or not!*

Along the southern banks of Strawberry Creek, Jericho "Save-The-World" Slabio gathered the members of the Guerillas for Free Speech, in a circle beneath a pergola at the entranceway to Anthony Hall, home of the campus humor magazine, *The Pelican*. On the front lawn stood a large bronze pelican, with its mouth agape and wings fully extended. The magazine staff had closed up early to listen to Zarzana, leaving Slabio and the Guerillas one of its two pergolas as a quiet, convenient place to caucus. Above the din of the crowd gathering at nearby Sproul, Strawberry Creek's happy gurgling soothed the nerves of the campus revolutionaries.

"This is a historic day for free speech," one Guerilla said gleefully. "Those trigger happy troops will play right into our hands."

"A riot that will define student rights,"another said.

"We'll show other university students how to bring down bourgeois, capitalistic, governmental institutions," a third said.

Exploiting his relationship with Anna, Slabio had finagled the plum role of introducing Pablo Zarzana. He had planned to seize the opportunity to advocate the goals of the Guerillas for Free Speech, tying them to Zarzana's politics.

This will be a perfect setting for Jericho Slabio and the Guerillas for Free Speech to make their mark on the world stage.

That was his thinking before the morning's brunch with Anna and her parents. Now, Slabio wasn't sure. What should have been a crowning achievement proved to be a disappointment.

The four had enjoyed an elegant buffet at the Claremont Hotel, high above campus. Slabio had not objected to the luxurious site, though the Claremont was a glaring symbol of capitalistic decadence. He had acquitted himself by returning to the buffet line three times, piling his plate high with foods he had only read about: fresh lox, oysters Rockefeller, Beluga caviar, and eggs Benedict. He identified Chateaubriand aloud, remembering the entree he had ordered at Bernie's with Ari Scott, and that pompous Garrick Nelquist

Slabio assumed Pablo Zarzana would have preferred to eat among the proletariat, at a plebeian restaurant like *The Radical Wienie*, a budget hangout on Telly. He was shocked that Zarzana was elegantly dressed in Italian fashion, right from the pages of *Esquire* magazine.

Shouldn't champions of the poor dress as if they belonged in the streets with the starving masses? he wondered.

Slabio felt out of place in Claremont's sumptuous environs, although he enjoyed the shocked glances of guests who read the inscription on his T-shirt:

"The Wealthy Suck."

Judging from the buffet feast, Slabio admitted that what the wealthy sucked was a far cry from the intent of his T-shirt message.

After Anna gave a glowing description of Slabio's importance in the campus left-wing movement, she became quiet, especially after he had asked the waiter to bring two more bottles of that French champagne, *"Dom"* something or other.

There had been no discussion of left-wing ideology, no sharing of struggles, no exchange of goals for future glory.

Mrs. Zarzana was polite, asking about the Guerillas for Free Speech, but she glanced, with raised eyebrows, at her daughter and husband, as Slabio outlined the goal of overthrowing "bourgeois, capitalistic, government institutions, by violence," beginning with the Cal school administration.

Pablo Zarzana had listened to his passionate presentation that became more boisterous with each succeeding glass of "Dom" something or other.

Zarzana interrupted him only once. In a soft Italian-accented voice that unnerved Slabio by its suddenness. Zarzana said, "Mr. Slabio, how certain are you about the necessity of violence to achieve your goals?" He looked directly at Slabio with a steadfast, piercing gaze of his dark brown eyes.

"As one who has suffered at the hands of right-wing Fascists," Slabio began, "you must appreciate the need for violence. America has a long history of violence, much of it committed by the wealthy and their puppets in the government they control. Violence is the only thing the American government understands." Slabio said.

When the Zarzanas excused themselves to prepare for the afternoon speech, Slabio was surprised to see a sadness in Anna's eyes. He was confused when she kissed him on the cheek and whispered, "Pablo will learn to like you."

What was there to learn?

His views about revolution were the same as her famous stepfather, weren't they? He had eaten the same food famous people, even famous Communist people, ate, had he not?

And what of her mother?

Anna had volunteered nothing about her mother's impression of him.

Not that critical, he concluded. *It was always the man's opinion that counted. If Pablo Zarzana approved of him, then surely his wife was bound to agree. The most important thing was that Anna adored him. She was the key to everything.*

As he marched, a bit woozy, down the hill toward campus, Slabio thought it was probably the effects of that *"Dom"* something or other.

Nothing to worry about.

Soon, he would share the spotlight with Pablo Zarzana, sending his own budding political career into an orbit with a life of its own.

Now, as Slabio outlined his plan to his confederates, his confidence returned. "The National Guard troops must be provoked," Slabio said. "Spit on 'em! Kiss 'em on the cheek! Do whatever is necessary to provoke 'em into brutality!"

Yes, nothing would stop him now. Everything was in place. Newspaper and TV coverage would be abundant. With the help of the reactionary National Guard, Jericho Slabio and the Guerillas for Free Speech would be internationally famous by tomorrow morning. And the revolution would begin!

Slabio sent his minions off to Sproul Plaza, amid alternating chants:

> *"What do we want?*
> *REVOLUTION!*
>
> *When do we want it?*
> *NOW!"*

He paused at the window of the Pelican Building, glancing at the mantle above the brick fireplace. He noted the engraved slogan:

> *"Be Good - If You Can't Be Good - Be Careful"*

19

MALE BONDING

It had been the moment Ari dreaded.

Standing before him, in the belfry of the Campanile, was the person Fate had ordained as his surrogate; the one who married Sofia after the War; the man who slept beside her for 13-years; the one who had raised Anna as his own; the man who was now Prime Minister of Italy, Pablo Zarzana.

Up close, Pablo was shorter than Ari, with thick, wavy hair that was prematurely silver. He was matinee-idol handsome, with a deep tan and dark brown eyes. Pablo was impeccably dressed in Italian fashion that made Ari, dressed in his casual, tweedy, professor garb, feel like a bum.

Pablo lit a small, thin, European cigarillo and exhaled smoke toward the Campanile's carillons.

"Professor Scott, it is my extreme pleasure to meet you," Pablo's handshake was firm, dry, unlike the sweaty palm Ari offered.

Earlier, Ari had stood among the huge throng gathered at Sproul Plaza to hear the first American address by the newly-elected leader of Italy. Lotta Ackshon, leader of the Campus Anti-Bra Committee, had made a glowing introduction of Jericho Slabio who, in turn, attempted to tie the Guerillas for Free Speech to the political philosophy of Pablo Zarzana. At the same time, Guerilla members tried to bait the National Guard into violent over-reaction. After five minutes of Slabio's stock harangue against the Cal administration, the crowd grew restless, issuing a smattering of boo's. Anna saved Slabio from self-embarrassment by gently tugging his sleeve, a discreet signal for "you've said enough."

Taking the hint, Slabio abruptly said, "It is my privilege to introduce the exciting new leader of the western world whose programs for social, economic and political change will be the model by which all other governments will be judged. Ladies and gentlemen, The Prime Minister of Italy . . . . PABLO ZARZANA !"

A thunderous roar engulfed Zarzana, as he glided to the podium, smiling, waving effortlessly.

"Pablo! Pablo! Pablo!" the crowd shouted.

Ari felt electricity in the air. He looked at Sofia and Anna standing at Zarzana's side, beaming with pride. Tears welled up in Ari's eyes. *Were they tears of happiness for Sofia and Anna? Or were they the tears of jealousy and defeat?*

Holding up his hands to quiet the crowd, Pablo said, in slightly-accented English, "You may wonder why I've summoned you today."

Affectionate laughter rolled across Sproul Plaza.

"For centuries, Italy's history is filled with stories of men traveling great distances to acquire knowledge they could not gain at home," Zarzana said. "Marco Polo left for China and returned 20-years later with the wisdom of the Far East. Christopher Columbus sailed westward to find a shorter way to India and returned in two years with the greatest discovery of the New World. Now, it is my turn, to visit your beautiful country and bring back, in only 20-days, the wisdom of America."

Sustained, enthusiastic applause drowned out the verbal insults the Guerillas for Free Speech heaped on the National Guard.

"I am pleased to introduce the true secret of any success I have enjoyed ," Zarzana said, "my lovely, loyal wife, Sofia, who is stronger than I will ever hope to be."

Cheers greeted Sofia, as she bowed graciously and waved.

"And my wonderful stepdaughter, Anna, a graduate student here at Cal," Zarzana said, amid a chorus of whistles.

"I would like to acknowledge someone I have yet to meet, but who, in his own way, is responsible for my personal happiness," Zarzana said, "a man who has stood for Higher Truth, the popular member of your faculty, who is Anna's birth father . . . Professor Aristotle Scott."

Ari was stunned. Zarzana was publicly acknowledging him! Tears streamed down his face. He felt light-headed, as students around him boosted him on their shoulders shouting "Ari! Ari! Ari!" From his airborne perch, Ari looked at the podium where Sofia and Anna were smiling, applauding. Spotting Ari, Zarzana waved a greeting that Ari reciprocated.

Ari did not remember much of Zarzana's speech, except for the frequent outbursts of applause from the adoring crowd. He was consumed by his own thoughts.

What a self-centered fool I've been. Instead of celebrating the wonderful life Sofia and Anna have enjoyed with Pablo Zarzana, I've been wallowing in the self-pity my own loss. What right do I have to impose my maudlin memories on those who live in present? I do not deserve to be mentioned in the same breath with this gracious man.

Now, Ari stood a few feet from Zarzana, as the sun slipped into the Pacific, beyond the Golden Gate. Miss Burdick was showing Sofia and Anna the Campanile's collection of dinosaur bones, while Sofia's two loves had their "man-to-man" talk.

Ari was tongue-tied, speechless.

"I do not normally smoke," Zarzana said, blowing another stream upwards, "but I have been so nervous about meeting you. I hope you won't mind this crutch. May I call you Ari?"

"You, nervous?" Ari blurted. "I'm the one who is an emotional wreck," he laughed, releasing pent-up tension. "You may call me Ari, only if I may call you, Pablo."

"I have a special place in my heart for Americans, Ari," Pablo began. "As a teenager, I was conscripted into the Italian army very reluctantly. I was against that mad man, Mussolini, and his stupid alliance with Hitler." He grounded out the cigarillo and placed the remnant in a handkerchief he placed in his jacket pocket.

"I surrendered to American troops, at my first opportunity. The GI's were supposed to turn me over to a military prison, but I got along so well with my captors, they released me to return home. I will never forget their kindness. Without American generosity, I would not have resumed my studies, met Sofia, and entered politics, eh?"

"I must confess, Pablo," Ari said, "I have been jealous of your life with Sofia and Anna. Yet, since my reunion with Anna, I must credit you with how wonderfully she has turned out."

"Now, it is my turn to confess, Ari. For the first few years of our marriage, I was so jealous of your *toure di amore.*"

"No, Pablo, don't . . ."

"Italian men are possessive, incurable romantics, in the affairs of the heart, Ari," Pablo said, shaking his head. "We suffer what you would call pride of authorship. I wish it were *I* who were with Sofia on your *toure di amore*. I wish *I* were the one who fathered Anna."

"Foolish notions of a foolish man, eh?" Pablo smiled. "One of Sofia's greatest gifts was the understanding that, in love, there is no room for *'I'* or *'Me.'* There is only *'we'* and *'us.'* "

Ari studied the face of the man who, a few hours earlier, had captivated the imagination of thousands of listeners. At this place, in this moment, Ari saw only the soul of the man Sofia married.

Ari felt a sudden peace, a release from burdens he had imposed on himself. He saw his life as a series of struggles for things that were never meant to be: life with Sofia, marriage to Cee Cee, now possibly, the loss of visitation with his children.

Reading Ari's mind, Pablo said, "Ari, we cannot control life and love. They have destinies of their own. But you and I are both blessed, for we have shared Sofia's love. Our lives have been enriched by that love. We cannot know what will happen tomorrow. We can only be thankful for how we have been blessed today. I was serious when I thanked you this afternoon. Without you, our destinies - Sofia's, Anna's, and mine - would have never been the same."

Pablo gripped Ari's hand firmly, then hugged him.

Ari thought he saw a glistening in Pablo's eyes.

"Fratello," Pablo said. *"Brother."*

"Fratello," Ari repeated.

The elevator door clanked open, admitting Sofia and Anna. Behind them was Hunch Hitowski, arriving for his evening carillon concert.

"You gentlemen have been enjoying yourselves,?" Sofia said, kissing Pablo lightly on the cheek. "Not gossiping behind our backs, eh?"

"In fact," Pablo said, kissing Sofia's forehead, "Ari and I agree we have much in common, especially the same excellent taste in women."

Anna gave Ari a hug, whispering, "Papa, I hope you like him."

"He is truly a great man," Ari said, without a hint of jealousy.

As darkness enveloped the campus, the Campanile's beacon illuminated the belfry where the four, standing in a circle, embraced: lovers, spouses, parents and child - all conjoined by history and love.

Above, Hunch swung gracefully rope-to-rope, ringing the carillons in the wartime favorite, *"Thanks for The Memory."*

20

SUBMARINE RACES

"What do you think, Lover-Boy?"

"Breathtaking, Ruby. I've never been up here before."

Beyond the Golden Gate, a harvest moon lingered over the black Pacific, and stars blinked knowingly. Above campus, on the eastern foothill, two sweethearts snuggled, within the concrete ring of the Big C. The golden Big C had been painted thousands of times - on occasion, an offending red by marauding Stanford students. Over the years, layers of paint had swelled the Big C's thickness several feet. On an adjacent hill, the deep blue glow of the purring Cyclotron was the only sound of this magical, romantic fall night.

The arduous hike up to the Big C was a destination for only adventuresome lovers who wanted to "watch the submarine races," as the uphill trek from campus took over a half-hour. Watching submarine races was the student euphemism for necking, and for tonight's submarine races, the two lovers had the Big C to themselves.

Ten's of thousands of pinpoint lights blinked before them: from the Marin headlands, across the luminous strand of the Golden Gate Bridge, to the small hills of The City, then along the gleaming necklace of the Bay Bridge, to the sprawling East Bay neighborhoods below.

Hugging his knees against his chin, Ruby Lips leaned back against the warmth of Lover-Boy's thighs encircling him.

"That's the problem with you secret queers," Ruby Lips said, thrilled by Lover-Boy's tumescence against his spine. "You waste so much time doing what is 'right and normal.' You never stop to enjoy the simple joys of life . . . and love."

Ruby kissed the back of Lover-Boy's hand caressing him.

"I wish I could live an honest life . . . like you, Lips; but I can't. Not with grad school and a career to worry about."

"Lover-Boy, no amount of college degrees and money will free you from the way you were born. Sure, you can live a double life; but, sooner or later, you'll have to confront the decision: 'to be or not to be' 'to thine own self be true.' "

"It's not going to happen in our life time," Lover-Boy said, stroking Ruby's neck. "The world's not ready to accept deviants like us."

"I prefer the term queer over deviant," Ruby said. "Deviant suggests depraved sicko's who lust after little kids. As an upstanding queer, I have absolutely no prurient interest in young children." He winked at Lover-Boy and said, "and I sure as hell hope you don't either."

Their romance had begun as a flirtation, when Lover-Boy slipped a note to Ruby, in the Men's Room of the Claremont Hotel, during the Gee Dees Halloween Presents Party, that read:

> *"Loved your moves.*
> *Meet you on the hotel veranda?*
> *Gay, too."*

Ruby had attended the party with the Dormie group that introduced Negro-style dancing to the music of the first black band to perform at a Cal, Big Berry and the Blackouts. Jonathan Aldon had brought the dances back from visiting his Oakland cousins; and the Dormies had practiced hours to simulate rhythmic moves to Big Berry's signature song, *"Louie, Louie."*

There, on the veranda of the Claremont Hotel, in the pale glow of a Halloween moon, the two had met and connected.

Wow! What a handsome guy, an Adonis, Ruby thought.

How incredibly sensual those pouty lips are, Lover-Boy thought.

Since Halloween, the two had met secretly in dark campus locations, protecting Lover-Boy's manly, public reputation.

Both had thought the novelty of finding each other would wear thin; but, as they exchanged hopes and shared fears, they found themselves drawn to each other spiritually and romantically.

"When do I meet your parents?" Ruby asked, half jokingly.

"I'd love to Ruby; but you know that's not in the cards. I'm destined to meet and marry a respectable female, probably a Gee Dee, who will make the perfect wife and mother. Someone who will never know my secret," Lover-Boy said with a sigh.

"Am I supposed to wait around while you set up this perfectly fraudulent lifestyle?" Ruby said. "I think you're the cat's meow, Lover-Boy; but I've got a life to live. And dishonesty is not part of my plan," he said, squeezing Lover-Boy's hand.

"I know," Lover-Boy whispered. "I wish the law recognized bisexual polygamy. That would be the perfect answer."

"Fine for you, babe, but not for me," Ruby said. "I don't want to share you or anyone else I care about, just because you don't have the balls to admit who you and what you are. I'd rather troll for sailors in the Castro than to put up with that garbage. I'd kick your sweet ass out of my life right now, if . . ." Ruby sighed, "you weren't so damned cute."

After a prolonged silence, Ruby added, "I guess frat rats aren't the only ones hung up on looks. For the first time in my life, I admit I'm addicted to looks . . . yours."

Lover-Boy smiled. "So am I. There's something about you that drives me nuts; but I can't put my finger on it."

"Your hands are doing fine," Ruby said, enjoying the soothing feel of Lover-Boy stroking his rear.

"There's something I have to warn you about," Lover-Boy said.

"That you're incredibly sexy?" Ruby said.

"No, I'm serious," Lover-Boy said. "Don't eat dorm dinner next Tuesday. I can't tell you why, but please don't."

"Not a problem, Lover-Boy. I'm leaving early for Thanksgiving. Wanna come home and meet my folks? They'll love you. You look so . . . how shall I say, so . . . normal?"

"Got my own family to deal with," Lover-Boy said. "My snotty uncle, aunt, and cousins from the Hamptons are flying in for Thanksgiving. Got to help my parents put on a good show for them."

"I'd love the chance to put on a good show for them," Ruby said, kissing Lover-Boy lightly on the cheek.

"And blow my perfectly constructed cover?" Lover-Boy said. "Let's just enjoy each other for as long as we can. No strings, ok?"

If he weren't so damned handsome, I'd just tell him to go to hell, Ruby thought. *But I'm as weak as any other horny Dormie. And what is this shit about next Tuesday's Dormie dinner? Better take this up with Casey Lee. He's the only level-headed person I can trust with my secret boy friend.*

"Ok, no strings," Ruby said, with little conviction. "Take off those damned glasses and kiss me, you sexy devil," he said, puckering his pouty lips.

In their embrace, neither noticed a copy of the latest of the McWilson science fiction series, *The Chelsea Chronicles,* tumble from the pocket of Lover-Boy's tweed jacket and cartwheel downhill, in the direction of the Campanile.

* * * *

El Cid sat erect on his charge pointing his banner-festooned lance toward the Marin headlands. From ground, the well defined steed stood 40 hands tall. Behind the statute loomed the outline of a smaller version of *Palais de la Legion d'Honneur*, the Palace of the Legion of Honor. The museum, with Rodin's *Thinker* prominently displayed in its courtyard, had attained international prominence as the setting for a pivotal scene in the Hitchcock movie, *"Vertigo."* However, for young lovers, the Palace's parking lot overlooking San Francisco Bay, was the primary attraction of the grounds, the perfect spot for "watching submarine races."

The young couple cuddled in the front seat of the late 1940's station wagon, a woodie, with broad wooden panels, trimmed in yellow and chrome. From hi-fi stereo speakers hidden behind the back seats, Johnny Mathis crooned, *"Chances Are."*

"Mmm, what is that perfume?" he asked, nuzzling the girl's neck.

"What I always wear, Chanel No.5."

"Couldn't tell," he winked. "I've never been this close before."

"And what is that musky aroma?" she said teasingly.

"Butch sprinkled some on me, as I went out the door. It's a hot seller in New York, a men's cologne called English Leather. Butch calls it 'instant nookie.' "

Blushing, the girl ignored the comment. "Isn't this romantic?" she whispered, kissing the cheek of the dark-haired boy.

"In a whimsical way," he said, stroking her luxurious blond hair.

"What's so funny about parking with ME at the Legion? Some boys would give their right arm for the privilege," the coed, said, in a tone of mock indignation.

"Boy, do I feel privileged," he said, grinning. "That's what's great about this spot. If your date is a cold fish, you can always root for your favorites watching the submarine races."

"Cold Fish? Try this one on for size," Kate Howell said, planting a long, wet kiss on the willing lips of Casey Lee.

The evening had begun as a celebration of Kate's completion of her training at Yearning Arms for part-time "hand-y"work in the Mardi Gras room. Although the pair had spent hundreds of hours, in intimate conversation, they had never been on a formal date; and Kate could not wait forever for Casey to ask her out.

"Why don't you show me San Francisco? I've only seen the insides of Bernie's, Blue Fox, and Ritz Old Poodle Dog," she said, referring to boring dinners she had suffered with dates in her freshman year. "Maybe I can meet your grandmother, Madame Lee?"

"Sure," Casey had beamed, warming to the idea. "I can give you a personal tour of North Beach." He hesitated, "but I don't think the time is right for you to meet Grandma. I've told her a lot about you, but . . . frankly, she doesn't think I should get involved with you."

"Involved? You know more about my thoughts, my secrets and my hopes than my parents. If we're not already involved, then I don't know what the word means!"

"Sorry, Kate. Grandma is very protective. She thinks I'll only be hurt. When you meet her, you'll understand."

"Promise, I'll meet her?" Kate said, emphasizing the word *Promise.*

"That's a promise. You'll meet her . . . sometime."

What Casey had not related was Grandma's fear that the sight of her grandson in the company of a gorgeous, blond coed would incite physical violence. Madame Lee recalled, as a child, drunken groups of young Irish boys bragging about their marauding forays into Chinatown looking for "Chinks" to assault for Saturday night "fun." She reminded Casey that it had not been that long ago that California law prohibited interracial marriage.

They had driven Rod Organ's woodie to The City for a dinner-show at Jumbo's 369 Club where the young calypso singer, Harry Belafonte, was performing. The line for admission was long, winding around the corner for more than a city block.

Royal and Jonathan had created perfect fake ID's, California driver's licenses.

A club host dressed in a tux - a stubby cigar and clipboard in one hand and a pencil in the other - worked his way through the throng, taking names and checking ID's. He was in his early thirties, with the blocky build of an ex-football player, wavy black hair and puffy eyes.

"No ID needed for you, baby doll?" The host looked Kate up and down approvingly. "Name?"

"Lee party," Kate said.

"A looker like you shouldn't be out by yourself. My name is Fredo. If I can be of service . . ."

"Party of two." Kate said cooly, slipping her arm through Casey's.

"You with the Chinaman?" Fredo said, puffing a dying stogie, blowing a stream of pungent smoke in Casey's direction, as he glanced at Casey's ID.

"I get it, baby doll." Fredo said. "From outta town, eh?" He flashed a smile of brown-stained teeth. "Hired a Chinatown guide, right? He's gonna blow *your* dough by showing you the world famous Jumbo's, right? Well, I ain't gonna disappoint you. Follow me."

"Listen, you . . ." Kate hissed.

"No," Casey whispered. "It's ok. Let's just get inside and enjoy Belafonte."

Angry stares and choruses of hisses greeted Kate and Casey, as they followed the host lumbering to the front of the line. Fredo elbowed his way through a group of milling waiters dressed in white dinner jackets, passing Jumbo's trademark, the girl-in-a fishbowl, an illusion created by the use of a series of mirrors reflecting a tiny image of a shapely chorus girl wiggling on a black velvet couch a floor below.

Fredo escorted them to a table, front and center to the stage. As Casey peeled off a five-dollar tip, Fredo handed Kate a business card and winked. "Call me if you want a real man to show you a good time."

Kate and Casey exited Jumbo's with "*Day-o*" ringing in their ears. The crowd had joined Belafonte for four encores of "*Banana Boat.*"

"What's next on the tour?" Kate asked.

"How about something atmospheric," Casey said.

"You're the guide," Kate said, sticking her tongue out at Fredo.

Casey and Kate sat next to the indoor pool of the Mark Fairmont Hotel.

Sheets of rain swept across the Tahitian Lagoon and jagged lightning bolts flashed above the turbulent white caps. Amid the crackle and boom, macaws and toucans screeched in rhythm to the tropical music of the J Quincy Black III combo and beautiful chanteuse, Kay Laughing, floating on a barge in the middle of the pool.

During a break between sets, Kate asked, "Why didn't you let me give that creep, Fredo, a piece of my mind?"

"Madame Lee raised me with the belief that there is a time and place to right slights, indignations, and wrongs. The line to Jumbo's 369 was not the place for me to pop Fredo in the mouth, although I admit, I was sorely tempted."

Kate placed her hand over Casey's. "I can't wait to meet your grandmother," Kate said. "She sounds like a truly great woman."

"You will meet her," Casey said. "and she is a truly exceptional."

At the end of the tropical rain storm, Kate whispered, "my turn to choose the next spot." She drained her champagne glass. "How about The Palace of the Legion of Honor. Muffy says it's a really beautiful place to check out the Golden Gate Bridge."

"The Legion, it is," Casey said, placing a five dollars under his glass.

I'm sure Muffy has checked out more than just the Golden Gate Bridge, Casey thought. *Don't have to worry about any awkward complications with Kate, though.*

"Mmmm," said Casey, coming up for air. "You are v-e-r-y sexy when you get mad."

"Why do you joke when I'm feeling amorous?" Kate asked. "Would you laugh if I asked you to make love to me? You know I'm on The Pill." Johnny Mathis segued into *"Wonderful, Wonderful."*

In their secret tete-a-tete's, in Casey's room, at the top of Dooch, Kate had confided she was a virgin and had divulged the pact with her Gee Dee sorority sisters to take The Pill until the end of the semester.

"Like most guys, my dong has a mind of his own," Casey said with a straight face. "My Sir Dong is telling me we should take you up on your offer. It would be, to use your term, a privilege to be your first."

"And?" Kate said, with a coy smile.

His exotic, brown eyes drive me crazy, she thought.

"Your parents raised you to save yourself for your husband," Casey said. "You say you've grown apart from them, but some things are so ingrained you can never escape them. Sex with me seems appealing now and boy, does it sound great, but you'll regret it. Maybe not today, maybe not tomorrow, but someday. I don't want to be responsible for any shame."

"Is this your version of the final scene from 'Casablanca,' or is this the voice of Madame Lee speaking?" Kate said, nuzzling against Casey's face.

"Little of both, " Casey said. "Grandma says society can never disregard the way one looks. You will always be the Golden Goddess, no matter what you say or do. . . ."

"It's terribly confining up here on the pedestal," Kate said.

". . . . and to some, I will always be a foreigner," Casey said.

"You're smart, sensitive, and handsome too," Kate said. "Anyone who gets to know you will learn you are an incredible person."

"Grandma says that's the problem with the world," Casey said. "It's much easier to pre-judge people by their looks than to find out what they're really like."

"That's the problem with you, Casey Lee. You think too much." Kate lowered her voice. "Have I ever told you how much I care about you?"

"Please, Kate, don't." He hugged her tightly. "Let's just enjoy each other for as long as we can."

"I've got a better idea," Kate said, tracing Casey's lower lip with an index finger. "You've shared Madame Lee's advice with me. Now, I'm going to tell you what my madam, Wanda Majic, said during our Yearning Arms training."

Kate pulled her face even with Casey's. "Madam Majic said the most intimate physical act is not intercourse. It's kissing with emotion. That's why she won't allow her girls to kiss their clients. She said kissing is too intimate for a business relationship."

"So?" Casey said, looking deeply into Kate's eyes.

"So, why don't we follow Madam Majic's maxim and become intimate. . . very intimate," she said, parting her lips, smothering his pliant mouth.

From the rear of the woodie, Ruby and The Romantics warbled, *"Our Day Will Come."*

Somewhere, beyond the Golden Gate, beneath the harvest moon, squadrons of submarines raced . . . undetected.

21

DOWN AND DIRTY

"Isn't it true, Professor Scott, you are a debaucher of innocent, young women?"

Bombastic attorney, Marvin Belly, was in his mid-thirties, portly, with thick, caterpillar eyebrows, and wavy hair. He wore a silver, Italian suit and a regimental striped tie.

"No!" Ari Scott said.

"Move to strike the answer as nonresponsive. Request the Court to instruct the witness to answer truthfully," Belly said, with a sigh.

The name plate on the bench read, 'Judge I.M. Holmrecker.'

"Professor Scott," Judge Holmrecker said, peering over a pair of pince-nez, "you have taken a sworn oath to tell the truth, the whole truth, and nothing but the truth, so help you, God."

"Yes, your Honor."

Judge Holmrecker sat hunched forward in his chair. His head was perched on the fist of an arm with his elbow propped on the bench.

"In case you didn't understand counsel's diplomatic question, let me pose it another way. Are you a fornicator of young girls? Yes or no, Professor?"

"No, your Honor," Ari said, in a whisper.

Marvin Belly continued, "Isn't it true, you fathered a child out-of-wedlock?"

"Yes, that is true," Ari said. "and my daughter, Anna, is now a lovely, young woman."

"I'm striking that last remark, on my own motion, as self-serving,"

Judge Holmrecker said, banging his gavel.

Belly's tone turned accusatory, "Isn't it true the mother of that child was a 19-year old teenager when you seduced her?"

"We were in love," Ari said, his mind flashing back to lovely memories of the toure di amore he had shared with Sofia Cappuccino.

"Objection, move to strike," Belly said.

"Sustained," Judge Holmrecker said, leaning toward Ari, "Answer Mr. Belly's question, Professor. Was the mother of your love-child, only 19 years old? Yes or no?"

"Yes, sir."

"So, now, you admit being a despoiler of young girls?" Belly said, with a smirk.

"Absolutely not!" Ari said, rising out of the witness chair.

"Sit down, Professor Scott; or I'll cite you for contempt!" Judge Holmrecker said, pounding his gavel.

"And," Belly continued, "as a man with bankrupt moral values, you are unfit to have visitation rights with your young, impressionable children. Isn't that true?"

"No! Never!" Ari shouted. "I am not an unfit father."

"I've heard enough of this degenerate nonsense," the Judge said. "I find Professor Aristotle Scott an unfit father and deny him all visitation rights."

"No. You can't," Ari said. "I have rights."

"You have no rights in my court," the Judge Holmrecker said. "Bailiffs, take Professor Scott to prison for the rest of his life!"

Ari struggled against hands wrenching his arms behind his back. He felt the sharp pinch of handcuffs, as he was dragged, like a sack of potatoes, from the courtroom.

I'll never see Marcus and Monique again! Ari thought.

In the distance, Ari heard a chorus of laughter from Marvin Belly, Esquire, and the Honorable Judge I. M. Holmrecker.

"No! No! You can't do this to me!" Ari shouted.

The room was pitch black, the only sound the hissing of steam heat from the bedroom radiator.

Ari sat erect, his body drenched in sweat, his heart palpitating, his breath labored.

4:16 a.m.

It had been a nightmare.

A week earlier, Ari had received a call from the Law Offices of Marvin Belly, Esquire, inviting him to an informal settlement discussion before the court hearing on Cee Cee's petition to deny Ari visitation rights. Ari had not hired an attorney, as he was confident he would be granted visitation rights.

Ex-cons had visitation rights. Why not a Philosophy professor with only a youthful indiscretion on his record? He thought.

Belly's office was housed in a turn-of-the century, brick building erected during the City's bawdy, Barbary Coast days. Books were stacked precariously on couches, files strewn, like playing cards, on Persian rugs. Standing guard over Belly's ten foot desk, a portion of a bar from a Speakeasy, was a full-size, human skeleton. Around its neck - like a miniature sandwich board - was a name tag that read, *"Herkie."*

"We can dispense with the pleasantries, Professor Scott," Belly said, puffing on a foot-long cigar. The attorney wore a silk shirt and suspenders embroidered with a vertical pattern of dollar signs.

"Professor, my client has instructed me to make you a settlement offer."

"You're referring to my ex-father-in-law?" Ari said.

"Your estranged wife, Cee Cee, is technically my client, but William Randolph Chandler is paying my bill." Belly blew a stream of gray cigar smoke a few inches above Ari's head.

"WRC acknowledges you have been a decent father to his grandchildren and believes the kids should continue their relationship with their dad, but . . ." Belly said, flicking ashes into the palm of Herkie's outstretched hand.

"But what?" Ari said.

"There is a certain something you must do, if you want to avoid a messy custody fight."

"And what is the 'certain something'?" A feeling of queasiness gripped Ari.

"Publish or perish is unpopular with the Cal faculty, right?"

"An understatement," Ari said. "There's going to be tremendous resistance from the Humanities professors. Even if the measure is supported by the science professors, the issue will split the faculty."

"WRC believes you and your buddies, Nelquist and Aural, can be peace makers, by publicly backing publish or perish. He would look kindly on this enlightened gesture and reciprocate accordingly, " Belly said, relighting his cigar.

"Reciprocate?" Ari said. "How?"

"You will have regular visitation rights and avoid going to court. As a bonus, you and your friends will be exempt from publish or perish. Of course, no one will know about your privileged status."

"This is blackmail," Ari said.

"A rather harsh term, professor," Belly said, behind a cloud of cigar smoke. "I'd prefer calling it settling the dispute amicably."

"And if I refuse . . .?"

"The trial will be messy," Belly said. "I guarantee it. I'm being paid big bucks to do to everything necessary to prove you're an unfit father. This means I'll have to dig up details of your old affair with Sofia Cappuccino. This will be embarrassing to you; to your daughter, Anna; to Sofia, and to her husband, Pablo Zarzana. As one who's championed the Higher Truth, you wouldn't want that on your conscience."

The thought of turning the *toure di amore* into a cheap, sordid affair sent chills up Ari's spine. Ari had avoided such a spectacle when disgraced Congressman Clayborn Muck and HUAC had abandoned its campus hearings. Now it appeared that his luck was running out.

"My integrity is at stake," Ari said. "I must defend it."

"Professor, be practical," Belly said. "Who's going to know or care about this minor concession. If you play ball, you get your visitation rights. Your life, and those of your faculty buddies, will go on, as if nothing happened. How can you lose?"

Practicality, Ari thought, *WRC's hallmark. Above all else, WRC was practical.*

Belly snuffed out the cigar, grinding the stub in Herkie's palm.

"Think it over, Professor. This is the best way to resolve a messy situation. Just call me, and it's a done deal."

Belly lowered his voice. "I'm going to give you some free advice, Professor. If you want to fight the Chandlers, for God's sake, hire a lawyer, a real tiger. If you don't, I'll kill you on the witness stand."

Marvin Belly stood and offered his hand. "Nothing personal, Professor. In my business, you win some; you lose some."

"Win some, lose some," Ari murmured, shaking Belly's hand.

* * * *

E Lyn "Ace" Chamberlin burst into Sam Paean's small, glassed office, waving a single sheet of paper.

"Sam, just received this from Bob Bateson, marked *"For Your Eyes Only."*

Bateson was Deputy Justice Administrator, Paean's inside source for courthouse information.

Paean read the hand-scrawled note and said, "William Randolph Chandler must really want to win badly. He used up plenty of IOU's to pull these rabbits out of the hat."

The note identified witnesses Marvin Belly intended to call to prove Ari Scott an unfit father.

"What can we do, Sam?" E Lyn said, stunned by the revelation. "Shouldn't we warn Ari about this?"

"As much as I'd like to help Ari with this inside information, I'd be breaching journalistic ethics, if I tipped him off privately," Paean said.

"We can't let Ari be ambushed by Chandler's backroom plotting," E Lyn said.

"If I print this as an eye-tem," Paean said, tapping the loyal Royal with a two-fingered stroke, "maybe Ari will figure out the clues."

"Terrific, Sam," E Lyn said, ripping the sheet of paper from the Royal. The eye-tem read:

> *"The custody battle between Cecelia
> and Aristotle Scott has turned nasty.
> Cee Cee's powerful daddy, WRC, has
> lined up an A-list of witnesses to help
> Marvin Belly, Esquire. destroy the
> reputation of the '36 Olympic metric
> mile champ. Can the Great Scott
> survive the blows of a tuxedo'd
> mammal, the bites of an Eastern pit
> bull, and the long daggers of the
> world famous alphabet head?"*

"Let's hope Ari will be ready," E Lyn said. "William Randolph Chandler smells blood, and there'll be buckets spilled in the courtroom."

22

GREETINGS FROM TWO LAKES

Two envelopes sat on Jonathan's desk. The pink one had flowery handwriting with the return address of

> *"Dawna Plumber*
> *Lake Lagunitas Apartments - #16*
> *Stanford University, California"*.

The smaller white one bore two separate kinds of penmanship. The return address of

> *"Four Winds Drive*
> *Clear Lake, Iowa"*

was the crisp, efficient printing of his mother, Gertrude Aldon, while Jonathan's name and dorm address was written in the short, slanted strokes of his father, Murle Aldon:

Both letters had been picked up by Butch four hours ago, but Jonathan had not opened either.

Next to the envelopes sat a small, wrinkled brown bag containing his prized possession, Buddy Holly's glasses. All three paper containers were reminders of his former life.

He recalled the last time he saw Dawna Plumber. It was the Clear Lake High grad party, and Dawna, who was enrolling at Stanford, had pressed his left hand firmly onto her right breast and flicking her tongue against his ear lobe, whispered, *"Oh, Jonathan, that feels so-o good.*

Maybe, we can get together. We have so much in common."

Despite Dawna's explicit sexual invitation, the only image Jonathan could conjure was her blue eyes bugging through her thick lenses.

I don't need experience THAT badly, Jonathan thought.

Jonathan had suppressed any thought of his parents since their last meeting at the Durant Hotel the morning after the Gee Dee's Halloween Presents Party. Gertrude and Murle Aldon had made a surprise visit to learn, first hand, why Jonathan had not kept the Three Promises he had made to secure their permission to enroll at Cal: join the Berkeley chapter of his father's fraternity, the P U's, faithfully attend Sunday service at the campus Methodist Church, and maintain good grades.

Why would Mother and Father write? Was it intended to restate their anger over his choice of remaining with the Dormies as a penniless waif? Had something terrible happened to Ziggy? To Uncle Mike or Aunt Pearl?

"Still too chicken to open them?" Butch asked, plopping down at the desk, hefting the envelopes, one in each hand. "They're only words, Junior. Remember the old nursery rhyme, about sticks and stones?' What more can your folks say that will be more hurtful than disowning you? And even, if that Stanford broad is as ugly as you claim, you don't have to hot foot your body down to Palo Alto.

"I say, open the damn things and be done with them. If it'll make you feel any better, you can always chuck 'em," Butch said, sliding open the large window facing San Francisco Bay.

Butch is right, Jonathan thought. *Anything short of illness or death to Ziggy, Mike, or Pearl would be a relief. And if Dawna wanted to see him, he could always offer a polite, no.*

"The card from the horny Stanford broad goes first," Butch said, handing Jonathan the pink envelope.

The seal broke easily. Inside was a greeting card bearing the face of *Mad Magazine's* Alfred E. Neumann with the notation:

> *"Miss you terribly, Jonathan!*
> *Hope to see you SOON !"*

"This fell out," Butch said, handing Jonathan a hand-written note

"Hi, Hi, Hi!

Greetings from across the Bay from your adoring Stanford Dolly! (Popular girls are called "dollies" here.)"

Jonathan could only imagine how Dawna had become so popular in such a short time!

"Hope your Cal experience has been as stimulating as mine down here on The Farm! My absolute favorite class is in the Hindu Dept. where I am the ONLY girl! We've been reading excerpts from the Kama Sutra and boy, do I enjoy the study groups! Can't imagine copies of the Kama Sutra being sold in Clear Lake!

Would love to get together so I can show you exactly what I've learned! Please call when you want to find out what Stanford dollies are all about.

Kisses and a Whole LOTS more
Dawna"

Taped to the note was a black and white photograph of Dawna, with her lips puckered and her nipples showing beneath a sheer nightie.

"Whoa, I take back everything nasty I've ever said about homely 'fuck privates,' Junior," Butch said, reading Dawna's letter over Jonathan's shoulder. "If some broad is willing to show you a thing or two jumping your bones, I say more power to your friendly tool." Butch snatched away the note and re-read it, drool dripping onto his spats.

Jonathan gently plucked the white envelope from Butch's other massive hand with a thumb and forefinger. He opened it by digging the tip of the forefinger beneath the seal and running his finger along the length of the envelope, creating a mountain range of jagged paper.

Unfolding the single page letter, neatly folded in thirds, he read aloud:

"Dear son:

It has been 30-days since our visit, time enough for your father and I to re-assess the sad events of that horrible day. No matter how much you have disappointed us, you are still our son. We cannot imagine how difficult it has been for you to survive without money. Have you lost much weight?

Your father and I will resume our financial support of your college education at Cal. (Frankly, I don't understand why you don't call it

Berkeley or UCB)

To show you how much we love you, we will compromise our expectations in the following manner.

First, we will not ask you to attend services at the Campus Methodist Church. We raised you as a God-fearing Christian and are confident you will eventually return to the church where you will be forgiven for your youthful transgressions.

Secondly, so long as you stay in school and graduate in four years, we will not demand that you maintain excellent grades. During our visit, P U alumni advisor, Mr. Krum II, told us his son, Dirk III, had only a gentleman's C average; and that the Cal degree, and not good grades, is the goal of all good fraternity men.

Thirdly, and this is the most important part of our proposal. You must leave the unhealthy environment of Dooch and join the P U fraternity. We are convinced that the Dormie influence is the cause of all your academic and personal problems. We raised you in a manner befitting your station in life, and we are convinced that your exposure to the riffraff of California society has corrupted your values.

Since meeting that nice Mr. Krum, his son Dirk, and the P U's, we are relieved that not all Californians are Beatniks and bums. You would be better served if you lived among your own kind, like the P U's! We have contacted Mr. Krum, and he assures us that his son and the P U's will accept your belated membership.

Enclosed is a check for $1,000 that should cover your dues and social expenses at the P U house.

With faith in the Lord on our side, your father and I are confident you will see the wisdom of our offer.

Love,
Mother

PS Son, as you will inherit Aldon Farms and continue the important work of producing premium hog meat to people of the world, consider your acceptance of this offer just the first of many wise business decisions you will make in your life.

Love,
Father"

"Wow," Butch said, examining the check. "I've never been this close to a grand before. A thousand bucks would free you up for more study time and to date that three star general, Pritti Diva. Tough deal to turn down, Junior."

Butch is right, thought Jonathan. *As a P U, I could still keep my Dormie friends. I could visit and hear about the latest Dormie RF's. Nothing would really change, except my address.*

It had been two weeks ago that Jerry Fart-ing, facing the same dilemma, had taken the path of lesser resistance by moving into the P U fraternity.

Maybe, joining the P U's wouldn't be such a bad idea, Jonathan thought. *Could the feud between the Dormies and the P U's be only a figment of Casey Lee's and Royal French's imagination?*

"I'll give you some privacy," Butch said, cinching up his spats. "I'm sure you'll make the right decision."

Jonathan stood at the open window, watching the last rays of the sun disappearing into the Pacific beyond the Golden Gate. He had won an important struggle. His parents had backed down from the Three Promises. He would no longer have to feel guilty about missing church or to suffer anxiety about not being a top student. He would be free to enjoy Cal and The City without worrying about every dollar. No more dressing up as Ruby Lips' mute, gypsy assistant. No more late nights helping Royal French crank out fake ID's. No more keeping Hunch's Campanile playing cabin sparkling clean.

What more could he ask for?

Jonathan sat at his desk and exhaled deeply. He removed Buddy's glasses from the crumpled brown bag, remembering the smoke and fire of the fateful plane crash. A piece of wooden shard dropped from the bag on which was scrawled, in child-like handwriting.

. . . Not Fade Away - Crunchy Munchy . . .

He had loaned the glasses to Crunchy Munchy during the Big C Sircus, and the ice-cream vendor had returned them, along with his message written on a wooden popsicle stick.

Jonathan removed a sheaf of stationary, lifted from the front desk of the Durant Hotel and, using a ball point advertising *Ovaltine*, wrote:

"Dear Mother and Father:

Your letter and check arrived today. Yes, a $1,000 would cure many of my problems. I have been working three part-time jobs to make ends meet and staying up late studying with my Dormie tutors. It has been the hardest time in my life. I have never felt such doubt and fear. There are times I think I want to give it all up and join the Navy, like Uncle Mike. But somehow, every morning, I tell myself I WILL make it through another day, and I have survived thus far, thanks to the incredible support of the Dormies.

You will find this hard to believe, but I cannot accept your generous offer. I am returning the check. I know you dislike my new friends and that, by Clear Lake standards, you consider them 'riffraff.'

However strange they seem to you, Dormies are perfectly normal Californians. They represent the wave of the future, raised in a large middle-class where anyone - no matter how humble his background, how homely his looks, or how exotic his national origin - can rise, with the help of a quality university education, to become a future business, political, and social leader.

I have developed a strong kinship with this middle-class value, where I can fail miserably and still have another opportunity to try again; where failure does not doom me for life; and where I am appreciated for the quality of my struggle. I'm sure you dismiss this as radical Berkeley Beatnik babble, but I have witnessed and lived this at Cal; and there is nothing more important or real than what is happening here.

My chief Dormie tutor, Michael Hu, agrees with you. He believes no one can change his destiny.

I disagree. There is something about this wondrous college environment that has changed my life forever. And wherever this Cal experience leads me, I will have no regrets.

One day, the rest of the world will realize that the California Dream is fueled and nurtured by the "riffraff," from all over the world, who come for a chance, even a second and a third chance, for happiness and prosperity.

I may eventually return to Clear Lake, chalking up my Cal days, as merely a youthful escape. But, until then, I am convinced that my Cal friends and experiences will be my best guides to my destiny.

Love always
- Jonathan

PS You raised me to appreciate how some things and people are inherently superior. Although there are other UC campuses - UCLA (Los Angeles), UCD (Davis), UCSB (Santa Barbara), UCSD (San Diego), UCR (Riverside), UCSF (med school in San Francisco), and a future one at UCI (Irvine) - there is only one Cal, the oldest and most prestigious of the UC campuses.

To Cal students, there is only one University of California, and it is located in Berkeley, so calling our campus 'Berkeley' or 'UCB' would be redundant.

This reasoning sounds haughty, if not snotty; but you taught me to understand there are times when Truth is both haughty and snotty. This is such a Truth."

Jonathan re-read his parents' letter again.

Folding it neatly into sharp angles to form a paper airplane, Jonathan gently launched it into the buffeting breezes of the East Bay evening. Amazingly, the airplane defied the physics of the prevailing winds and dove in a beeline, crumpling into a jagged mass, in the dorm parking lot, three stories below, and swirling among the vortex of dead leaves.

23

BRING ME THE HEAD OF OSKI BEAR

The ursine figure staggered out of the P U patio, past the babbling water fall, and stumbled onto the moonlit corner of Channing and College. The creature was barely 5-foot-6 inches tall, his diminutive stature accentuated by the oversized, cartoon, paper mache head with large ears, double-eye holes and permanent, smiling face which had been described as a "shit-eating" grin. His gold letterman's sweater, baggy blue pants, white gloves, and floppy tennis shoes were sopped with the sweet scent of beer doused on him by throngs of Cal fans celebrating another rousing football victory, this time over "Wazoo," Washington State University.

It had been too much to expect that, after the upset of the hated USC Trojans, the Joe L. Capp led Bears would win even more games. But more miracles had occurred in Strawberry Canyon, and the under-sized Bears had run off four straight Pacific Eight wins, including today's win over the WSU Cougars from the Palouse country of eastern Washington.

One final win, in the Big Game against Stanford next week, and Cal would have its first winning season in a decade.

At the post-Wazoo P U party, Oski had downed 12-brews by placing one end of a clear, plastic tubing into a cup of beer, stretching the length of the tubing through one of his eye holes, inserting the other end into his mouth, and ingesting the contents in one sustained gulp. In a quasi-inebriated stupor, Oski had almost forgotten his vows of silence when voluptuous Muffy Peachwick had plopped into his lap to share a beer.

Drink, don't talk, Oski reminded himself. *But, man, that Gee Dee babe, Muffy. is one hot number! How I'd love to boink that Amazon in blissful silence!*

Better move on, Oski told himself, remembering he had promised to check out the souvenir goal posts the Dormies had torn down after the SC upset. Oski usually traveled with two others who were more body guards than escorts; but they too had been caught up in the post-game hoopla of the P U party and did not notice their charge leave.

Out in the street, Oski inhaled the cool, evening air hoping rocking side-to-side would steady himself. He had trained for moments like this, when hours of beer drinking clouded his memory and impaired his balance.

Not to worry, Oski thought. *Dooch Dorm is only a block away, and I can stagger, if not crawl, down to the Dormies for at least three more beers.*

Behind him, Oski heard the lyrics of Lloyd Price's *"Stagger Lee,"* from a slow approaching vehicle. The Bear mascot was leaning against the street lamp, catching his breath, when a red station wagon emerged from the darkness, pulling alongside. Inside were six students dressed in red sweatshirts and white hats.

One of Wazoo's colors is red, Oski recalled, burping.

"Oski, how's tricks?" one occupant said, from a rear side window.

Oski nodded and gave a thumbs up sign.

"How about a beer, Oski" another said, extending a bottle of beer from an open window.

What the hell, another brew-ski's not gonna hurt, Oski thought, uncoiling his clear, plastic tubing, noting the offering had an import label. *Who can afford expensive foreign beer?*

Suddenly, the occupants of the station wagon spilled onto the street corner, surrounding him. It was then that Oski first noticed the white lettering on the cardinal-colored sweatshirts:

"Leland Stanford Junior University."

Stan-furd!

Reacting instinctively, Oski dove between the legs of the one closest to College Way.

If I can make enough noise, the Dormies will hear me, he thought, suddenly forgetting his vow of silence.

"Get him," the leader shouted, diving after the Bear mascot. Oski found himself buried under a swarm of grunting, grabbing, and swearing Stanford red.

The more Oski resisted, the more he felt like a deflating balloon. His ability to breathe was slipping away into unconsciousness, as his lungs labored, gasping for air.

A bad nightmare, Oski thought, twisting against the avalanche of grappling hands. *What the hell do they want?*

The answer came in the sickening rush of fresh night air engulfing him, allowing him to cough haltingly, as the mob retreated, piling into the station wagon, and zooming away, amid a chorus of hoots and laughter.

Dazed, prone, Oski felt nauseous, naked, and violated.

No! No! he thought, pounding his fists on the street. Within seconds, the station wagon's tail lights disappeared, westbound on Channing.

They've kidnaped my head!

The following week should have been filled with traditional, colorful activities leading up to the Cal-Stanford Big Game. Instead, it was now a moribund period of mourning. "Blue Monday," the Monday day before Big Game where everyone on campus wore Cal blue and gold, and anyone caught dressed in Stanford red was publicly humiliated, was quietly observed. Students jammed Professor Roderick Seakin's annual Big Game science lecture where, dressed as Archimedes, he magically turned, with an animated swirl of a swizzle-stick, the color of beaker, from offending Stanford red, to loyal Cal blue.

The campus community packed Dwinelle Plaza for Professor Jacob Aural's SRO candlelight eulogy to the memory of Cal Coach Andy Smith's 1920's undefeated "Wonder Teams." Greek living groups went through the motions of decorating their houses in anti-Stan-furd themes, with the prizes awarded at the Bon Fire Rally at the Greek Theater, the night before Big Game.

Yet, a discernible pall of sadness engulfed the Berkeley campus on learning that Oski's head had been stolen. Without his "shit-eating grin," the mascot would be absent from Big Game. It was a disaster tantamount to Cal stealing the war bonnet of Prince Harry Hotfoot, Stanford's full-blooded Indian mascot.

It was distressing enough that Stanford held the Axe, symbol of the previous year's Big Game winner. Now, the $tan-furd Indian$ also had the head of Oski Bear, the symbol of Cal irreverence.

Insult to Oski's decapitation was a photo in the San Francisco *Sentinel* showing Stanford's Rally Committee joyously holding the Axe, while Prince Harry Hotfoot, brandished Oski's head like a prized scalp, above the headline.

"Stanford Indians Behead Bear Mascot"

In his gossip column, Sam Paean posted an eye-tem from a Stanford campus source that foretold of a death in the Cal family.

> *My almost alma-mater lost Blue & Gold face*
> *when marauding Indians scalped Oski's top.*
> *The Shadow Knows Oski's smiling face will be*
> *roasted in front of 10,000 Red & White clad*
> *Stan-froo students - 8 p.m.- at the Annual*
> *Bonfire Rally at bone-dry Lake Lagunitas . . .*

The Cal Alumni Association offered a $500 reward for the safe return of Oski's head to which a Stanford grad sniffed, "$500 or $5,000, both are meaningless to us."

Although eschewing a call for violence, the usually pacifistic *Daily Californian* issued a call for "extraordinary measures" when an educational institution exercises "self-defense" against "barbaric hooligans."

* * * *

Two figures, dressed in black, faces hidden behind ski masks, emerged from the Jacaranda grove and dropped to their knees. The roar of unseen thousands could be heard over the tune *"All Right Now,"* which the Stanford band played incessantly whether things were all right or not, a musical habit analogous to the USC band droning endlessly with its signature song, *"Conquest,"* whether SC was winning or losing.

The evening darkness had not hampered the two from finding Lake Lagunitas. Daytime visitors were always at a loss for bearings, as all the buildings of the Stanford campus shared the same faux Spanish mission design, were similarly pink, and crowned by adobe tile roofs.

Royal French pulled up the sleeve of his left arm, glanced at the luminous numbers of his combat watch, and signaled to Mo McCart, by flashing the five fingers of his right hand twice: ten minutes before the start of *"Operation Stinky Chief RF."* RF stood for Rat Fuck, the irreverent phrase used to describe a prank or trick, carried out in retaliation or revenge against a rank injustice.

The pair crawled on their stomachs, to the rear of massive, wooden bleachers temporarily erected in a large circle below banks of battery-powered flood lights. The tinny plink-plink-plink of beer cans landing on the 50-foot mountain of lumber echoed to the reverberations of shouts and applause of thousands of Stanford students at the bonfire rally at Lake Lagunitas, once a respite for early Californian Indians.

For Royal French, this exercise in college skullduggery triggered deep-seated nightmares of life and death, of clandestine missions he had undertaken in countries whose names had no meaning to the average American: *Vietnam, Cambodia, Laos.*

After the fall of the French in Indo-China in 1954, Royal had been a member of an elite, secret US Army unit sent to Southeast Asia "to stem the tide of Communism." For three years, Captain Royal French had led local anti-Communist guerilla forces in espionage forays, search-and-destroy missions, and assassinations ("terminations with extreme prejudice"). Royal commanded unwavering loyalty from his Liliputian-sized trainees, not because of his imposing 6-foot-9-inch height, but despite it, as his recruits could not believe a white man, of such size, could escape detection, much less death, in jungle warfare. On his part, Royal did not care to count the number of times he had killed with his bare hands, all for naught, as he had concluded that American forces would never defeat dedicated, Asian adversaries who did not commit to well-defined battle lines.

The reward for his bloody service had been a government-paid tuition to a university of his choice. Born and raised in Santa Monica, nearby UCLA would have been a logical choice. He could have earned a gentleman BA, as a Bruin, and accept the offer for a movie career from his childhood buddy, an up-and-coming movie star, Robert Readyford, with whom Royal had raced cars in the early Fifties. But Royal had picked Cal to escape the destruction of the small town feeling of the beach-centered Southern California of his youth, by the emergence of the LA freeway system.

Royal soon learned an irony of life is that one can never escape one's past. Bonding immediately with the iconoclastic Casey Lee, an Oriental, the likes of which he had never met in Southeast Asia, the two had taken the socio-politico advancement of the middle-class Dormies as their undergraduate mission. Despite the high level of intelligence prevalent on campus and the rational thought that was supposed to be the campus paradigm, time and again, the Dormies' struggle for dignity and respect depended on the imaginative survival skills Royal had honed in the jungles of Southeast Asia.

On his part, Mo McCart knew there was no logical reason he should be in this precarious position, other than loyalty to his Dormie friends. If he were caught, his position as a starting member of the Cal football team, would be seriously jeopardized for tomorrow's Big Game. The Cal team needed him on the field if they were to have any chance of beating the hated Stan-furd Indians, but the Dormies needed him even more.

It had been an unlikely road to Cal. Mo had been adopted by a deaf couple in the small San Joaquin Valley farming community of Turlock. To communicate with his parents, Mo learned signage, at an early age. Despite his massive size and natural aptitude for football, Mo had been a straight A student, his athletic talent balanced by a keen intellect nurtured by his parents' commitment to education.

Mo had turned down a coveted football scholarship to Notre Dame and instead enrolled at Cal where he was doomed to anonymity, playing for a losing football team. But Mo's parents had instilled in their man-child a mature sense of perspective, that athletic glory was fleeting, but education was a rewarding, life-long process.

Now, despite three years of football losses, he had not regretted his decision. Mo loved the campus and his Dormie friendships. Witnessing his adoptive parents struggle for dignity, Mo understood his roommate, Ruby Lips's battles in a homophobic world.

8 p.m.

The bank of flood lights went dark, replaced by the flickering of 10,000 candles accompanied by the rhythmic beat of unseen tom-toms and the hissing of bead-filled rattles. A deafening roar enveloped a procession of red and white clad Stanford Rally Committee members carrying two trophies of immeasurable value: The Axe and a silver tray large enough to transport a whole, roast pig. On the platter was the battered, shit-eating grin of Oski Bear.

Royal nodded to Mo, as a sustained chorus of war whoops greeted the thin, wiry form of Indian royalty, dressed in a full-length, feather war bonnet and tan buckskin pants, pranced into Lake Lagunitas, accompanied by a phalanx of Stanford Band members. The Indian Chief's upper torso and face were striped with red and white war paint. Around his neck, he wore a shell choker necklace and a beaded shirt bib.

Prince Harry Hotfoot danced feverishly in front of the six story tall pile of lumber, dancing and chanting lustily:

"HI-YUM, SKOOK-UM,
TILLY-KUM, MOKUM,
HI-YUM, SKOOK-UM,
HOY! HOY!

HI-YUM, SKOOK-UM
TILLY-KUM, MOKUM
HI-YUM, SKOOK-UM,
HOY! HOY !"

Keep it up, "Prince Harry Hotfoot, " Royal thought. *We need only ten more minutes of delay.*

Unbeknownst to the undiscerning eyes of Stanford students who could not tell an authentic Native American from a phony dime-wooden variety, the Prince Harry Hotfoot who danced so charmingly before them was Rod Organ wearing layers of brown body makeup, re-creating an Indian ritual he had used as a member of the Boys Scout, Beaver Patrol.

Earlier, Dormie commandos had snatched and chloroformed the real Prince Harry Hotfoot, relieved him of his ceremonial garb, and left him bound and gagged in the garbage dumpster of the "Rich & Marie Dishop's Gourmet Oasis," a popular Stan-furd beer and burger joint.

8.05 p.m.

Jonathan Aldon and Dawna Plumber entered her third floor apartment overlooking Lake Lagunitas, 50-yards away. The couple had returned from a tandoori dinner at Dawna's favorite Hindu restaurant, Dancing Shiva. Jonathan had felt over-dressed. Dawna was dressed in sandals and red, halter-top dress that fell immodestly to the middle of her thighs. The sheerness of the dress advertised the fact that Dawna was bra-less.

"Jonathan, I'm so-o-o happy you would come all the way to Palo Alto to see me," Dawna said, encircling his neck in her arms. "I've had the biggest crush on you since grammar school, and now that we've escaped our small-town prison of Clear Lake, we can satisfy our deepest yearnings." She tossed her thick, bi-focals on a nearby couch and planted a wet kiss on him.

"Mmmm," Jonathan mumbled, unable to form words, as Dawna's tongue twisted his into a pretzel. The muffled, primitive sounds of tom-toms and bead-filled rattles coursed through the closed, sliding glass door to the apartment balcony.

Releasing her oscular grip, Dawna said, "Let's go to my room and make ourselves comfortable. I want to show you some positions from the Kama Sutra that will drive you absolutely wild!"

Clasping her hand on his, she led him in the direction of her bedroom. "My roomie, Carolee Sheef, is at that stupid Bonfire Rally and won't be back for hours." She pointed to the outline of the massive pile of lumber towering over the apartment. "We can set our own bonfire, Jonathan."

Passing the front door of the apartment, Dawna did not notice Jonathan quickly twisting open the deadbolt.

Outside the fire escape of the apartment crouched two ski-masked figures dressed in black, carrying dark duffel bags. If there had been witnesses, they would have noted that the taller of the two wore white spats over his black shoes, and the shorter one seemed to have almond-shaped eyes.

It had been Butch who remembered Dawna's address at Lake Lagunitas from the mash note she had sent Jonathan a few weeks ago, and now, Jonathan was doing his duty for the RF.

Climbing quietly into the hallway, the duo heard the deadbolt lock click open. Ten seconds later, Butch and Casey Lee carefully admitted themselves into the apartment.

From the bedroom, a voice cooed breathlessly, "Oh, Jonathan, let me teach your hands how to talk to my nipples."

The duo eased themselves into the small balcony, quietly closing the sliding glass door behind, quickly emptying the contents of the duffel bags: kite-size strips of balsa wood, clear, plastic dry-cleaning bags, small, birthday candles, fast-bonding glue, rubber bands, and tiny aluminum canisters.

Using glue, they fastened pairs of balsa wood strips at right angles. The two created four crosses, gluing the corners of each, equal distance, at the open end of the plastic bags. They attached bundles of birthday candles to the center of each cross and fastened aluminum canisters an inch from each bundle of candles.

8:10 p.m.

One at a time, Butch stretched the closed end of the clear, plastic, dry cleaning bags above his head, while Casey ignited the bundle of candles from below, filling each bag with expanding hot air that soon converted the plastic bags into a miniature, hot-air balloons. Launched one minute apart, the four home-made dirigibles were buffeted by the prevailing westerly South Bay breeze toward the mountain of lumber, 50 yards away.

8:15 p.m.

Rod Organ, as Prince Harry Hotfoot, had done his part in delaying the lighting of the bonfire. Royal tugged Mo's sleeve, pointing to the night sky where a parade of four burning crosses floated on collision course with the lumber mountain. The flotilla of hot-air balloons fell from the sky in fiery balls, crashing into the mountainous pile of lumber, as the candle flames melted burning through the balsa wood strips and igniting the aluminum containers.

Transfixed by the aerial sight, Stanford students assumed the Rally Committee had devised an ingenious way to start the bonfire. The true nature of the Dormie RF was revealed when the chemical contents of the canisters burst into clouds of blinding, cough-inducing stench.

Tear Gas Bombs!

Wearing Army-issue gas masks, Royal and Mo dashed through the noxious smoke, noise, and confusion toward their goals. Using his football skills, Mo bowled over three Stan-furd Rally Committee members like skinny tenpins and ripped away The Axe, while Butch snatched Oski's head from the silver platter, and tucked it under his arm. Like raging bulls, the two commandos stampeded through the coughing, screaming crowd toward the darkness of the Jacaranda grove.

"Get 'em!" many shouted. "They've got the Axe!" others screamed.

Too late, Froo-froo's, Royal thought, running rear guard for Mo. Flashing martial arts skills he had not used since his duty in Southeast Asia, Royal dispatched a dozen of the Rally Committee, with his feet, sending them sprawling into the dusty lake bed of Lake Lagunitas.

Royal caught up with Mo in the Jacaranda grove, and the two huffed, side-by-side, as a mounting chorus of voices behind them shouted, "Surround 'em!" "They went into the grove!" "There's no way out."

Nearby, an auto with its front lights dimmed, careened out of the darkness. Pulling along side, churning a cloud of dust, was a woodie. Inside, Rod Organ, still in war paint, shouted, "Rod's Indian cavalry to the rescue! Pile in guys!"

Looping around the darkened Jacaranda grove, Rod Organ powered the woodie past hundreds of disoriented Stanford students. Two blocks later, the woodie screeched to a halt in front of the Lake Lagunitas Apartments. Two figures, dressed in black, sprinted toward them. Butch and Casey squeezed into the rear of the woodie.

"Where's Jonathan?" Royal asked.

"He's freeing himself from the octo-pussy charms of that horny Stand-furd broad from Clear Lake," Butch said.

Thirty seconds later, Jonathan, tripped and shuffled through the front door of the apartment, his gait entangled by slacks and belt shackled around his ankles.

Behind him, Dawna Plumber, clad only in panties, shouted, "Wait, Jonathan! I haven't shown you my favorite, 'Humping Turtles!'

"Hurry, Mr. Fashion Plate," Mo shouted, pulling the half-dressed Jonathan into the back seat.

"Jonathan deserves a Purple Heart," Rod said, flooring the woodie.

"How about a Purple Dick?" Casey teased.

Rod gunned the woodie toward Camino Real and the safety of the Bayshore Freeway.

"Great RF, Dormies." Casey said, reaching toward the back seat. "What a bonus! Let me touch the Axe."

The 15-inch steel axe, trimmed in red and white, with its shortened wooden handle was permanently mounted on a walnut plaque, below which were recorded the scores of each Big Game engraved in silver. The Axe had made its first appearance during a Cal-Stanford baseball game in 1899; and since 1930 had been awarded to the winner of the annual football game. Over the years, both Cal and Stanford students had initiated intricate schemes to steal The Axe and parade it before the sold-out throng before the start of The Big Game.

"The $500 reward for Oski's head should give Hunch's Campus Snow King candidacy a jump start," Casey said.

From the radio, the familiar voice of All-Pro's voice, on KALX, radio announced cryptically, "Now, a special dedication to the BRAVE commandos conducting 'Operation Stinky Chief RF,' here are the harmonic sounds of the Platters with *"Smoke Gets In Your Eyes."* GOOD LUCK on your mission, DORMIES!"

From the front seat, Butch said, in a tone mimicking Dawna's breathless voice,

"Oh, Jonathan, let me teach your hands how to talk to my nipples."

As Jonathan blushed Stan-furd red, from its perch on Royal's knee, the paper mache head of Oski Bear smiled at Jonathan with his shit-eating grin.

24

TWO-FACED

"You won't believe who was in the Mardi Gras Room today!" Joan Dildeaux said.

"Dil-dee, when it comes to sex, nothing surprises me," Muffy Peachwick said, filing her finger nails.

"But Father Gregory?" Joan squealed. "The last time I went to Mass, Father Gregory preached about the 'noble sacrifice of self-control.' "

"Do as I say, not as I do," Muffy said. "Speaking of strange, I had this Cal Engineering professor who wanted conversation. I mean, all he wanted to do was talk. When I reminded him he had paid for a hand-job, he said he'd give me a really big tip if I'd just listen to him. So off he goes about how meaningless life was, how his elderly parents didn't understand him, how the love of his life had jilted him in grad school. Wanda Majic should charge extra for counseling services."

The four Gee Dees, Kate Howell, Joanie Dildeaux, Muffy Peachwick, and Dandy Cane, were seated in the kitchen of Yearning Arms, comparing notes on their new, part-time jobs as quasi-courtesans.

"I had this Berkeley business man who cried like a baby after he dropped his drawers," Dandy said. "He said my Little Bo Beep outfit reminded him of his granddaughter."

"Men are obsessed with their penises," Kate Howell said. "Every guy apologizes for the size of his Thing, but they all look the same to me."

"Be discreet, ladies," Wanda Majic said, entering the kitchen, accompanied by Sascha. "You are discovering a universal truth."

The madam of Yearning Arms poured herself a cup of steaming tea. "The secret to success in this business is massaging the male ego, as well as massaging the male organ."

"They seem to be two sides of the same coin," Muffy said.

"They're both sick," Sascha said, plopping into a chair. She was dressed in her cat lady costume. Through her feline mask, one eye gleamed orange, the other green.

"Kate, do you know a guy named Dirk?" Sascha asked.

"Dirk Krum III?" Kate said, "He's President of the P U fraternity across the street."

"A real sick-o," Sascha said. "I don't mind guys having fantasies when they're getting their rocks off, but this is TOO much," she said, sliding the object across the kitchen table.

Huddling, the quartet issued a collective gasp. Staring at them was a life-size, black and white portrait of Kate's face.

"Dirk had me wear this photo of your face, over my cat mask, while I serviced him," Sascha said, disdain in her voice. "He kept moaning, *'Oh, Kate! 'Oh, Kate! 'Oh, Kate!'* "

"Going to vomit," Kate said, excusing herself, feeling bile rushing up from her stomach. Joan followed in quick pursuit.

"Dirk Krum is such a friggin' jerk-off!" Muffy muttered, sailing the photograph of the Golden Goddess into the garbage can filled with used condoms.

25

THE SEXY SIX

"Stop, Organ! You can't do that!" Mo McCart shouted.

"Sure, I can. No one's around. Watch my dust!"

Instead of turning left where Telly dead-ended into Bancroft, Rod Organ aimed the yellow and chrome woodie due north, jumping the curb, careening past Ludwig's Fountain, zooming past Sproul Hall, and screeching to a halt under the central arch of Sather Gate.

"Jeez, I've just upchucked my dorm dinner," Butch moaned, "why the hell are we stopping here? We've got work to do."

Erected by Mary Sather, in honor of her deceased husband, a prominent alumnus, Sather Gate was the historical main entrance to the campus. Four beveled masonry columns, each topped by a large, glass globe encased in a meridian; two longitude bands, and a bronze shaped flame supported three, sculptured bronze arches. The middle arch, accented by laurel leaves, bore Cal's insignia: a book, a star, and the motto, *Fiat Lux,* Latin for *"Let There Be Light."*

It was past midnight, and Sather Gate's four globes cast an ethereal glow above Strawberry Creek gurgling nearby.

"Only take a minute," Organ said, exiting. "C'mon, guys, give me a hand. Form a pyramid on top of the woodie."

Crouching side-by-side, on their hands and knees, across the width of the woodie's roof, the largest of the six, Mo, Butch, and Royal formed the base. Jonathan and Casey straddled the trio, balancing themselves in the next row. Rod then gingerly boosted himself to a standing position at the apex of the quivering pyramid.

"Hurry," Butch said. "We can't hold you up forever."

"I think the roof's gonna buckle," Mo gasped.

"Almost," Rod said, teetering above them "There! Done!"

Organ lowered his body between Jonathan and Casey, onto Mo's broad back, motioning the second row to slide off.

"Give Royal and Butch a hand," Organ said, collapsing on Mo.

"Back's killing me, Organ," Mo groaned. "I'll give you two seconds to get off," Mo groaned.

Beneath Sather Gate, the sextet paused, gazing up at Organ's handiwork. There, perched at a jaunty angle, on one of Sather Gate's globes, was the shit-eating, grinning head of Oski Bear.

"Smile, Dormies," Rod said, flashing a Brownie Hawkeye camera. "We'll need proof to collect the $500 reward from the Cal Alumni Association."

"An uplifting sight for the early birds," Organ said, revving up the woodie's engine.

"Oski will have his head back for The Big Game, " Casey said.

"But those poor, spoiled Stan-furd-ites won't have their precious Axe," Royal said, with a mischievous chuckle.

* * * *

"Are you sure it's here?" Casey whispered.

"It's here, somewhere," Jonathan said. "Butch and I found it using Super Sleuth's map of secret campus entrances."

The six were on their hands and knees pushing aside piles of decaying leaves, along the north wall of venerable South Hall.

"It was near this bush," Butch said, running his hands along a thin layer of dirt. "Aha, found it!"

The others huddled around, as Butch slipped his fingers under the edge of a metal plate.

"Gimme a hand!" Butch said.

Mo dug his fingers under the opposite edge. "Ok, lift," he grunted.

The other four joined in twisting the plate from its mooring, revealing a rectangular opening.

"Only a short drop," Jonathan said, disappearing into the dark hole.

The others followed with their treasure.

Jonathan traced his hands over unseen contours of irregular shapes and angles. "There's a light somewhere," he said, recalling the prior visit with Butch.

"Here," Butch said, snapping a string of an overhead bulb.

In the dim light of an ancient, ten watt bulb, they squinted through layers of graceful cobwebs. Standing end-to-end, as Jonathan and Butch had related, were eight marble panels, nude bas reliefs of four men and four women, missing from Sather Gate since its completion in 1913. Mrs. Sather had been shocked by the representation of human nudes and ordered the panels removed from beveled masonry columns of Sather Gate. Until the Jonathan and Butch stumbled across the panels during Fall Class Registration, they had been presumed lost or destroyed.

"Perfect," Casey said. "If the nude panels have been in this spot for 46-years, nobody's gonna find the Stan-furd Axe."

"How long are we going to keep this secret?" Mo asked.

"Let's see," Royal said, "Since there are six of us, let's swear we won't divulge the location of the Axe until either Cal or Stan-furd wins six Big Games in a row."

"We'll take the secret to the grave, Royal," Organ said. "No way either school will win or lose six in a row!"

Of the 60-football games played prior, Stanford had won 26, Cal 24, and ten had ended in ties.

"So be it," Casey agreed. "We pulled off Operation Stinky Chief RF against heavy odds, so we agree that it will take six, straight Cal wins or six straight losses before any of us talks."

"One for six, and six for one," Jonathan said.

Standing in a tight circle, the marauders joined hands.

"Here's to the secret of the Dooch Sexy Six," Royal whispered.

"To the secret of the Dooch Sexy Six!" the sextet said in unison.

The Stan-furd Axe was now buried treasure!

26

MISS FOUR B'S, ESQ.

Warm finger rays of dawn slowly penetrated the cool, early morning mist, caressing the iridescent plumage of nature's burnished death robe spreading luxuriously across the Berkeley foothills. The Campanile issued a reassuring gong-gong greeting to another autumn day. Fall, a time for deep reflection, as Nature bids a brilliant, glorious adieu to all things deciduous.

Mona Morgan leaned against the creaky railing of the redwood deck, following the glowing taillights of the limousine, as it snaked past the Berkeley Rose Garden. Behind her, the living room fire crackled to the strains of Mantovani's orchestral strings performing *"Love Is A Many Splendored Thing."*

A many splendored thing?

Yes, she thought, hugging the terry cloth robe tightly to her body. These magical nights of passion made her feel as if she were the center of the universe.

But Love?

Mona had never enjoyed the luxury of giving herself to any man, much less this one, the one who complicated her life, the man who had given her fits, the one she affectionately called "Fitz."

What claim do I have on his life?

Fitz was a married man. A recent *Saturday Evening Post* cover story described him as "a happily married man with a bright political future."

Fitz was ebullient about his chances for the 1960 election. When his New England rival, Congressman Clayborn Muck's attempt to exploit

HUAC hearings at Cal had backfired, Muck's chances of being a viable vice-presidential candidate had evaporated, leaving the door open for Fitz to explore his own chances for a spot on the national ticket.

Who am I to treat our monthly trysts as anything more than a discreet fling between adults who should know better? Thank God for the new birth control pills, Enovid, Fitz had brought from Boston, she sighed.

An unplanned pregnancy was the last thing she and Fitz needed in their already convoluted lives.

Mona Morgan was 36-years old, single, and by 1950's standards, an "old maid," but not from the lack of feminine beauty. Mona had white porcelain skin, auburn hair, in an elfin, pixie cut, and deep emerald eyes. She had a figure that a male admirer described as "Monroe-esque."

Her voluptuous figure made her the center of attention, but it was not the kind of attention she craved. She intimidated most men, especially male attorneys, some who referred to her, behind her back, as *"Miss Four B's"- "Beautiful Ball-Buster Barrister."*

Where was the respect from her male peers?

Mona had been successful in securing substantial divisions of community property for her female clientele in divorces from their wealthy husbands. Perhaps helping women obtain their fair share of marital assets was hitting too close to home.

Were male lawyers fearful she would represent their spouses in their own future divorces?

Now, she had the opportunity to prove her courtroom skills against the notorious Marvin Belly, in *Scott v. Scott*, the divorce trial of the year. Mona had never represented a husband, but it had been a stroke of genius for Aristotle Scott to retain her. Ari had reasoned a female attorney would be more effective in challenging Belly's witnesses because of their inexperience in dealing with a female lawyer.

Mona padded across the deck and into the kitchen and poured herself another cup of coffee.

Who were Belly's celebrity witnesses?

She ruminated over the tantalizing clues Sam Paean had planted in his column.

The *"blows of a tuxedo'd mammal"* was an obvious reference to Ari Scott's faculty opponent, Professor Werner Von Seller, the Prussian Penguin. The *"bites of an Eastern pit bull"* could refer to Congressman

Clayborn Muck, but what would Muck gain in returning to San Francisco after his embarrassing exit? If Muck were to testify, he would be expecting something in return from Cee Cee's father, William Randolph Chandler. But what?

The most intriguing clue was Paean's cryptic reference to the *"daggers of a world famous alphabet head."*

Head of what? Which letters of the alphabet? One thing was certain. William Randolph Chandler was pulling out all stops for his daughter's trial.

Who had WRC lined up as his ace-in-the-hole? Someone very powerful, with damaging information, but *Who? and What?*

Without the identity of the mystery witnesses's, Mona's task of protecting Ari's interests would be daunting. Yet, despite the obstacles, this was one case Mona Morgan, Esq, *"Miss Four B's" -"Beautiful Ball- Buster Barrister,"* could not afford to lose.

27

FLIES BOTH WAYS

Above the soothing sounds of the six foot waterfall splashing in the P U patio, the Seeburg KD200 Select-O-Matic blared the tortured lyrics of *"Tragedy"* by the Fleetwoods.

"So, we dressed Jefferson up as a delivery boy," Chip Fist chuckled, pointing to the P U freshman president. "Then we sent him into the Dooch kitchen with a 50-pound bag marked 'flour.' "

"When I got into the kitchen," Warring said, picking up the story, "It was easy. The dietician told me to pour the contents into a huge kettle where she was cooking something called 'gravy and dumplings,' so I dumped the entire bag of laxative," Warring said, blushing at his triumph.

"Tonight, there'll be lines of Dormies waiting to sit on the can," Fist said, snapping his fingers in glee.

A perfect revenge on Casey Lee and the Dormies, Dirk Krum III thought, a sneer forming across his face.

"Not to put a damper on things, Dirk, but I'm not sure that was the thing to do," Chauncey Remington, P U Graduate Advisor, said, lighting his briar pipe.

"But Dirk's scheme was perfect," Fist said. "We stuck it to every one of those rotten Dormies."

"We have to remind the scum across the street who really runs this campus," Krum said.

"I agree," Chauncey said, "but there are better ways to get that message across than doing something that's going to foster violence.

"Look at history. In every revolution, the rulers are killed or ousted by the sheer weight of numbers. Look what happened in the French, Russian, and Chinese Revolutions. In each, the masses were aroused and rose up against those in power and violently threw them out."

"I wouldn't call those Dormie freaks a revolution," Krum said, spitting into the crackling fireplace.

"Maybe, Dormies are a revolution," Chauncey said, pooching two circles of wobbly, pipe smoke. "If William Randolph Chandler is not elected Governor, the legislature will be hell bent on helping middle-class and nontraditional students enter Cal. In time, the sheer numbers of non-orgs would weaken the power of the IFC.

"We've got to use our political power to insure our dominance without stirring up the masses." Chauncey continued, "Apathy is our greatest ally. Let the sleeping giant lie. History has taught us the few can always control the many, so long as the few do not unnecessarily antagonize the many.

"Let's hope the price of keeping the Dormies in their place is not an uncontrollable uprising," Chauncey said, relighting the briar, then picking up the latest edition of McWilson's science fiction series, *The Chelsea Chronicles.*

"What if this is a hoax, and dorm food isn't poisoned?" Royal French said, arching his 6-foot-9 inch frame into the pose of a praying mantis.

The hastily-assembled strategy session was convened by Casey Lee, after Ruby Lips confided that a "reliable source" had learned of the P U scheme to lace Tuesday Dormie dinner with a laxative to induce mass diarrhea. Ruby had withheld the identity of the "reliable source," and Casey discreetly did not ask.

Summoned were Royal, Ruby and Eng-ineers Dick Phuncque and Harry Hormone Lennings.

"Dormies can't afford to eat out, so they'll have to take their chances with dorm food, poisoned or not," Casey said. "I'm worried about the capacity of our sewer lines and how we should respond."

"The Dooch sewer lines should be ok," Harry Hormone said. "They were designed to accommodate simultaneous flushings; but, if all 32-toilets were flushed continuously, over a long period of time, say for 30-minutes, there could be a back-up problem."

Harry Hormone Lennings was short and round, with a pimply face, topped with short-cropped light brown hair. He wore thick glasses and carried a slide rule on his belt like a sword. Hormone was the only Dormie Eng-ineer working on a degree in Sanitation Engineering. He had earned the nickname, Hormone, because of his habit of analogizing human events to the secretion of hormones.

"If the University had known what our dietician serves, it would have built a stronger system." Royal said. "We've had Beef Barf-aroni, Rubber Chicken, Petrified Lasagna, Mystery Meat; and, in honor of the holidays, 1000-year-old Turkey that could rupture any sewer system."

"Don't forget Halibut from Hell," Casey added.

"How much worse can dorm food get?" Phuncque said. "We've developed cast iron stomachs. Maybe a laxative would give dorm food some flavor."

"The point is," Royal said, "if those P U ass holes are going to great lengths to make us sick, we should return the favor. They've got to learn that for every unsavory P U action, there will be an equally unsavory Dormie response. Turning a cheek or in this case, flushing a toilet - is not going to stop Dirk, the Turd, from venting his spleen on us."

"Agreed," Ruby said. "But what should we do?"

"Hormone," Casey said, "Let's take a look at your map."

Kneeling, Hormone spread a 8-by 6-foot flowchart on the floor.

"Thin lines trace each Dooch toilet to the sewer below Channing Way," Hormone said. "From Channing, the sewer joins other lines to the sewage treatment plant in west Berkeley."

"What would happen if the Channing sewer were blocked?" Royal asked, a smile spreading across his face.

"Gravity would prevent it from backing up, all the way to the Dooch toilets," Dick Phuncque said. "Dooch's first floor is 15-feet above ground level, and each floor above is 8-feet tall."

"True," Hormone said, examining the sewer map. "Effluent would seek a new path, one with less resistance, meaning, if it couldn't make it into the Channing sewer, it would flow in a different direction."

"Which direction?" Casey said, suddenly understanding Royal's tack.

Pointing to the map, Hormone said, "There is a sewer line from the P U house to the Channing sewer line."

"Is the waterfall in the P U patio hooked up to that sewer line?" Royal asked.

"Sure," Hormone said, "directly to that sewer line."

"So, if the Channing sewer were blocked," Ruby said, "the backup would flow toward the P U house?"

Hormone nodded.

"What would cause the Channing sewer to be blocked?" Royal asked.

"Hmm. Other than some physical obstruction . . ."Hormone said, "increasing the rate of flow into the Channing sewer would do it."

"How could that happen?" Casey said.

"Interesting," Hormone said, scratching his chin. "According to the map, there is a knob controlling the rate of flow into the Channing sewer located under the kitchen in the dorm dining hall." Hormone paused, deep in thought. "If the control were turned to maximum, and all 32-Dooch heads were flushed continuously, say for 20-minutes, the sewer would be overwhelmed and cause a backup toward the P U house."

"Would it back up all the way into the P U waterfall?" Casey asked.

"Sure, the waterfall is only six feet tall," Hormone said.

"You are a sewer genius, Hormone," Royal said.

"For academic reasons, I'd like the privilege of turning the control knob to maximum," Hormone said, a serious look on his face. "The result would be like the triggering massive secretions of hormones from all the glands!"

"The pleasure is yours, Hormone," Royal said.

"A shitty Eng-ineering feat I'm going to enjoy," Phuncque said.

"We need a name for this RF," Casey said.

"How about Flush-Your-Blues-Away RF?" Royal responded.

Slithering, slathering slime. Putrefying, polluting poop. Oozing, oscillating offal.

Sludge from the back up of the Channing sewer spewed from the P U waterfall as a trickle, engorging into a stream, then gushing as a tidal wave, pushing past a patio door, engulfing the wood-paneled living room with dark, foul muck, flooding the fireplace, leeching into the bowels of the Seeburg KD200 Select-O-Matic.

Inside the House of Beauty, an incessant knocking aroused Kate Howell and Joan Dildeaux from deep slumber.

"Kate! Dil-dee! Wake up!" Muffy Peachwick shouted.

Cracking open the door, Joan eyed Muffy sleepily. "This better be good, Muffy-kins. What the hell's going on?"

"You girls must be out of it. Can't you smell it?"

Clearing her nostrils, Joan inhaled deeply, ingesting a noxious scent that jolted her awake. "Whew! What is that?"

Behind Joan, Kate sniff, sniff, sniffed, then recoiled, pinching her nostrils with her fingers. "Whew! Where is it coming from?"

The trio, dressed in pajamas, tiptoed to the window overlooking Channing Way. From the third floor of the Gee Dee House, everything looked normal.

"Let's get a little air," Joan said, pushing open a window.

"Yuck, it's worse outside," Muffy said, placing the crook of her elbow against her nose.

"Look! Over there!" Kate said, pointing toward the P U patio.

Despite the darkness, the three could see black muck plopping from the P U waterfall, spreading across the patio, pushing into the living room.

"I'll call police and fire," Joan said.

"I'll phone the P U night line," Kate said. "Someone's got to be up."

"Or dead from stink inhalation," Muffy added.

The headline of the *Daily Californian* blared:

"P U Stink!"

The article attributed the sewer flooding of the P U house to an unfortunate "act of God." A Berkeley Public Works inspection found "no defects or problems with the sewer system."

The next day, Jefferson Warring and the P U pledges wearing surgical masks, stood knee-deep in sludge, shoveling crappy flotsam, into a dumpster. Across the street, Dick Phunque and Harry Hormone unfurled a banner from Dooch's seventh floor balcony emblazoned with the childhood slogan Jonathan Aldon had coined:

"Shit Flies Both Ways!"

28

CUBAN JACK

The mammoth wooden hands of the Campanile's four clocks groaned forward to the Roman numeral VI.

1:30 p.m.

Jonathan stepped out of the elevator, stopped, puzzled by the plume of thick, pungent cigar smoke snaking from the Campanile offices.

Miss Burdick will not be happy, he thought.

As chime mistress, Miss Burdick supervised the operation of the Campanile with a kindly, but firm hand. For over 40-years, her rules were the Campanile's rules, and smoking anywhere within the bell tower was not permitted.

Jonathan had finished his daily cleaning of the playing cabin of the belfry and had planned to spend the next two hours studying in the quiet sitting room of the Campanile's library.

Who's here? Only dignitaries are allowed, Jonathan thought, as he entered the sumptuously appointed sitting room.

The walls were ringed with rows of black and white photographs of famous people who had toured Miss Burdick's domain - every President from Teddy Roosevelt to Ike Eisenhower, members of world royalty, and celebrities - all frozen in polite, cultured smiles, next to the diminutive, silver-haired woman who had dedicated her life to the Campanile.

The source of the cigar smoke sat in an easy chair facing the western window that afforded a view of the Bay and the Golden Gate.

Jonathan rapped gently on the door. A handsome man with a full head of dark, chestnut hair struggled to stand. He wore a button-down white shirt, with a loosened rep tie. His jacket covered the stack of daily newspapers on the redwood coffee table.

"You must be Jonathan," the man said, extending his hand in a firm handshake. "I'm Jack," he said.

The stranger's voice was slightly strident with an accent Jonathan could not place. "Miss Burdick said you were due any minute. What a lovely place for peace and solitude."

Jack beamed a smile that made Jonathan forget the cigar smoke.

"Miss Burdick is giving my brother a tour of some of your ancient dinosaur bones. I understand the Campanile's got one of the largest collections in the world. Hope you don't mind my intrusion."

"No, sir," Jonathan said, noticing the outline of a corset beneath the dress shirt. "Please sit down, sir. Every visitor of Miss Burdick is a special guest of the Campanile."

"Thank you, son. Please join me," Jack said, easing himself into the leather chair. "Back acts up now and then. Old war wounds seem to have a mind of their own."

Seating himself next to Jack, Jonathan noted the piercing gaze of eyes that seemed to read his mind.

"Miss Burdick is especially fond of you," Jack said, in that curious accent. "She told me you're a bright, charming student."

"The truth, sir," Jonathan said, avoiding Jack's gaze, "is I may flunk out by the end of the semester."

"Grades aren't everything," Jack said, taking a long, deliberate drag of the cigar. "My brothers and I all went to Harvard where it's almost impossible to flunk out."

"My father went to Harvard," Jonathan whispered.

"Your dad would understand," Jack winked. "My brothers and I were average students. We were always distracted by sports, women, and parties. In fact, my baby brother partied so much he had to drop out and finish at a public university."

Jonathan warmed to Jack's directness.

"Jonathan, one of the great things about Cal, is it gives everyone, rich or poor, a chance for a quality university education. Harvard will never admit anyone but blue bloods and the filthy rich."

"Which were you?" Jonathan said. "Blue blood or filthy rich?"

"My family's more filth than blue blood." Jack said, handing a cigar to Jonathan. "Try one, real Cuban."

Butch had recounted to Jonathan the thrill of smoking a real Cuban cigar his uncle had given him on his 16th birthday.

"I thought Cubans were illegal," Jonathan said.

"They are now, but these are pre-Castro Cubans. I've got a humidor closet full of them." Jack produced a cutter and snipped the end of the cigar. "This is an authentic Naifyez-Weldez Cuban. Jaime Naifyez and Juan Weldez were great cigar makers until that bastard Castro confiscated their business. Be a sport, try it."

"Sure, why not," Jonathan said, accepting the slender, dark smoke.

"Lick the wrapper first," Jack said, striking a match, placing the flame beneath the cigar."

"Draw slowly, Jonathan. Let the flame jump to meet the Cuban."

Jonathan followed Jack's instructions, holding the cigar with both hands, puffing greedily.

"Whoa, slow down, Jonathan," Jack chuckled, waiving away clouds of gray smoke. "Take it easy. No need to imitate a speeding train."

Jonathan felt his face flush. After a few puffs, he felt lightheaded. His lungs, first irritated, were now relaxed, as he leisurely drew smoke.

"What brings you to Cal, sir," Jonathan said.

"Call me Jack."

"Sure, eh . . . Jack," Jonathan said, now filled with an unexplained sense of euphoria.

"Garrick Nelquist is an old Navy buddy of mine. He asked me to give a little talk at Wheeler Auditorium at 2 p.m., as a guest of the Political Science Department. Would you like to come?"

"Love to," Jonathan said, puffing smoke toward the ceiling, "but I've got to study. The thought of going back to Iowa is depressing."

"Iowa?" Jack said, chewing on the end of his Cuban. "My colleague, Bourke Hickenlooper, is from Iowa."

"What a small world," Jonathan said. "My father was Cerro Gordo County Chairman for Senator Hickenlooper's re-election campaign."

"A good man," Jack said, hissing smoke, ". . . for a Republican."

"What's the topic of your talk?" Jonathan said.

Jack appeared startled by the question. "The usual political bull shit that's thrown around as an election year approaches."

"Yes, the usual, political bull shit," Jonathan echoed, now feeling almost drunk from the Cuban.

"What are your plans after graduation," Jack asked. "You'll make it through school. I can feel it."

Jonathan was energized by Jack's sense of confidence.

"I don't know," Jonathan said. "I'm on the outs with my parents, so I won't be returning to their hog farming business."

"Why don't you consider a career abroad, helping people of other countries?" Jack said, relighting the stub of his cigar. "America will be taking a leading role in improving the quality of life of the less fortunate of the world. We'll need dedicated young people to be part of this new global order, this New Frontier of the Sixties."

The lilt of Miss Burdick's laughter announced her return. She was accompanied by a handsome man, younger than Jack, with thick, wavy, dark-brown hair that drooped over his forehead.

"I see Jack's has been leading youth astray again," brother Bobby said, in that same high-pitched accent. "Shame on you, Jack."

"Miss Burdick, thank you for the informative tour," Bobby said, retrieving Jack's jacket, helping his brother into it.

"My immense appreciation for your gracious hospitality," Jack added.

Handing a Brownie Hawkeye camera to Jonathan, Miss Burdick said, "You can do the honors. You boys will be right at home on my wall."

After Jonathan had photographed Miss Burdick with the brothers, each bussed her on the cheek, causing her to flush a beet red.

Shaking Jonathan's hand firmly before the elevator doors of the Campanile clanged shut, Jack said, "Think about a career abroad, Jonathan. The world awaits American public service and dedication."

"I won't wash my face for a week," Miss Burdick said, sounding more like a starry-eyed Cal coed than the matronly, chime mistress.

Extinguishing the butt of the Cuban in a metal waste basket of the sitting room, Jonathan noticed today's *Daily Californian,* sitting on the coffee table, with the headline:

"JOHN F. KENNEDY TO SPEAK AT WHEELER
Senator May Seek 1960 Presidential Nomination"

29

DAOWAGA GHOST

"Bitchin,' it's the most beautiful thing I've ever seen," Waz said.

"Nothing in New York comes close," Butch said.

"There she is gentlemen," Casey said, "what Mark Twain described as the fairest sight in the world."

"Much wider than the Amazon," Living Buddha said.

"Maybe, we can find the water used in Kerrs," Jonathan said. referring to the rare beer, with the cult following, Kerrs, brewed from the water of natural, artesian springs of the area.

Their vehicle had pulled onto a small outcrop, on the side of the winding, two-lane road. Nearby, a sign read,

"Elevation 7328 feet above sea level"

Below, nestled in a thick, blanket of snow, was the jewel of the Sierras: 12-miles wide, 26-miles long, and 72- miles around her shores.

Millions of years ago, creeping glaciers gouged an acorn-shaped abyss between two towering mountain ranges, creating an alpine lake, 5,600 feet above sea level.

Washoe Indians who first visited the area believed the lake sacred and conducted spiritual rituals along its shore giving the lake basin the name, "Da-ow-a-ga," meaning "edge of the lake." In a report to President Zachary Taylor, General John C. Fremont wrote he and scout Kit Carson had discovered the lake on Valentine's day, 1844. Fremont and Carson mispronounced the Washoe name, shortening it to its first two syllables, "Da-ow" which phonetically became "Ta-hoe."

Flanked by the Northern Sierra Nevadas on the west and the Carson Range to the east, Tahoe lies on a north-south boundary, two-thirds of her waters in California, one-third in Nevada. A logical border should have been a straight north-south axis; but, for an inexplicable reason, after traversing three-quarters of the lake, the state line veers 45 degrees southeast, creating a dog leg to its southern shore.

It was the winter break. Casey Lee had invited the out-of-state Dormies - Jonathan, Butch, Waz, and Living Buddha - to join him at his grandmother's Tahoe summer home. Madame Lee had dispatched her stretch limo, and aide, Calphung Quock, to drive the Dormies from Berkeley to the Lake.

Madame Lee's spacious two story, six bedroom, four bath, Alpine house sat on a sprawling meadow, amid groves of quaking aspen and Jeffrey pine, next to Lake Tahoe's placid waters.

For Butch, Waz, and Jonathan, the snow was a reminder of family and home east of the Rockies. For Living Buddha, the white landscape was a wondrous change of pace from steamy jungles of Brazil.

Under Calphung's watchful eye, the Dormies played Frisbee in knee-deep drifts of swirling powder and built snow figures, complete with sex organs, in sexual positions of *flagrante delicto*.

Late one evening, as Jonathan, Butch, and Waz snored before the warmth of the living room fire, Living Buddha said, "Madame Lee must be a remarkable woman. As a child in Shanghai, I was told the poor dirt farmers of Canton were inferior Chinese. Since coming to Cal, I have learned that Cantonese families, like yours, have greatly improved their lives in California; but to own property like this summer house? And to send young employees like Calphung, to British schools in Hong Kong? For a woman to do so?" Living Buddha's face bore a quizzical expression.

As recent as a decade ago, California law allowed Caucasian land owners to insert restrictive covenants in deeds prohibiting the sale of land to "people of the Negroid and Mongolian races."

.   "I dare say, Madame Lee is truly an extraordinary person," Calphung said, "in more ways that you can imagine."

Smiling, Casey nodded in agreement.

If Living Buddha had hoped this would loosen information about the mysterious Madame Lee, his effort failed, as Casey and Calphung turned their attention to stirring the dozing Dormies.

On Christmas day, Calphung orchestrated kitchen labor preparing a traditional turkey dinner with all the trimmings. Fueled by a case of rare Kerrs beer Calphung had procured from a local source, the Dormies competed in noisy, animated rounds of Charades.

Early the next morning, Casey rousted the Dormies, marching the sleepy group through the dark, across the snow-covered meadow, to Madame Lee's dock. There, they boarded a varnished wooden boat - a 1948 Chris Craft Sportsman Runabout - piloted by Homewood local, Ted Grebits, a handsome man, in his 40's, with salt and pepper hair, ruddy complexion, and a meticulously maintained moustache.

Grebits guided the Chris Craft smoothly to the middle of the lake and idled the engine, allowing the boat to bob gently on the watery border between the two states. The wintry air was crisp and still, the stars twinkled, signaling a respite from the series of storms disgorging snow on the Sierra Nevada and Carson Ranges.

Bundled in snow caps and ski jackets, the passengers warmed their hands on steaming mugs of coffee and hot chocolate.

"This better be worth getting up in the middle of the night for," Butch yawned. "Wake me when the sun shows up."

A few minutes later, the first rays of dawn streamed over the rim of the Carson Range, splashing Homewood in pink, canary, orange, and transforming the black waters of Lake Tahoe into a brilliant spectrum of indigo hues.

"Different shades of blue represent different depths of the Lake," Grebits explained, pointing to the smooth glassy water of the Lake now gleaming in various hues of blue: slate, navy, cobalt, lapis, royal, turquoise, azure, and powder. "The deeper the depth, the deeper the blue."

"Tahoe is the second deepest lake in the country, tenth deepest in the world," Grebits said, with a tone of reverence.

"The temperature on the Lake bottom is near freezing." Grebits lowered his voice in a conspiratorial tone. "Scientists have located powerful underwater currents that haven't been fully charted. Now and then, something amazingly well-preserved is fished out of the Lake."

"Like freezer meat?" Butch said, arching an eyebrow.

Grebits nodded. "A fisherman, trolling for Mackinaw, reeled in the body of dead woman."

"How long had she been dead?" Jonathan asked.

"Hard to say," Grebits said, "but her skin was smooth, and she wore clothes of a pioneer from the Gold Rush of 1849."

Jonathan gave a low whistle. "A 100-year old corpse!"

Grebits continued. "Locals believe everyone who disappears in the water is taken, by the underwater currents, to a certain area deep in Lake Tahoe, where their bodies are preserved forever."

"My gawd," Waz said, "an underwater graveyard."

"Maybe that explains why the state line veers to the southeast," Living Buddha said, in his Latin-accented voice. "Nevada didn't want any of the dead popping up on its side of the Lake. Frozen bodies would be bad for casino business!"

"Refill, gentlemen?" Calphung asked, holding a fresh pot of coffee, in one hand and a thermos of hot chocolate, in the other.

"What's the cross?" Butch said, pointing to a snowy, perpendicular indentation on the peak of a tall mountain, on the California side of the Lake, suddenly illuminated by the morning sun.

"That mountain is called Tallac, and the cross is known as the T of Tallac," Grebits said. "The two troughs forming the T are so high, the snow there never melts. Tahoe winters are so cold the Washoe Indians couldn't live here, so they came to Tahoe only in the spring and summer, after the snow melts, like certain flat landers who own property on the Lake." Grebits gently jabbed Casey.

"Better head back before the wind picks up," Casey said, poking Grebits in return. "I'd hate to see your beautiful Chris Craft take a pounding from the waves."

"We might wind up in that underwater grave yard," Waz said.

Turning the Chris Craft around, Grebits aimed it westward toward Homewood. The Hercules engine growled a throaty roar, as the boat skipped across the water at top speed.

"What's that?" Jonathan shouted, pointing to a grey, cotton ball haze, several miles away, skimming effortlessly on the water.

"It's the ghost of the SS Tahoe Steamer," Casey said.

"Ghost, my ass," Butch said, "It looks real to me."

"A rare atmospheric condition that occurs only in winter, not exactly fog, not quite a cloud," Grebits explained.

"What's the Tahoe Steamer?" Waz shouted.

"Look closely," Casey said, handing Waz binoculars. "In the middle of that cloud is an outline of an old boat, the Tahoe Steamer, once known as the Queen of the Lake. Fifty years ago, that boat was Tahoe's only public transportation."

"I think I see it," Waz said. "It's got a black, smoke stack."

"Yes," Living Buddha said, taking a turn with the binoculars. "It's moving fast, rocking from side-to-side."

"Chaps, are you certain it's a mirage?" Calphung said. "I dare say, the SS Tahoe looks quite real."

"It was in the dead of winter of '34," Grebits shouted over the engine's roar, "when the Tahoe Steamer disappeared without a clue. No oil slick, nothing."

"Now, stuffed with stiffs from that underwater graveyard," Butch chuckled, peering through the field glasses.

"Legend has it," Casey added, "the ghost of the Tahoe Steamer reappears, every winter, carrying people on missions of mercy."

"Ghost, optical illusion, mirage, atmospheric phenomenon, whatever you want to call it, there is definitely a boat moving in that cloud," Jonathan said, putting the binoculars down.

Grebits slowed the Chris Craft, allowing the Dormies to watch the floating cloud carrying the ghost of the SS Tahoe Steamer accelerate and disappear into the half-light of the December morning.

30

HURRY, BILLY

"Brrr," E Lyn Chamberlin said, shivering in the alpine air.

Despite the blinding rays of the sun emerging behind the Carson Range, the temperature was freezing.

E Lyn was bundled in a ski outfit she had last worn on a trip to Mammoth with Jani Kay Fong in 1955.

Not the latest for the fashionable ski bunny, E Lyn thought.

She and Sam Paean had left, on such short notice, there was no time to slip into Joseph Magnin's to find new winter wear.

"Wish we could have stayed in and cuddled, Sam."

"To find an eye-tem. . " Sam Paean said, pulling down his Tyrolean hat and turning up the fur collar of his overcoat.

"You gotta sight-em," she finished the sentence for him.

In the months since their romance bloomed, Paean had used the justification to explain every whim; and to her credit, E Lyn had been a helluva good sport, unlike Paean's former wives.

Paean's first wife, a long-stemmed chorine, had considered his column, *"Sam's Paean to The City,"* a royal pain in the ass. The second, daughter of the French Counsel General, dismissed the column as the "grist and ooze of San Francisco Gone." Number three, a young society matron, called his work the "dots and whats of snots" clawing their way up the moneyed slopes of "(S)Nob Hill."

Yesterday, the pair had crossed the barren agricultural counties of Solano, Stanislaus, Yolo, through Paean's hometown, Sacramento - "Sacra-Tomato" - he called it, and braved the snow that fell above

Placerville, formerly known as Hangtown because of the swift justice meted to Gold Rush outlaws. The drive from The City to the Sierras had taken eight hours, the last five with tire chains shackled to Paean's new Caddy, a promotional gift from McDermott Motors. It was 7 p.m. when the Caddy lurched into the darkened driveway of the Tahoe Tavern.

They don't make hotels like this anymore, E Lyn thought, gazing at the four-story, turn-of-the century resort with its rows of dormers, spacious second floor porches, and a tall medieval steeple with a lookout and weather vane.

They were greeted by Dante Pomering, the Tavern's effusive manager, an ex-reporter for the *Sentinel*. With long, white hair and deep, pink complexion, Dante was a dead ringer for Santa.

"Merry Ho-Ho, Sam. Got the place to yourselves," Dante said, lugging their suitcases. "Don't know how long we can hang on. Folks from The City don't come up anymore. Most spend their vacation time on the coast, in Carmel, Monterey, and Santa Cruz."

"There'll always be a loyal following for the Tavern," Paean said, with less than full conviction.

Paean noted the Tahoe Tavern, once the grande dame of Tahoe resorts, was showing her age. Broken wooden shingles dotted the hotel exterior, and the wind whistled dissonantly through cracks of her facade.

The Sixties will be here in a week and the winds of change are also blowing in the Sierras, Paean thought.

After checking them in, Dante gave the couple a tour of the Tavern, replete with a rambling, oral history of her fabled past.

E Lyn marveled at the amenities that had made the Tahoe Tavern the favorite of wealthy San Franciscans between 1901 and 1940 when trains, not autos, were the prevalent mode of transportation.

The wood-beamed main lounge had the quintessential feel of an all-male club with its frayed oriental rugs, cracked, straight-backed leather couches, and creaky, rocking chairs scattered before the eight foot fireplace. A buck's head, with five point antlers, craning above the fireplace hood made the room an inviting refuge from the winter storm.

The Casino Ballroom with its coffered ceilings, angled beams adorned with Chinese lanterns and a polished tongue and groove dance floor, hinted at a grandeur of a bygone era. At the far end of the Ballroom, framed by lattice work, was the stage where touring Big Bands once performed. In a corner, above stacks of wicker chairs, was

an enlarged, black and white photo of a steam ship, a plume billowing
from its smoke stack, with the T of Tallac in the background.

Emblazoned on the ornate picture frame was the inscription:

"SS Tahoe Steamer 1896-1934"

The two had Christmas dinner alone at a table set with linen and
sterling silver. Above, chandeliers fashioned from deer antlers cast a
glow from the distant past. Seated next to a picture window, they
watched snow flakes drift gently through the pine, fir, and cedar trees.
Through the darkness, they could make out white tendrils of icicles -
several stories tall dripping from dormers and overhangs above the
Tavern's long, empty veranda.

Dante had assigned them the Bridal Suite with its room-sized
bathroom and roaring fireplace. Tired from the long drive and sleepy
from copious amounts of cocktails and wine, they had fallen asleep in
each others arms, until the wake-up call from Dante, at the uncivilized
hour of 6 a.m.

Downing cups of coffee, they dressed quickly, then waded through
snow drifts covering the abandoned train tracks that used to haul
members of The City's society to the Tavern, and reached their
destination, the deserted pier, where passengers once boarded the SS.
Tahoe Steamer.

Earlier, E Lyn's investigation had turned up the name of Howard
Muse, as the owner of Grand Designs, Inc., with a post office box
address at Stateline, Nevada. Paean had asked for help from an old
drinking buddy, Billy Hurry, owner of the popular casino, "Hurry's,"
on the Nevada side of the Lake.

Two days before Christmas, Billy Hurry had left Paean a phone
message with instructions:

"Meet at the old Tahoe Tavern pier
7:30 a.m. on December 26, 1959."

"What are we waiting for?" E Lyn said, rubbing her gloved hands for
additional warmth.

"It should be here momentarily," Paean said.

"What is the 'it' that should be here?" E Lyn said.

"I think I see it now," Paean said, squinting at the Lake.

Shading her eyes with her gloves, E Lyn said, "The only thing I see is a low lying cloud."

"Anything unusual about the cloud?" Paean asked.

"It's moving pretty fast," E Lyn said.

"What else? Do you see a ghost?" Paean said.

"Ghost? A ghost of what, Sam?"

"There's a legend about a ghost ship on the Lake," Paean said.

"Something's in the middle of that cloud!" E Lyn said, "and it's headed right for us."

"Good, then you've answered the question," Paean said.

"A ghost ship? C'mon, Sam be serious."

They edged to the end of the pier, watching the cloud billowing toward them. At a quarter of a mile, E Lyn thought she could distinguish the shape of a smoke stack. At 100-yards, she could see the shape of a narrow hull.

"Sam, do you see what I see?"

"E Lyn, I think I see a ghost."

At 25-yards, the cloud enveloped them in a grey, pea soup, thicker than any San Francisco fog. As the vessel edged up to the pier, a hand waved from the pilot house.

A roped gangway dropped to the pier, and a deck hand dressed in turn-of-the century, naval uniform waved Paean and E Lyn aboard. Above the loud hissing and puffing of the engine, the deck hand shouted, "Step lively, folks! Welcome, aboard."

Alighting gingerly on the narrow, wooden deck, E Lyn looked at a figure in the pilot house, spinning the boat's wheel counter-clockwise, moving the boat away from the pier. Beneath the pilot house window, a circular white, life preserver was emblazoned in red,

"SS Tahoe Steamer"

* * * *

"You really had E Lyn going," Paean said, laughing, chocking on the steaming cup of coffee.

"Ok, so I fell for the ghost story hook, line and sinker," E Lyn said, admiring the wood- paneled walls and polished brass.

They were seated at a round table with a nautical map of Lake Tahoe varnished onto its smooth surface. The comforting warmth from the engines suffused the pilot house. Across from them sat a thin man with clear blue eyes, hawk nose, and pre-maturely silver hair. He wore white pants, a Navy blue, double-breasted jacket, white shoes, and a white sea captain's cap with a shiny, black leather bill. On his lapel was a name tag, *"Capt. Joseph Palming."*

"E Lyn, may I introduce the ghost of Joe Palming, Captain of the SS Tahoe . . . alias Billy Hurry."

"A mighty comely lass, you are," Billy Hurry said, shaking E Lyn's hand. "Welcome aboard the SS. Tahoe Steamer."

"How's the restoration going?" Paean asked.

"Almost done, Sam. Project's been a bit of a pain in the ass."

Billy Hurry explained to E Lyn that, for ten years, he had been secretly constructing a replica of the SS. Tahoe Steamer that had mysteriously disappeared somewhere in Lake Tahoe during a moonless night in the winter of 1934. To discourage gawkers and kibitzers, Hurry had been building the boat, in an indoor facility, on lakeside property, at Cave Rock, near his casino.

"I restore old cars, too; but this boat's my pet project," Hurry said. "I take it out only in winter when the tourists are gone."

"And the floating cloud?' E Lyn said.

"I've created my own little fog machine by using equipment I installed in the bilge that blows dry ice out through special port holes," Hurry explained. "I wanted to keep the lid on the details of the restoration until I was finished. That's how this ghost tale got started. Some of the locals know, but they enjoy putting on the flat landers."

"Tell us about Howard Muse," Paean said, changing to the reason for their Tahoe trip.

"Eccentric, but harmless," Hurry said. "Met him in the casino a decade ago. Dressed like a bum, but he was a high roller throwing piles of money around, drinking my best scotch, and flirting with my prettiest dealers."

"We became friends," Hurry said. "Rode my restored cars around the Lake and discussed the meaning of life. I could tell something was bothering him, some dark secret, something from his past. One day, he told me what was nagging him. From that day on, Muse stopped gambling and drinking and became one of California's most successful, but unknown, business men."

"What secret? What kind of business/" E Lyn said, scribbling in her notebook.

"Can't tell you," Hurry said, shaking his head.

"Why not?" E Lyn said.

"The casino owner's code," Paean explained. "Billy Hurry sees all, knows all about everyone who comes to his casino; but he guarantees anonymity for everyone who gambles at Hurry's."

"So, how are we going to find out about Howard Muse's connection to Grand Designs Inc.?" E Lyn said, closing her notebook.

"You'll have to ask him yourself," Billy winked, motioning the helmsman to slow the boat.

Swiveling in his seat, Billy spun a circular knob."No need for the fog machine here," he said.

"Are we meeting him on shore?" E Lyn said.

"Sort of," Billy said.

"Out on the Lake?" she asked.

"Sort of," Billy said again.

"What are the other choices?" E Lyn said.

"How about an island?" Billy said.

"In the middle of Lake Tahoe?" E Lyn said.

"Let's go topside," Billy said. "I want to show you something unique to the Lake Tahoe."

31

MYSTERIOUS MR. MUSE

Paean, E Lyn, and Billy Hurry stood on the bow of the ghost of the SS Tahoe Steamer, as fog from the dry ice-cloud machine dissipated. The soft plop of snow falling on the Lake's waters echoed above the murmur of the boat's idling engine.

The Tahoe Steamer had entered the narrow opening of a small, narrow bay with waters gleaming a deep blue-green hue. Above, from the crest of a peak a double-tiered waterfall cascaded down to the Lake. At the far end of the bay, in a grove of yellow pines, stood an imposing Scandinavian stone mansion. On a small dock buried under snow, a sign read: *"Closed for the winter."*

"Emerald Bay with its Vikingsholm, Eagle Falls, and island," Hurry said. "Muse will meet you at the Tea House." He pointed to a stone, fort-like structure sitting prominently on the top of the isle. "I'll have you rowed ashore and come back for you in an hour."

"Howard Muse is meeting us there?" E Lyn said, eyeing the steep slope leading up to the Tea House.

"I told you he's a bit eccentric," Hurry said. "But you're the ones who wanted to meet him, so he makes the rules."

They landed on an outcrop where the emerald water had melted the snow. Paean and E Lyn gingerly negotiated the snow-covered, rocky hill single file, one large rock at a time. Half-way up, they saw a figure emerge above the wall of the Tea House. As the pair drew closer, they saw a hatless man dressed in buckskin and knee-length boots with long flowing silver hair and a wispy white beard. As the two reached the summit, the man extended large, calloused hands, pulling first E Lyn, then Paean, into the entry way of the Tea House.

Catching her breath, E Lyn noticed a canoe below, beached on the back side of the island.

Howard Muse was tall, big-boned, with broad shoulders. Paean noted a well-chiseled face beneath the facial hair. Muse studied Paean and E Lyn intently, as he motioned his visitors to sit on large, smooth rocks arranged in a circle. He poured them hot coffee from two thermos bottles.

"Thanks for meeting with us, Mr. Muse," Paean said, making introductions.

There is something familiar about Muse, Paean thought, *but I can't put my finger on it.*

"Hah," Muse grunted. "Thank Billy Hurry. If it were up to me, we wouldn't be talking."

Taking a sip of coffee, Muse said, "Hurry says your word is good, so there's something you'll have to promise, or I leave."

"First, Miss, put your tablet away, you can't take any notes."

Paean nodded, and E Lyn placed the notebook back into the pocket of her ski parka.

"I'll answer all your questions, but listen carefully. You agree not to print any of it," Muse said, directing his deep-set eyes at Paean. "Not a single, printed word, understand?"

"But what's the use of . . .?" E Lyn said.

"I think I do," Paean said. "I promise not to print a word of what you say, but nothing prevents me from using the information, correct?"

Muse broke into a grin. "Paean, you understand me perfectly."

"What is your role in Grand Designs Inc.?" Paean said.

"Money is wired to me," Muse said. "I deposit it in the company account, and the company buys downtown San Francisco real estate."

"Do you know the money is used to buy up pieces of Chinatown for the building of a hideous pyramid, a skyscraper that will leave residents homeless and ruin San Francisco's skyline?" Paean said.

Muse flicked a piece of mud from his boots, and said, "I'm not happy about it; but yes, I know."

"Why don't you just stop?" E Lyn said.

"I can't. It's part of the deal," Muse said.

"What deal?" Paean asked.

"Ten years ago," Muse said, "I was paid a lot of money to disappear but make myself available for special transactions."

"How much is a 'lot of money'? E Lyn asked.

Muse paused, then whispered, "One million dollars."

Paean issued a long, low whistle. "And your patron?"

"My brother," Muse hissed. "I was a weak bastard. I should have said no." Muse slammed a fist on his knee. "Instead, I made a deal with the devil."

"What's wrong with a million bucks just to leave town and run this corporation?" E Lyn said.

"Because family honor, pride, and love should have been more important than any amount money, even a million!" Muse shouted, his face reddening.

Paean thought he detected tears welling in Muse's eyes.

"And your brother is . . .?" E Lyn said, holding her breath.

Muse looked at the pair, hate in his eyes, and slowly spit out the answer. "He's better known as WRC . . . ."

The recognition struck Paean even before Muse spoke his sibling's name. Now, the similarities of the brothers were striking. Both were tall, big-boned, with broad shoulders and the same well-chiseled faces, deep-set eyes, and hair color.

The inescapable truth was that Howard Muse's brother was . . . "William Randolph Chandler," Muse said, closing his eyes, slumping against a rock.

As they spoke, the wind picked up. The brilliant early sunrise had been eclipsed by the thin, advancing clouds of the next storm.

Howard Muse told his story.

The San Francisco Gazette had been founded by Walter Chandler, who amassed a fortune in the Nevada logging business and moved to San Francisco where he founded the newspaper. My mom, Jenn K. Ogens, had been a young secretary at the Gazette when she caught the eye of Walter Chandler.

\Mom became Walter's girlfriend, naively believing he would divorce his wife and marry her. There were endless reasons why Walter couldn't divorce He could not leave while his son - William Randolph Chandler - was a child. His wife would not consent. He would lose the Gazette in a divorce.

Over time, Mom accepted her station, especially after I was born. Not wishing social embarrassment to Walter Chandler, Mom gave me her middle name, as a surname, and told me my father had died in an accident before I was born.

Walter Chandler supported both families - the one ensconced on Nob Hill and the secret one leading a quiet existence in the Peninsula neighborhood of Burlingame.

Walter sent my half-brother, WRC, to Stanford; and me to Cal. When Walter Chandler died in 1940, WRC was 19, I was 18. WRC knew all about me, but I didn't know about him until later.

In 1950, Mom became seriously ill and, believing she would soon die, she revealed the identities of my real father and half-brother. It was at that time WRC, with an eye toward future public office, promised to pay all of mom's medical costs for life - with an annual visit by me - and pay me one million dollars to leave The City and to never acknowledge my relationship to the Chandlers.

I was the one who said 'yes,' but I was so worried about Mom's health, I didn't have the guts to turn WRC down."

"Wow!" E Lyn gasped

Paean was stunned by the revelation. "Why did you decide to come to Tahoe?" he asked.

"A natural decision," Muse said sarcastically. "The Chandlers made their fortune raping the forests of the Carson Range. When I accepted WRC's money, I felt   stripped of my dignity - like the Carson Range stripped of its trees."

"That's when you met Billy Hurry?" Paean said.

"I met Billy during a time I tried to throw the blood money away, drinking and gambling," Muse said.

"And the name, Muse?" E Lyn said.

"When Billy talked me out of my vices, we spent countless hours throwing around ideas of how Billy could turn his little casino into a world class operation rivaling anything in Vegas," Muse said.

"You became his muse?" Paean asked.

"That's how I came by my name," Muse said, smiling.

"Billy said you are a successful, but unknown, business man," E Lyn said. "What do you do?"

"This is where I get a small measure of revenge against my half-brother, WRC," Muse said. "I've always loved beer but never found any American brands that suited my taste, so Billy talked me into setting up my own little brewery producing small quantities of my own premium brand. Amazingly, the beer has developed a cult status among beer drinkers, especially college students."

"And the revenge . . ." Paean said.

"The beer is named after my mother's middle name. The K In Jenn K. Ogens stands for Kerr," Muse said. "I own the Kerrs Beer Co.."

Damn it, Paean thought *I can't report this scoop!*

"My brother knows I'm behind Kerrs, and it pisses him off to no end," Muse said. "Every time there is a favorable mention in the news, at a bar, in polite company, WRC must roil, knowing that his bribe is perpetuating my mom's name."

"Where do you brew Kerrs?" Paean said.

"That's one of the reasons Kerrs is hard to find. I can't brew many cases at my secret, *au naturale* site."

"Where . . .? You know my lips are sealed." Paean said.

"Here's where Billy Hurry really helped me out," Muse said. "As a kid, Billy found a secret cave, up there, behind Eagle Falls, large enough for me to crank out 10,000 cases a year."

"So, when a Kerrs label says '*Great water makes great beer*,' you're not kidding?" E Lyn said.

"It's absolutely the water," Muse said proudly, pointing up to the double tiered falls above Emerald Bay. "The same water flowing from Eagle Falls into Emerald Bay."

The frustration of learning Howard Muse's secret weighed heavily on Paean. He was bound by his promise not to *print* a word of it. But Muse also agreed that he could somehow *use* the information. But how?

Muse sensed Paean's dilemma.

"There's not a damn thing you can do about it, Paean," Muse sighed. "Everything Grand Designs Inc does is perfectly legal. You can protest to high heavens against the pyramid; that it will ruin The City's skyline; that it's going to displace the poor of Chinatown; but it's going to be built. When it's completed, WRC plans to move his newspaper into the building and call it "Chandler's Great Pyramid of News.""

"As influential as you are," Muse said, "you can't stop it. There are many who will welcome the tallest skyscraper west of Chicago. Your opposition is doomed, Paean."

Paean was overwhelmed by Muse's simple logic. *"Sam's Paean to The City"* had been the arbiter of good taste for so long, Paean had taken for granted that any cause he trumpeted would prevail in the court of public opinion.

Muse was right. The newly arrived, the nouveau riche of The City, would rally around a modern, colossal building whose size alone would be a tasteless symbol of "world class" status.

The thought of William Randolph Chandler putting his stamp on The City's skyline made Paean nauseous; but the possibility that the state's political landscape would also be altered by Chandler, as Governor of California, was too much for Paean to stomach.

Something had to be done to stop Chandler. But what?

32

KISS OF LADY LUCK

"Ka-Chung! Ping-ping-ping-ping!
Ka-Chung! Ping-ping-ping-ping!"

The tinny cacophony of small spinning reels of chance rang incessantly like unanswered phone calls. A grey pall of tobacco smoke drifted above like an inclement weather front. Below, scantily clad cocktail waitresses, in push-up bras and spike heels, winked "thank you's" for "tokes," or tips. Pit bosses pretending to be working, ogled a long line to the Ladies Room. Nearby, at the postage-size, cabaret bar, a Dean Martin impersonator warbled *"Volare."*

New Year's Eve at Billy Hurry's Stateline Casino was Halloween, Mardi Gras, St. Patrick's Day, and April Fool's Day all rolled into one.

At the craps tables, stick men barked,

"Nina, Field, Nine! Who wants the hard ways?
Back up on the C and E? We need a shooter!"

Dentyne-gnawing, peroxide blondes, in strapless evening gowns, cheered on stogie-chomping cowboys, in Stetson hats, throwing chips indiscriminately onto the green felt craps tables.

At Blackjack tables, dealers cajoled,

"Gonna sit on those pair of 8's? Split 'em?
Show some guts, Lady! Double down!"

Sen-Sen sucking society matrons, awaiting final Nevada divorce decrees, waved foot-long cigarette holders like magic wands and pondered wagering decisions.

At the roulette table, the croupier intoned,

> *"Round and round the wheel goes,*
> *where she stops nobody knows!"*

Ski bums with wind-burned faces and white-ringed racoon eyes, nursing long neck bottles of beer, scattered chips on the numbers of chance, as the white ball jumped in and out of the spokes of the wheel.

10:30 p.m.

A black stretch limo edged up to the entrance to Hurry's Casino and discharged its well-dressed passengers. Exiting, the five men smoothed their coats and straightened their ties

Huddling the group, Casey Lee whispered, "We've practiced all week; so keep cool. Let's win a pile of money for Hunch!"

Earlier, the plot had been hatched at an after-dinner bull session at Madame Lee's summer home, inspired by another case of rare Kerrs beer provided by Calphung Quock.

"How much dough do you think it'll take for Hunch to be elected Campus Snow King?" Waz said, punching a hole in a can of Kerrs with a triangle-shaped "church key."

"We got a nice head start with the $500 reward for returning Oski's head," Casey said, "but the P U's will come up with money to offset our lead. I think it'll take another $1,500. That's $2,000 total."

Butch whistled. "$1,500 bucks is room and board for a two Dormies for a semester."

"My Oakland cousin's band will donate all their proceeds to Hunch," Jonathan said, referring to the concert Big Berry and the Blackouts had agreed to perform.

"That's another $250 ," Casey said.

"Suzette Mew Mew's autograph signing should bring about that much too," Butch said, "even, if we give half to the Campus Crusade for Cats. "

"Need another $1,250," Casey said.

"$250 from hot dog feeds, raffles, and car washes," Living Buddha said.

"Kate said the Gee Dees have 'something special' planned that may raise another few hundred bucks," Casey said.

"Leaving us about $750 short," Waz sighed.

"Only $650 short, chaps, " Calphung said, dropping a $100 bill on the coffee table. "Let's call this a donation from Madame Lee. She gave me this for any 'emergencies.' "

"The last $650's gonna be a bear to raise," Waz said.

"I've got a sporting proposition," Calphung said, draining the last of a Kerrs. "Since you weren't counting on Madame Lee's $100 anyway, why don't we go to Billy Hurry's and convert that $100 into the $750 you need."

"Gambling?" Jonathan said.

"Why not?" Casey said. "If we lose, we're not any worse off."

"But how can we beat the casino?" Waz said.

"If we practice, we can win at Blackjack," Living Buddha said. "Tahoe casinos use only a single deck, and I can keep track of all the cards dealt. If we're patient, we can increase our chances of winning as much as five percent."

During the next few days, Living Buddha taught the Dormies the Portuguese words for numbers 0 to 20 to designate the number of 10's and aces left in the deck. He also demonstrated a series of silent signals: touching his nose, clearing his throat, and blinking.

"What about the other games?" Butch said. "We shouldn't put all our casino eggs into one basket."

"I think we can make money at casino craps," Jonathan said, remembering his Uncle Mike's story of how Grandfather Miles Aldon had used the profits from the dice game to start Aldon Farms. "If Living Buddha hypnotizes me, I think my subconscious memory will tell us how to bet."

Between Christmas and New Year's, the Dormies remained inside, practicing Blackjack and throwing dice on the floor before the roaring fireplace.

Using his diamond pendulum, Living Buddha hypnotized Jonathan, gently sending the freshman into his subconscious to retrieve details of the story Uncle Mike had related about the secrets of shooting craps.

Slowly, details of craps betting strategies surfaced in Jonathan's subconscious. Winning on 6 and 8 paid 7 to 6; 5 and 9 paid 7 to 5; and 4 and 10 paid 9 to 5. 7 was a losing number, except on the first roll of a series, during which both 7 and 11 were winners.

Casey had doled out a $20 stake to each Dormie from Madame Lee's "emergency" money." At a minimum bet of a dollar, the Dormies should last at least two hours before the casino odds would take its toll, unless the Dormies caught a lucky streak."

Calphung, the only one of legal age, would roam, table-to-table, picking up winnings and placing them in a burlap sack. To avoid casino security, the Dormies donned disguises.

The quintet entered Hurry's Casino in their new hirsute looks: Casey with a Groucho Marx; Jonathan in a blond Vandyke and Buddy Holly's glasses; Butch with a full Smith Brothers cough drop beard; Waz in a waxed handle-bar moustache; and Living Buddha in a wispy Foo Manchu.

They paused a hallway, glancing at the "Celebrity Wall of Fame," filled with photos of Billy Hurry and famous guests. Nearby, a photographer flashed a picture of the casino owner posing with a couple. The woman, E Lyn Chamberlin, recognized the bearded Dormies and elbowed Sam Paean.

Approaching the new arrivals, Paean said, "Billy, may I introduce some famous San Francisco Beatniks," directing Hurry's attention to the bearded five.

"How about a picture of the North Beach Five for your 'Celebrity Wall of Fame?'" Paean asked, winking at the Dormies.

"Why not," Billy said, extending his hand. "Welcome to Hurry's. Quite an honor. We've never had real Beats here before."

"Carlos Marx ," Casey said, extending his hand.

"John, the Baptist-poet," Jonathan said, grinning.

"Wadsworth Wazinski," Waz said, bowing.

"Butch-ero Smith," Butch said, nodding.

"Simon Boulevard," Living Buddha said, in his Latin accent.

Surrounding Billy Hurry, the "North Beach Five" said, "cheese" to the photographer.

A security guard appeared and whispered in Hurry's ear.

"Excuse me, gentlemen. Gotta say hi to a high roller. I'll send Paean copies of the photo. Good luck and Happy New Year!"

"Happy New Year," the Dormies echoed.

Paean broke into a broad smile.

"I think your disguises will work, guys; but please don't get arrested.

I don't have money to post bail!"

E Lyn blew them a kiss, as she and Paean hailed a cab for the drive back to the Tahoe Tavern.

11 p.m.

Betting conservatively, the Dormies had made $30 playing Blackjack. Living Buddha's photographic memory of the cards dealt was the difference, as he signaled Butch - speaking Portuguese and tapping his nose, coughing, and blinking - from his position at "third base," the last seat, next to the dealer. Meanwhile, at the craps table, the action had been "choppy," with an equal number of wins and losses. Jonathan's betting scheme was keeping Waz and Casey even.

Above the clouds of cigarette smoke, Lady Luck suddenly smiled on the Blackjack table. A new dealer had been rotated in, a beautiful brunette, with a dynamite smile, wearing the name tag: *Kandace Kaltwell.*

For the next 20-minutes, Living Buddha and Butch could not lose. Kandace dealt them several consecutive hands of 20 with a few "blackjacks" for good measure. When hands were crummy, their decisions were correct. When they asked for a card, "a hit," they drew small cards bringing their totals closer to 21 than Kandace. When cards were bad and they declined a card and stood, Kandace obliged by "busting," going over twenty-one. When Calphung signaled "let's go," Living Buddha and Butch each left Kandace a generous $5 tip.

The total in Calphung's burlap sack was $200!

Picking their way through the throng, Butch and Living Buddha heard a roar. Following the noise, they approached a craps table where Waz and Casey jumped for joy, as Jonathan methodically stacked chips in racks before them.

Waz had the dice; and, after each throw, Jonathan scooped up winning chips. The pit boss nodded and a bosomy cocktail waitress delivered complimentary glasses of beer for the Dormie craps players.

"Don't get distracted," Living Buddha said.

"Forget the booze, just shoot!" Butch shouted.

Neither admonition could be heard over the shouting and clapping of a crowd that was now ten deep around the table. Waz and Casey each chugged half their beers, as Jonathan inventoried winning chips.

As the dealers paid off other players, Calphung appeared at Jonathan's side, and emptied several trays of chips into the burlap sack.

"You blokes have your $750," Calphung said. "I'll lock the cash up in the limo," he said, disappearing into the crowd.

The cocktail waitress appeared with another round of beers for the Dormies. Lady Luck continued to smile, as Waz hit number after number. Sevens materialized only at the start of a series and disappeared until the start of a new series. In between 7's, Waz repeatedly hit all the numbers Jonathan had placed bets on: 6, 8, 5, 9, 4, and 10.

Emboldened by the beer and the lucky streak, Jonathan let the bets double up. Instead of picking up profits, Jonathan now joined the Dormies in chugging and cheering, as the stacks of chips on the green felt table grew.

The noise was deafening. Bets from unseen bettors flew through the air, bouncing amid the towers of chips. Two additional pit bosses appeared, joining the beleaguered dice boss in officiating the identities and amounts of the myriad of bets on the table. The Dormies shared their beers with Butch and Living Buddha, as the cocktail waitress brought a third round of drinks.

"Whoo-eey!" Butch shouted. From the original $1.50 bet on 4, 5, 6, 8, 9, and 10, he now counted $120 on 6 and 8; $100 on 5 and 9; and $100 on 4 and 10.

Waz hit 4, then a 6, a 10, another 6, then a 5, as Jonathan continued to increase the stacks of chips on the numbers.

"Over a $1,000 bucks on the table!" Butch shouted, hugging Living Buddha and Casey. "C'mon, Waz, roll those bones!"

There was a sudden hush, as Waz flicked the dice. Miraculously, a die landed squarely on top of a stack of chips, as the other die bounced off the table.

"Too tall, no call!" the croupier yelled.

"Bad luck," one bettor moaned.

"Same dice! Same dice!" the crowd roared.

"Same ones," Waz echoed, taking another swig of beer.

Each of the three pit bosses examined the dice before the stick man, using a curved, bamboo stick, pushed the lucky dice back to Waz. The pit bosses whispered among themselves and suddenly pointed at Jonathan. One pit boss motioned to unseen persons in the crowd.

Waz picked up the dice gently, blew on them, as the crowd regained its noisy intensity. As he raised his hand to toss the dice, beefy, uniformed security officers appeared at the pit bosses' side and shouted, "this game is suspended!"

A security officer pointing at Jonathan, said, in a firm, defiant voice, "You boys are under arrest for gambling under age!"

The stunned crowd turned toward Jonathan.

From above, Lady Luck was now weeping.

Chugging the free beers had loosened the glue on Jonathan's chin. His Vandyke beard was floating in beer foam!

"B-O-O-O'S" filled the air, as security officers muscled their way through the crowd, ripped off the Dormie disguises and snapped handcuffs on Jonathan, Casey, Waz, Butch, and Living Buddha.

As security led the Dormies away, the crowd applauded loudly and yelled, "nice hand, boys," and "pick on someone your own age."

Relieved, the pit bosses swept the mountain range of bets off the table. Balloons descended through the smoky clouds, as the Dean Martin imitator sang, *"Auld Lang Syne."* Male gamblers hugged and kissed every female in sight while dealers yawned.

At a distance, Calphung Quock had witnessed the turn of fortune.

My goodness! The situation has gotten rather sticky!

33

FLYING THE COOP

"Never entertained celebrities before," Will Bartone, said, clanging the creaky, cell door shut.

Bartone had been Sheriff of Zephyr Cove for 20 years and before that, deputy for ten. He was 61-years-old, with a ruddy complexion and short-cropped silver hair. On the tip of his broad nose was perched a pair of reading glasses.

To commemorate New Year's Eve, Bartone wore his formal law and order outfit: a starched white shirt, brown vest with his sheriff's badge, a black string tie, and well-shined cowboy boots. An ancient Colt 45 and holster were strapped to the side of his protruding gut. On the wall hung a white cowboy hat.

Guests at the Zephyr Cove Jail were usually out-of-state drivers and casino drunks. In the Stateline area, there was no crime to speak of; and Will Bartone liked it that way - made his job more social, more neighborly. During the day, locals dropped in for friendly gin rummy games, even Billy Hurry, allowing Bartone and the regulars a crack at recouping a few bucks from the owner of Hurry's Casino where locals gambled away their pay checks.

The Zephyr Cove Jail was a wooden shack erected in the late 1800's during the hey day of the lumber industry - a time when Walter Chandler had stripped the Carson Range bare of its virgin timber.

In the 1930's, Bartone's predecessor, Sheriff Timmy McGinnis, had renovated the jail, erecting a shingled facade around the front and sides, so visitors passed through two entrances, the new outer door and the original shack door. The bars of the jail cell were a row of rusted iron rods, seven-feet tall, and the interior three walls were planks of ancient knotty pine.

The jail cell-office of Will Bartone was toasty warmed by a wood-burning stove that emitted an intense heat The pendulum of a clock tick-tocked above Bartone's head. From the antique Victrola, Glenn Miller's orchestra played *"Moonlight Serenade."*

Gawd-All-Mighty, what a strange group of college Joes, Bartone thought, taking stock of his five guests.

A pair of Orientals - one who speaks damned good American, the other who sounds like Cesar Romero.

Two East Coast kids - a big New Yorker with a five o'clock shadow, wearing spats; the other one, skinny with a Jersey accent.

And a clean-cut kid who's a dead ringer for Tab Hunter!

The convicts sat on a chipped wooden bench carved with the names and dates of former prisoners. Jonathan placed Buddy Holly's glasses inside his jacket pocket and shed his jacket.

"Billy Hurry's security said one of you boys held the dice for almost an hour!" Bartone said, looping the key ring over a wooden peg on the wall. "Which of you was the hot shooter?"

Waz raised his hand.

"Wish I'd been there. Might have made a few bucks," Bartone said, squatting on a cracked leather chair, placing his boots on top of the oak desk. "Understand you made 52-straight passes! Imagine, 52-passes! *Tahoe Tribune* will be here tomorrow for an interview and take your picture. You'll be famous, son!"

"What will my folks say?" Waz moaned. "They sent me West for a sheepskin, not a rap sheet."

"Jeez," Butch sighed. "How's this gonna affect my plans for law school?"

"Destiny, Living Buddha said. "An exotic entry in our biographical data."

Jonathan envisioned his face, behind bars, appearing in the *Clear Lake Mirror-Reporter* with the caption,

"Ex-Scion of Aldon Hog Farming Family, A Nevada Criminal!"

"C'mon, boys, relax," Bartone said, in a comforting tone. "Under-age gambling is a misdemeanor. Count yourselves lucky. If you boys had raked in all those chips on the table, you would have been guilty of a felony. As it is, You can pay a fine, and the whole thing's over."

"How much?" Butch said, arching his eyebrow.

"A $100 bucks each," Bartone said. "Tomorrow, after you've been booked, you can call your parents and have them wire the dough by Western Union, and you're free to go."

The phone on the lawman's desk rang.

"Sheriff Bartone, speaking."

Bartone listened intently for several minutes before speaking.

"Calm down, sir." Bartone said. "Lucky's no one's been hurt. You and the Missus are probably in shock. Just sit tight. I can get down to Sand Harbor with a tow truck, in about 30-minutes. Just stay in the car and keep your flashers blinking."

There was a pause as the caller spoke.

"You're welcome, sir, Bartone said. "Wouldn't want you telling the folks back home the Sheriff of Zephyr Cove didn't take good care of our foreign visitors, in your hour of need."

There was another pause.

"And a cherrio pip-pip to you too, sir," Bartone said.

Throwing on his overcoat and grabbing the white cowboy hat, Bartone said, "Damned busy New Year's Eve. English couple ran off the road. Dumb foreigners trying to drive around the Lake, in the middle of the night. Fella sounded like that British actor, David Niven."

Bartone opened the door to the stove and tossed in several dry pieces of wood into the raging inferno.

"This should keep you boys nice and warm until my return," Bartone said, exiting. "Better get some shut eye. Sunrise will be here before you know it."

The Dormies rattled the cell, then stood in silence, faces pressed against the metal bars. The sound of wind whistled through the knotty pine walls above the tick-tock of the wall clock and Glenn Miller's "Moonlight Serenade."

"There's gotta be a way out of here," Waz said, kicking the cell door.

"The lock's old and rusted," Butch said, peering through the ancient key hole. "We should be able to bust right through this piece of shit."

"PSSSST! PSSSST!"

The quintet looked around the cell.

"PSSSST. Can you chaps hear me in there?" said a familiar voice.

"Over here. Behind you chaps, in the corner."

Spinning then crawling, the Dormies found a large knot hole, on the bottom of the wall beneath the bench.

"CALPHUNG, you sneaky son-of-a-gun," Butch said, wiggling an index finger through the hole.

"How did you . . .?" Jonathan said.

"Elementary," Calphung shouted, above the howling wind. "I just called the Sheriff from a 5 cent pay phone and pretended my car went off the road on the Nevada side of the Lake."

"Bitchin' RF," Waz said. "How're you gonna get us out of here?"

"First things first, gentlemen," Calphung said. "You'll have to find a way to disengage the cell lock."

"Got an idea," Casey said. "Who's got a match? We can probably burn through the rusted key hole."

"Wait, I've got something better. I'll be just a moment," Calphung said, crunching his way into the darkness.

"Hurry," Waz shouted.

A few minutes later, a scraping noise announced the arrival of a red, cylindrical object jutting through the knot hole.

"Tally ho, boys," Calphung said.

"A car flare! You're a genius, Calphung," Butch said. "Get that limo revved. We'll be out in a few minutes."

"Gimme that," Waz said, striking the flare, dropping it to the ground. "Don't touch it until the sparks die out."

All five recoiled, as the flare spit a shower of blinding sparks, creating plumes of pungent smoke. They waved their jackets like bull fighters at the fiery, smoky outburst.

"Oh, shit," Butch said, coughing, picking up the remnant of the flare, "the flare's going out. Not hot enough to burn through the key hole."

"Waz, drop your drawers," Casey said, suddenly recalling the Meter Mel's God-given talent.

"Blue Flame Champ!" Jonathan said, nodding in agreement.

"Waz, bend your bare ass close to the cell lock," Butch said.

"Don't know if I can do it in this cold air," Waz said, dropping his pants to his ankles. "I've got goose bumps on my butt."

"Don't choke now," Butch said, gently placing the flare's shrinking flame between Waz's derriere and the cell lock.

"Cut us a mother of a fart," Casey urged.

"I'm trying," Waz said, grunting, wiggling his butt in front of the dying flame.

"Hurry, Waz! It's almost out!" Butch said, placing the end of the flare directly into the keyhole.

"Got one coming," Waz said, in a tortured, grunting whisper.

The Dormies held their breaths, praying for a blast of blue flame.

"We need a giant cut of cheese!" Living Buddha shouted, watching the flare spit its last few sparks.

"PH-O-O-O-O-T," a stream of methane hissed at the flare's last ember, igniting a blue flame engulfing the key hole.

Butch shook the cell door in a rattling embrace. "THERE!" he said, snapping open the door. "Waz, I could kiss you."

"Let's go," Jonathan said, scooping up the jackets from the floor.

"Think I got a hernia," Waz said, slowly pulling up his pants.

"The hell with your hernia, let's get out of here," Butch said.

The five dashed to the inner front door of the jail.

"Locked on the outside," Casey said, jiggling the door.

"Out of my way," Butch said, lowering his shoulder, ramming his 6-foot-5 inch frame into the ancient door, ripping it from its hinges.

"Ah, modern technology," Living Buddha said, clicking open the deadbolt of the outer front door.

Scrambling down the steps of the hoosegow, the jail birds saw the outline of the limousine in a cloud of exhaust.

"Now, that's my idea of a ghost inside a cloud," Waz said, as the group piled into Madame Lee's limousine.

"Carry on, Calphung," Butch said, in a mock British accent.

"With dispatch," Waz said, reaching into his pants pocket.

"I'll never say an unkind thing about the Cantonese again," Living Buddha said, breaking into a grin.

"Cheerio pip-pip, gentlemen," Calphung said, spinning the limousine out of a snow drift

"*For old acquaintance be forgot,*" Butch crooned.

"*And never brought to mind,*" Calphung and Living Buddha, chimed in with their respective accents.

"Here, frosh," Waz said, dropping two cubes into Jonathan's palm. "Souvenirs of the Dormies night at the casino.

"We'll toast a cup of kindness, dear," Waz warbled nasally.

"Wow," Jonathan said, rolling the pair of dice in his hand.

"For Auld Lang Syne," the Dormies sang.

"HAPPY NEW YEAR, 1960!" Butch burped.

Now, I've got two historic items, Jonathan thought, searching the inside pocket of his jacket: *Buddy Holly's glasses and the dice that made 52 straight passes at Hurry's craps game!*

"Oh, no!"Jonathan gasped, a wave of panic washing over him.

Buddy Holly's glasses were gone!

* * * *

Sheriff Will Bartone surveyed the remains of the Zephyr Cove jail.

"Holy shit," he whispered, "I've been duped!"

The front door was ajar, and snow drifts had collected in the alcove. The broken, inner door resembled a beached raft. The cell door was open, with a circular, black heat mark around the key hole. A carpet of dusty, white ashes covered the cell floor.

Then, he noticed it under the wooden bench, dropped in haste when the five boys had flown the coop. Bartone picked up the pair of glasses and dropped them in an envelope marked *"Evidence."*

The locals will never believe this, he thought. *Fifty-two straight passes at Billy Hurry's and the only break out in the history of the Zephyr Cove Jail. And, all I've got to show for this mess is a damned pair of black hornrim glasses!*

Bartone sealed the envelope and tossed it into the bottom drawer of his oak desk and slammed it shut.

Helluva way to start the 1960's, he thought.

34

ART'S REVENGE

"PHOEBE APPLETON RAPED AND MURDERED!"

The *Daily Californian,* front-page headline screamed the shocking, violent crime as students returned from the Christmas-New Year winter break. The gruesome tale included a photograph of a smirking Professor Werner Von Seller standing beside a tall wooden fence, pointing to a sign that read:

> *"By order of the UC Regents:*
> *Future Residence of USC*
> *Teaching Assistants -*
> *Publish or perish program"*

Phoebe Appleton Hall for the Advancement of Female Studies was a circular, three-story, Victorian-Gothic brick and stone building, adorned with tresses of thick ivy, squatting directly east of the Campanile. Donated by one of Cal's early woman benefactor's, The Womb, as she was affectionately called, provided feminine balance to her mate, South Hall, the stately brick and ivy Second Empire style building immediately west of the Campanile. Both had been constructed in 1873 as part of the original group of buildings on the Cal campus.

The couple, Appleton and South, had aged gracefully through the first half of the twentieth century, watching first, the erection of the Campanile in the open space between them; and later, the new generation of buildings sprouting around them, to accommodate a growing student population during the Roaring Twenties.

On this first day of school, January 4, 1960, nothing remained of The Womb - not one brick, not one stone, not one lock of ivy. There was only an eight foot, wooden fence circling the gaping pit where the building once stood.

Angry students and faculty maintained around-the-clock pickets at the site of the unspeakable crime. All Pro produced an evening *KALX Appleton Memorial Show* attended by thousands of students holding a candlelight vigil for the departed spirit of Phoebe Appleton Hall for the Advancement of Female Studies.

From his perch high up in the Cyclotron, Werner Von Seller took a long drag from his sterling silver cigarette holder glowing with the remnant of a Gaulois. Von Seller squinted through his monocle at the flickering pin pricks of lights adjacent to his handiwork.

It had been so easy, Von Seller thought.

His benefactor and ally, WRC and his cronies on the Board of Regents, had passed an emergency directive, permitting Von Seller to

> " . . . *requisition any and all necessary campus facilities and resources for the establishment of suitable housing for the Graduate Student Teaching Assistants hired from 'that great private institution of Higher Learning, the University of Southern California,' to implement the educational program, publish or perish . . . "*

A stroke of genius, Von Seller thought. *What better site to house the USC graduate TA's than the symbol of female intrusion into the male dominated university, Appleton Hall.*

What right did rich widows have in donating campus buildings for the "advancement of female studies?" Female studies? The term was an oxymoron, Von Seller thought.

Let them train to be secretaries, school teachers, and hospital nurses where they belong! Most girls attended Cal to snare a suitable husband, to get an MRS degree. How dare they use a Cal education to compete with men! If girls truly wished to serve mankind, they should ply their God-given talents at Yearning Arms!

During the winter break while students were pursuing frivolous pursuits like skiing and holiday parties, Von Seller had supervised the wrecking balls that laid waste Appleton Hall on Christmas eve.

Merry Christmas, Cal girls! Von Seller had chortled

The radio blared the forlorn lyrics of *"The Big Hurt."*

"That was the plaintive voice of Toni Fisher," All Pro oozed. "Speaking of The Big Hurt, this IS All Pro broadcasting LIVE at the former site of Phoebe Appleton Hall for the Advancement of Female Studies.

"Our next guest is NONE OTHER than the Golden Goddess herself, KATE HOWELL! What are your thoughts about this CAMPUS DISASTER?"

The Golden Goddess, pretty little thing, Von Seller thought. *What vacuous thoughts could this classic example of mindless female pulchritude offer?*

"The women of this campus will NOT tolerate this assault on our dignity," Kate said. "We have THE RIGHT to control the destiny of our education AND our bodies. No amount of misogynism by oppressive, male faculty members, like Professor Werner Von Seller, will deter us from attaining our goals! You can destroy our brick and stone, ivy-covered symbols, but you will NEVER destroy our spirit!"

Choruses of cheers from KALX radio echoed through the Cyclotron.

Von Seller snapped off the radio and lovingly placed an LP on the turntable spindle. He increased the volume to full, as Wagner's *Die Walkure*, suffused the Cyclotron.

Misogynism? Where did Kate Howell learn that two-bit, left-wing word? Wait until the publish or perish TA housing is built and filled with blue-eyed, blond SC men with chiseled jaws and muscular physiques. Kate Howell and Cal girls will be falling over one another trying to get the attention of those handsome SC Trojans. Yes, you will rue criticizing the wisdom of Werner Von Seller!

* * * *

"What do you think about giving Phoebe grey pubic hair?" Muffy Peachwick asked, squinting at the outline of the female nude.

"Muffy-kins, you're so gross," Joan Dildeaux said, applying final touches to her portion of the female anatomy. "I've never seen my grandmother naked. Your guess is as good as mine."

"I sure hope I don't grey when I'm middle-aged," Muffy said. "It might put a damper on my sex life."

From the darkness, a high-pitched female voice giggled. "My Big Sis is s-o-o outrageous," freshman Dandy Cane said.

"Sex, Sex, Sex," Joan said. "Is that the only thing you ever think about. Nobody over the age of 50 has sex. Why are you so concerned?"

"Maybe you're gonna give it up when you're a grandma, Dil-dee, baby," Muffy said, "but I plan on screwing my brains out until they drop me into a pine box."

"Great," Joan said, dabbing the female figure lightly, "you can donate both your brain and vagina to science. I can see your gravestone:

'Here lies one of the world's great lays,'

Mimicking Muffy batting her long eyelashes, Joan said, "or maybe:

'Here lays one of the world's great lies?' "

"Tsk, tsk, girls," Kate Howell said, "let's not get testy until we finish this work of art."

The four Gee Dees stepped behind the bank of flashlights held by two dozen Dormie Eng-ineers, and admired their handiwork. They were dressed as commandos, in black berets, black sweat shirts and black peddle-pushers with black grease paint on their faces.

"Nice work, ladies," Casey Lee said.

"Thanks for the opportunity," Kate said, giving Casey a hug , waving to the tall, thin figure a few paces behind.

"What say, Lizard?" Casey asked.

"Absolutely bitchin'," Lizard said, displaying the lascivious tick that gave Bobby B. Jean his nickname, Lizard - undulating his six inch tongue around the outer edges of his lips.

Boy, these Gee Dees smell great, even in the dark, Lizard thought.

The project had taken shape after Kate complained to Casey she and the Gee Dees wanted to express their anger over the destruction of The Womb. Listening to Kate vent, Casey had conceived the idea of the RF that would be an artistic and political statement.

Who was better qualified to design and supervise this effort than the

Dormies'resident *artiste extraordinaire*, Bobby B. Jean, alias Lizard? The Dormie reptile had attained campus notoriety for his art with his bold decoration of the Dooch tent during the Big C Sirkus, supervising the splashing of Life Saver candy colors: lime, lemon, pineapple, orange, and cheery - onto canvas.

Lizard's great-grandfather, Calois, had been from a family of noted tailors in the old Roman outpost of France, Aix-en-Provence. At age 18, young Calois had joined the rush of Europeans seeking their fortune in the California gold fields. Landing in the small fishing village of San Francisco in 1849, the young gold seeker, in fractured English, gave his name, in the European fashion: surname first, given name second, and middle name last. The Frenchman, *Calois, Jean Bleu*, became the American, *Calois Blue Jean.*

Reaching the gold fields of the Sierra Nevadas, above the bustling river city of Sacramento, young Cal Blue Jean saw the need for clothing strong enough to survive the rigors of gold panning. Utilizing skills gleaned as an apprentice in the family business, Cal fashioned pants from bolts of blue canvas used for making tents. In a stroke of inspired practicality, he fastened pieces of canvas with copper rivets that resisted tearing and ripping. The new pants were an instant hit with miners willing to pay top dollar for the blue pants that gained a reputation for long wear, bearing the name of its young designer: Blue Jean.

When the Sierras had been stripped of gold, Cal Blue Jean moved his thriving business to San Francisco where he built a factory to fill world-wide orders for his now legendary Blue Jeans. The popular pants made Calois Jean Bleu a very wealthy man. Marrying a daughter of the Crocker railroad clan, Cal Blue Jean built a home among the wealthy families who inhabited Pacific Heights. There, three generations of Blue Jeans flourished, renown for their philanthropy and civic involvement.

The Blue Jean family assumed young Bobby would join the business, but Lizard had his own ideas. Art was his true calling.

Yes, he would dutifully obtain a degree from the Cal business school, but he would be an artist, a famous painter.

He had artfully disguised his identity by refusing to join his father's Cal fraternity and dropping Blue from his name, in favor of the initial B. Living in blessed anonymity among the Dormies, Lizard had attained his goal, pursuing art without the burden of the family name.

Now, as Lizard surveyed his artistic masterpiece, an 8 by 30 foot reclining nude, symbolizing the spirit of the departed Phoebe Appleton Hall for the Advancement of Female Studies, he preened.

All great artists craft their careers in this manner, he thought, *with bold, imaginative public statements of art.*

This reclining nude of the Phoebe Appleton was his.

In his stylized view of the famed benefactress, Lizard had outlined Phoebe with voluptuous curves, replacing her silver bun with red tresses flowing over her shoulders. Lizard directed the painting of dark eyes flashing with rebellion and pouty lips hinting of sensual pleasure. In keeping with the spontaneous nature of his use of colors, Lizard had supervised the Gee Dees painting of Phoebe's voluptuous, luxurious body with swirls of lime, lemon, pineapple, orange, and cherry, reflecting the emerging San Francisco style known as psychedelic art.

2 a.m.

The painting had taken four hours to complete. The Dormie Engineers had gladly stood, flashlights-in-hand, the entire time o-g-l-I-n-g and d-r-o-o-l-I-n-g as they watched the quartet from the House of Beauty:

s-t-r-e-t-c-h-i-n-g . . .

b-e-n-d-i-n-g . . .

s-q-u-a-t-t-i-n-g . . .

s-t-o-o-p-i-n-g . . .

w-i-g-g-l-i-n-g . . .

in graceful movements of their artistic exercise.

Lizard strode to his masterpiece and quickly painted, in the foreground, the prone carcass of a dead, black and white penguin with a monocle and silver cigarette holder lying nearby.

Jutting from the flippered mammal's torso was a dagger, an artistic exclamation point, on which Lizard neatly inscribed,

"Art survives the cruelty of science."

35

THE P WORD

The history of Free Speech overlooks an incident that occurred on the Cal campus in early 1960, foreshadowing the tumultuous events of the Berkeley Free Speech Movement of 1965.

It began as a provocative mention in the San Francisco *Sentinel* gossip column, *"Sam's Paean to The City:"*

> *"Only in Berserk-ley: A campus*
> *scandal raised its ugly head*
> *when a quartet of lovelies from*
> *Gamma Delta sorority wrote an*
> *X-rated song, an ode to the male*
> *sex organ, to raise money for*
> *Campus Snow King and Snow*
> *Queen. The naughty title is a P*
> *word. Is it the P word with only*
> *one vowel? Is it the P word with*
> *one vowel used twice? The P*
> *word with two different vowels?*
> *Or the P word with six letters?"*

Paean's juicy eye-tem was followed up by a full-length article in the next day's issue of the *Sentinel*, with the screaming headline:

"CAL CAMPUS GIRDS FOR PRICKLY ISSUE"

"The Berkeley campus is a-dither over the announcement that four members of the Gamma Delta sorority, the Gee Dees, calling themselves the Woody Wood Pecker-ettes, have penned racy lyrics to a tune about the male sex organ. They plan on singing the song at a fund raising event for the Annual Campus Snow King and Snow Queen Contest. (The title of the one word, turgid ditty begins with the letter P and rhymes with the current Number One song in America that begins with the letter V)

The fact that lead singer of the quartet is campus queen, Kate Howell, and that another member is popular coed, Muffy Peachwick, has aroused debate over the propriety of the Pecker-ettes intention to publicly performance of their P word song.

When the news first leaked, the Inter-Fraternity Council denounced the idea as an activity unbecoming of members of a Greek sorority dedicated to "female civility and propriety."

IFC President, Dirk Krum III, declared, "this is BULL ----! Sorority girls should not be diddling with P---- in public!"

When asked for a response to Krum's criticism, a member of the Pecker-ettes (who requested anonymity) called Krum a different five letter P word. (This P word has one vowel and four consonants)

It is rumored that the Gee Dee Morals Committee and MAD (Mothers Advisory Detail) are contemplating suspension of privileges and removal from active status of the offending quartet.

In a prepared statement, Chancellor Haynes said, "This is a classic case of blowing something little into a something big ."

Campus radical, Jericho "Save-The-World Slabio, head of the Guerilla For Free Speech Party, said, "It's about time prim and proper sorority girls discover what 'real' men are all about."

The American Civil Liberties Union (ACLU) intruded itself into the swelling controversy by offering free legal services to protect free and unfettered use of anatomical body parts in music. Said an ACLU staff lawyer, "We will mount stiff opposition against anyone seeking prophylactic legal action against these courageous, young women's quest for free speech and expression."

An informal, noontime poll, taken at Sproul Plaza, yielded the following results, to the question:

'Should the Pecker-ettes be allowed to sing the P word song ?'

200

The Results:

> 20% *Favor*   *(mostly female)*
> 40 % *Oppose*   *(mostly male)*
> 39 % *Undecided*   *(half male/half female)*
> 1% *Didn't know the meaning of the word*

It was noteworthy that Sproul Plaza denizen, Ludwig Von Schwaren, remained curiously silent on the issue.

The singing group intends to charge a dollar admission for its performance, with all proceeds going to their Campus Snow King and Snow Queen contestants: Joan Dildeaux and Hunch Hitowski.

Dildeaux, a member of the singing group, characterized the lyrics as "thoughtful, penetrating." Lead singer, Kate Howell, downplayed the controversy by noting, "the P word is in the dictionary." Muffy Peachwick, said, "the lyrics definitely have a female bent." The fourth member, freshman Dandy Cane, said, "It (the lyrics) should choke every clear thinking girl on campus."

ASUC President Ralph Van de Kamp said the Academic Senate which historically has been an organ of the Greek system will "wrestle with the subject" at its next meeting.

Veteran Senate member, Zeeko Parlo, summed up the collective mind set of the governing body by noting, "There's no real consensus. We're still chewing on it."

The Sentinel will provide coverage of the performance, as well as a critical review of the linguistic use of the P word.

-By Jani Kay Fong - Sentinel Cub Reporter

36

HOLDING COURT

Only at Cal, Butch Tanenbloom thought, surveying the full-house in Harmon Gym.

Butch waved at his roomie, Jonathan, and the Dormies who had turned out for the first team practice of the 1959-60 basketball season.

The noise that began as polite applause, as the varsity basketball players entered single file, suddenly exploded into a thunderous roar, as the deeply tanned, debonair-looking, silver-haired man dressed in a herring bone sports jacket, emerged from the bowels of venerable Harmon Gym.

At 50 years old, Pete Mewell was already a coaching legend: a winning record of 80% with basketball talent a rival coach charitably described as "a bunch of slow white boys," whom Cal fans affectionately called "Mewell's Mules."

Pete Mewell sauntered to center court, basking in the adulation of an appreciative student body. Adjusting the podium microphone, Mewell said, jovially, "Written notes will be dispensed with today."

The crowd responded with foot-stomping that triggered a tsunami of vibrations rippling through the ancient, wooden bleachers.

Jeez, Butch thought, *where else would students turn out to hear a basketball coach's pep talk?*

Butch Tanenbloom had been a *Parade Magazine* first team, high school, All-American. At 6- foot-5 inches tall, Butch was stronger than most guards and quicker than most forwards. With his versatility, Butch could play point guard, shooting guard, small forward, and power forward. At his Brooklyn high school, he had even played some games at center.

Butch had been heavily recruited by all the major basketball powerhouses: U Conn, Cincy, Duke, Ohio State, and UCLA, but when he arrived for his Cal campus visit, he had been enchanted with the eclectic, electric campus atmosphere and the temperate weather that made his native Flatbush seem like the South Pole. Standing in the Botanical Garden above the Big C, gazing across the magnificent view of San Francisco Bay, he had proclaimed, *"California, here I come."*

Coach Mewell addressed his team, but for the students in attendance, he was speaking to them.

"Gentlemen, welcome to Cal basketball. We must never lose sight of the most important reason we are here, to receive a quality education," Coach Mewell began. "We are student-athletes - students first, athletes second.

"Our top priority is to do well academically and graduate. We cannot play basketball forever, but we can reap the benefits of a Cal education throughout the rest of our lives.

"My colleague, Professor Aristotle Scott, also Coach Scott of the Cal track coach, is renowned for his philosophical teachings of A Higher Truth. Basketball teaches us higher truths we can put to use in our lives.

"First, the only control we have in life is the quality of our effort, every waking moment of the day. Secondly, there is no substitute for self-discipline. Thirdly, basketball is a team sport. There is no room for "I" in T-E-A-M.

"Gentlemen, we are neither the most gifted, nor the most talented ball players, although a certain freshman brings a rather impressive scrapbook of press clippings."

For one of the few times in his life, Butch blushed.

"I assure you, we will assemble a very competitive squad," Coach Mewell said. "We will accomplish this by playing disciplined, team basketball. We will learn that by working as parts of a greater whole, we will defeat many teams who have far superior, individual skills. If nothing else, we will learn to play unselfishly, to value the common good, rather than individual glory.

"As a member of this team, we will be expected to hustle, to give 110% effort at all times. We will contest every shot. We will dive for every loose ball. We will fight for every rebound. Most importantly, we will defend every inch of the floor with all the energy our bodies, hearts, and minds can muster."

"On offense, we will make taller teams come out from under the basket. When they do, we will use single, double, and triple picks, back door plays, and pick-and-rolls to neutralize height advantage. We will, if necessary, hold the ball and play keep-away to keep the score low, within reach.

"On defense, we will use full-court press, zone-traps, sagging man-to man, diamond and one, triangle and two, every possible means to disrupt our adversary's rhythm and poise. Some call these junk defenses; but, as in life, beauty is in the eye of the beholder.

"To accomplish this, we must not only be disciplined, we must also be in perfect physical condition. I will join you, as we will run up and down the Big C hill, full-tilt, every day, three times-a-day. We may lose to superior talent, but we will never lose because of fatigue.

"We will master fundamentals, so that we will never beat ourselves with sloppy play. We will think pass, first; shoot, second. We will learn to protect the ball while dribbling and make crisp, smart passes. We will learn the art of moving without the ball. We will master footwork to out-maneuver taller, stronger players.

"Our tactics will not be popular, frustrating opponents who may demand the NCAA to implement a shot clock limit, but our goal will always be: total, disciplined, team effort.

"Professor Scott teaches us that the Higher Truth always leads the conscientious, thinking person to certain inescapable conclusions of morality. As a member of this Cal basketball team, you will learn that the values of discipline, of unselfishness, of team play will yield not only victories, but also a sense of well-being that comes from giving of self and receiving, in return, the joy of the greater good. *Go Bears!*"

7,200 Cal students rose as one and responded in unison, *"Go Bears!"*

37

A TAIL OF TWO TWISTIES

It was not quite the best of times, not really the worst of times.

Super Sleuth had spent an enjoyable morning following the curly-haired redhead, Lotta Ackshon, President of the Campus Anti-Bra Crusade, who had captivated the Dormies at Pablo Zarzana's speech. He had picked up her tail as she trekked through Dwinelle Plaza where each fraternity claimed a ringed-tree to congregate. Super Sleuth marveled at how she ignored the salivating stares and whistles of fraternity boys admiring her breasts jiggling in a braless red T-shirt.

An anatomical wonder, Super Sleuth thought. *Can't wait to add her address to Royal French's campus map.*

It was this symbolic capture of beautiful women that gave Super Sleuth a sense of social accomplishment. Any campus horny could lust after a female from a distance, but to tail her, as an unnoticed shadow, was an art form.

He had been tracking Lotta's reflection in the window of Cathy Simpson's Fine Fashions For Young Ladies, when a toot-toot of Waz's Vespa motorbike interrupted his hot pursuit.

"Sleuth," Waz said, "Casey's got an important mission for you. Hustle up to Dormland."

Shit, Super Sleuth swore to himself. *Just when Lotta Ackshon seemed to be heading home.*

When Super Sleuth learned the request had originated from Professor Ari Scott - who disproved of Jericho Slabio dating his beautiful daughter, Anna Cappuccino - Super Sleuth was ready for the task. He fondly recalled tailing Anna from campus to her room at I-House (International House) and, in doing so, had discovered HUAC's Chief Investigator, Seymour Graft, peeping into her room from a nearby black walnut tree. Super Sleuth's stealthy observations eventually led to the discovery of the scheme among HUAC Chairman Clayborn Muck, Professor Werner Von Seller, and the P U's to smear the reputations of Ari Scott and his colleagues, Garrick Nelquist and Jacob Aural.

Super Sleuth had been thrilled to be of service to Professor Scott, whose philosophy class in Higher Truth had been a favorite lower division course.

Possibly Professor Scott would show his appreciation by arranging a date with his beautiful daughter? That would be too much to hope for, Super Sleuth concluded. *Even if Anna went out with him, there would be the daunting task of speaking face-to-face with a real, live, gorgeous female. What the hell would I have to say? No, it was easier to enjoy the vicarious world of the chase than the uncertainty of the confrontation.*

Super Sleuth had picked up Jericho Slabio's tail around noon at Bancroft and Telly where Slabio urged anyone within hearing distance, to "escape the shackles of university propaganda," and to "resist frivolous temptations of campus life."

Slabio had ended his harangue promptly at 1 p.m. and made the rounds of left-wing health food hangouts: Luis Kelli's Nirvana Donuts, D&D Organ's Unbearable Lightness of Being Ice Cream, D'Niece Jones's Existential Pizza, Pam Tyler's Escargot-To-Go, David-Shirley's BBQ Pighvarre-On-a-Stick, and LO. Welter's Radical Weenie - where he was showered with free offerings befitting Cal's celebrity radical.

Jeez, the guy eats a lot, Super Sleuth thought, watching Slabio put away a bag of escargot-to-go and a third Radical Weenie.

I gave up tailing Lotta Ackshon to shadow Slabio in a food frenzy?

Marty Silverstein, aka Super Sleuth, could not recall when he did not prefer to be invisible, to be an observer rather than a participant. In his youth, his parents entertained legislators, lobbyists, and political hangers-on in their palatial mansion facing the state Capitol in Sacramento. His father, Franco, an international diamond merchant, was scholarly and urbane, with a twinkly smile and a wicked, sly sense of humor. His mother, Blanca, was a red-haired dynamo, animated and charismatic, with a shrill laugh that shattered crystal. Anyone desiring the Governor's ear, on any issue, had to have the blessing of Blanca Silverstein, the most powerful woman in California politics.

Although imbued with perfect manners, young Marty was painfully shy. When paraded before guests, he nodded and shook hands with men, addressing each. "sir" and bowed to women calling each, "madame." Marty preferred to witness his parents' social events from the spindled balcony overlooking the grand ballroom, where he secretly absorbed the cacophony of spirited debate, whispered gossip, and tinkling glasses.

From his perch, Marty learned to survey the room focusing on one guest at a time, detecting a signature phrase, catching a nervous tick, or observing a social proclivity. Some were Marty's favorites: silver-haired Governor Goody who patted ladies' fannies after two drinks; patron of the arts, F. Gail Tufmama, who wore tons of makeup and kissed young men on the lips; and suave liquor lobbyist, Tony Canady, who poofed melodic farts only Marty could detect.

As a teenager, Marty's shyness was tested by his sudden interest in girls. Unlike high school buddies who admired topless females, in surreptitious copies of *Playboy*, Marty ogled the budding charms of real, alive girls, by anonymously shadowing them. He soon perfected techniques that would earn him the nickname, Super Sleuth. Staying in graceful, perpetual motion stuffing hands into pant pockets, hunching his shoulders, and lowering his eyes into beady slits, Super Sleuth shuffled effortlessly in the silent flat-footed glide of a phantom.

Now, as Super Sleuth watched as Slabio inhaled a fourth Radical Wienie, wiped his lips of mustard, and strolled into the Fall evening. Following Slabio along Telly, Super Sleuth glimpsed the distinctive outline of Lotta Ackshon making a turn on Durant Way.

7 p.m.

Shadowing Slabio had yielded *nada,* nothing helpful to Professor Scott. Slabio was probably headed for home anyway.

Tomorrow would be a more productive day. Yes, tomorrow. In the meanwhile, it wouldn't do any harm to see where Lotta Ackshon lived, Super Sleuth thought. *What the hell!*

Making a 90-degree turn, Super Sleuth tailed the delightful outline of Lotta Ackshon wiggling down Durant Way toward the Bay.

A few blocks later, Super Sleuth watched Lotta plucking keys from her faded blue jeans at the entryway to the Berkeley City Women's Club, medieval castle, designed by Julia Morgan that echoed Morgan's architecture at Hearst Castle in San Simeon.

Now, we're talking, Super Sleuth thought.

From experience, he knew behind the Berkeley Women's Club was a tree towering above the six-story structure. Scurrying to the rear of the building, he scanned the windows.

There, on the third floor.

Super Sleuth saw a light switch on. Reaching for a branch, he pulled himself up to the crotch of the tree. Slowly, he inched his way to a crook level with the third floor. Super Sleuth settled in, rolling up his jacket for a cushion.

He blew lint from the lens of his pocket binoculars and focused them on a Spartan living room, devoid of furniture, with oriental rugs scattered about hard-wood floors. The walls were covered with posters from the *Kama Sutra* depicting pairs in Byzantine, conjugal couplings. At the bottom of each poster was a description of the coital act.

Gotta be a joke, he thought, *these exotic sex positions require couples to be contortionists!*

Oh, my, Super Sleuth said to himself, as Lotta Ackshon came into view, totally nude. As her bra-less T-shirt hinted, Lotta was bodaciously well-endowed and deserving of her nickname, Miss Treasure Chest.

She's a true redhead, he noted.

Super Sleuth heard the soft clang of a fire escape ladder disengaging. Training his binoculars below, Super Sleuth saw the profile of a male tiptoeing up the fire escape. At the third floor, the male quietly tapped the window of Lotta Ackshon's apartment.

What happened would be an indelible memory on Super Sleuth's career. The visitor quickly doffed his clothes on the fire escape and was naked with a fully engorged organ by the time Lotta opened the window, admitting him. Flopping on the oriental rugs, the two grappled in a series of frantic couplings that left Super Sleuth breathless. With each animated position, Super Sleuth scanned the posters, locating the name of the position assumed.

He watched, in astonishment, as the couple serpentined into what one poster described as *"Monkey and Swan Heaven."* The duo then repositioned into an embrace Super Sleuth concluded was a replication of *"Mouse Swallowing Elephant."* Turning upside-down, for a better view, Super Sleuth interpreted the subsequent jumble of limbs as

"Spider and Centipede Embrace."

Duty calls, he told himself. Producing a miniature camera loaded with infra-red film, Super Sleuth clicked the images of serpentining bodies, slithering and humping in physics-defying congress.

Casey Lee owes me a large favor for this, Super Sleuth thought, snapping a photo of the couple, two undulating human pretzels, segueing into *"Pig and Cow Ecstasy."*

38

REDWOOD REDOUBT

In the half-light of the quarter-moon, the shadowy figure resembled a bowling pin, careening down the eastern foothill. Werner Von Seller waddled as fast as his stubby legs allowed, traversing the steep, barren slope below the Cyclotron. He had jettisoned the remnant of the Gaulois and tucked the sterling silver cigarette holder and monocle safely into his coat pocket. Von Seller extended his arms, like a fighter plane, as he had done so many times as a child in pre-War Berlin, leaving balance solely to his innate sense of feel.

If life were so simple, he thought, now slaloming past the Big C, like a dive bombing German Junker.

The phone call came late last night from Lumken, William Randolph Chandler's personal secretary. Von Seller recalled the efficient, stern, blond male, in his mid-thirties - *Austrian, no doubt*, Von Seller had thought - who sat next to WRC, jotting down every word during their only meeting at the Chandler mansion in San Francisco.

"Professor Von Seller. Mr. Chandler desires a report on the status of the publish or perish program," Lumken said, in his Teutonic-accented voice.

"Certainly," Von Seller replied.

But where? We can't risk being seen in public.

As if reading his mind, Lumken responded, "We will meet tomorrow, at midnight, in the secret room of Senior Men's Hall."

What a genius, Von Seller thought, now zooming past the top rim of the Greek Theater.

Libraries close at 11 p.m. No one will see him entering the Redwood Grove next to Senior Men's Hall.

How generous! WRC is still willing to give me a chance to prove myself!

Von Seller was still smarting from the disaster of Pablo Zarzana's Sproul Hall speech. Jericho Slabio's Guerillas for Free Speech had tried to provoke the National Guard into violence; but that traitor, Colonel McReynolds Jones, had refused to unleash his troops. Instead of a riot, a wire service photo of Slabio inserting a daisy into the barrel of a soldier's rifle, was sent around the world by AP and UPI with the caption,

"Berkeley Flower Power"

Worse, Pablo Zarzana's speech was not inflammatory. He called for "co-operation and collaboration among peoples of all social strata;" "a sharing of democratic ideals;" and "economic reform through equal participation."

For a Communist, Pablo Zarzana sounded like any generic Democrat or Republican! This was not the stuff revolutionary dreams were made of.

There had been serious egg splattered on his face that must be removed by a glowing progress report on his publish or perish duties.

Yes, soon, WRC will forgive me for my misstep at Sproul, Von Seller thought. *Publish or perish will be in place in a few weeks, and WRC will reap the political benefits of my loyalty.*

It was not William Randolph Chandler's immense wealth and power that impressed Von Seller. No, it was WRC's ability to perpetuate one face in public and advocate an opposite position in private.

Von Seller had displayed this same quality to survive the quicksand of changing political fortunes. He retraced his recent flirtation with political disaster when he cast his support for Congressman Clayborn Muck and HUAC, only to see Muck disgraced by the public imbroglio that followed. It had taken great political skill for him to distance himself from Muck and HUAC.

Flapping his elbows, the Prussian Penguin slowed his fluttering descent, waddling around Kleeberger Field, crossing Gayley Road, and passing Cowell Student Hospital. Stubbing his foot in the darkness of the Redwood Grove, Von Seller rolled the last few yards to the entrance of Senior Men's Hall.

Built in 1905, Senior Men's Hall was a large, wood cabin sitting on the south bank of Strawberry Creek, half-way between the Men's and Women's Faculty Clubs. The Hall was constructed with large redwood logs, with intact bark, its pitched roof supported by post trusses resting on log pilasters. The spacious main room was the center of activity, but behind the large fireplace was a room with its own arched fireplace, the secret meeting place of the OGB, the Order of the Golden Bear.

From the early 1900's, Senior Men's Hall had been maintained by the Order of the Golden Bear, a secret men's honor society comprised of student leaders, faculty, administrators, and alumni, dedicated to promoting the Hall as the *"center for molding of public opinion through free discussion."*

Since joining the Cal faculty, Von Seller had not been invited to join the OGB.

An obvious oversight, he concluded; although, had he been invited, he would have had reservations about the *"free discussion"* part of the Order's mission of molding public opinion.

Von Seller dusted off the patina of pine needles accumulated by his pratfall. He tiptoed the seven steps to the entrance and depressed the creaky, rusted latch. The massive redwood door opened, as Lumken had promised. Quietly closing the door, Von Seller squinted in the darkness, inhaling the strong, pungent smell of the forest permeating the Hall.

This is the way Mother Nature should be used . . . for the whim and benefit of Mankind.

He had been disturbed by recent news that so-called environmental groups were forming to preserve redwood timber lands from cutting.

Misguided fools! How could magnificent structures such as Senior Men's Hall, be constructed, if redwoods were left to grow, instead of harvested for honorable human monuments?

Von Seller slowly felt his way in the dark. His hands groped outlines of chairs, tables, benches, and shelves, all fashioned from redwood. At the far end of the room, he collided with the clinker bricks of the arched fireplace. Following Lumken's instructions, he side-stepped to the left, until he was greeted by the musty scent of a moldy bear skin. He slipped his hand behind the mounted fur hide and found the handle to the hidden jib door, admitting himself into the secret meeting room of the OGB.

"Come in, Professor," the familiar voice of WRC said. "Please sit down."

Taking a seat at the head of a massive redwood table illuminated by a single candle, Von Seller squinted in his monocle. The eye piece had collected a field of lint during his downhill sprint, but he could see well enough.

Facing him at the other end of the table was William Randolph Chandler dressed in a three-piece tweed suit. He hunched sideways with his head resting on the fist of an arm with its elbow perched on a knee. In the flickering candle light, WRC's silhouette against the far wall resembled Rodin's, *The Thinker*.

A fresh box of Gaulois lay before him.

WRC thinks of everything, Von Seller thought, breaking open the box of cigarettes. He plucked the sterling silver cigarette holder from his pocket and inserted a Gaulois. Picking up the candle, Von Seller lit the French cigarette and drew deeply. Blowing a stream of smoke, Von Seller noted a figure standing in a darkened corner of the room.

WRC addressed Von Seller, without looking directly at him. "You've met Lumken," Chandler said, nodding toward the muscular figure standing in the shadows.

Von Seller nodded at WRC's male secretary.

"Sorry, I'm a bit late," Von Seller said. "The walk took longer than I thought." He plucked pine needles from his sleeve.

"Let's get down to business, Professor," WRC said. "Did you have any doubts the Regents would pass the publish or perish program?" Chandler asked.

"Absolutely not, sir!" Von Seller said. "You assured me you had enough votes on the Regents to pass any measure." He blew a stream of Gaulois smoke toward the pitched ceiling.

"When you explained publish or perish was the best way to punish the Cal faculty, especially your left wing son-in . . . pardon my error. I meant to say, your *former* son-in-law, I was convinced you possessed the wisdom to be the next Governor of California."

"Thank you for your confidence, Professor," Chandler said, "and what news do you have of your progress?"

"The program is progressing marvelously," Von Seller said in his most enthusiastic voice. "Of course, I have not completed all the work; but pursuant to your instructions, I have hired 100 Teaching Assistants from your alma mater, the University of Southern California, including a few members of the SC football team that was robbed of a victory by Cal this past year. They'll enjoy punishing Cal students with irrelevant and unreasonable classroom assignments, as Cal professors are struggling with their publishing demands."

Von Seller was referring to Cal's recent upset of SC when a call of nature helped the Joe L. Capp led Bears to a 20-18 victory over the Number One ranked Trojans.

"What assurance, Professor, do I have that most of the faculty will fail their requirement to publish or perish?" Chandler asked.

"Ingenious, I must admit," Von Seller said, placing a new Gaulois into his sterling silver cigarette holder. "I have assembled a list of academicians from across the country, whose patriotic allegiances are to the House Un- American Activities Committee, to serve as judges."

"I'm impressed," Chandler said. "If you are successful in getting most of the Cal faculty fired, how do you wish to be rewarded?"

Von Seller had already given the question serious thought.

"If it would please you, I thought an appropriate reward would be for you to appoint me Chancellor of the Cal campus. This would be a way to rid the campus of the left-wing influence of that pompous Chancellor Roger Haynes."

Von Seller was surprised by the silence that followed.

Had he been too greedy?

"Of course, I would be grateful for whatever reward Governor Chandler felt would be appropriate," Von Seller said, backpedaling. The last thing he wanted was to appear presumptuous.

"I will give your efforts every consideration," Chandler said.

Von Seller hissed a stream of smoke in relief.

"And, if I should need more assistance?" Chandler asked.

"Ask and your every wish will be my command," Von Seller said, bowing his head in reverence.

"Even testifying at my daughter's custody trial?"

"It would be my pleasure to do anything to rid the Cal faculty of left wing elements such as your *ex*-son-in-law, Ari Scott."

What a wonderful opportunity, Von Seller thought. *With all the press coverage, my testimony will enhance my stature as an advocate of patriotic atomic research!*

"Perfect," Chandler said. " I'll look forward to seeing you at the trial.

And you must never . . ."

Von Seller finished the sentence for WRC, ". . . acknowledge that we ever discussed these issues. If confronted, you can be assured, I shall deny everything."

"Thank you, good evening," WRC said, ending the meeting.

Exiting into the cool Fall evening, Von Seller wondered. *For all I've done for him, WRC could have offered me a ride back up to the Cyclotron in his limousine! Damn the rich and powerful, anyway! They never appreciate those who have contributed to their success. I will never suffer this condition. When I am Chancellor of the Cal campus, I shall never forgot anyone who has helped me along the way!*

Tucking his monocle and cigarette holder back into his coat pocket, the Prussian Penguin began the long uphill waddle. It would be 2 a.m. by the time he reached his beloved Cyclotron, still time to smash a few more atoms.

"*Chancellor Von Seller,*" he said to himself. *The title has a lyrical, Germanic-sounding ring of authority to it. Yes, Chancellor Werner Von Seller of the University of California - Berkeley,* he said to himself.

He could hardly wait.

39

FREE SPEECH HARMONY

It was <u>not</u> a dark and stormy day - just a dank January day, foggy and chilly enough to dissuade coddled Cal students from loitering for more than a few minutes. The varsity basketball team was on the road for a Pac 8 game, so there was no logical explanation for the line that queued up at 4 p.m. and stretched two blocks down Bancroft, almost to Telly, for an event that would not begin until 7 p.m. Despite the inclement weather, Crunchy Munchy pushed his bicycle-wheeled ice cream cart up-and-down the line, selling Eskimo Pies at a brisk pace.

A discreet sign, at the entrance to the site of the performance, Women's Gymnasium, announced:

*"World Debut of the
Woody Wood Pecker-ettes
Backed By Big Berry and the Blackouts"*

<u>Admission: $1.00</u>

Across the street, fraternity boys, dressed uniformly in tan khakis, white button-downed oxford shirts, and tan wind-breakers, marched in a circle, in front of K Carter's Boys Store, chanting,

"NO, On Public P !"
"NO, On Public P!"

216

Some carried placards:

> *"Keep the P in Your Pants"*
> *"Nice Girls Don't Talk About P"*

No one could recall an event that provoked members of the IFC to demonstrate for or against any issue.

Peeking from an upstairs window of the Women's Gym, the objects of the crowd's fascination, watched in wonder.

"Oh, my God! Look at all those people!" Dandy Cane said, with a squeal. "I'm gonna pee in my pants."

"Must be over 500," Joan Dildeaux said, squinting through her bi-focals. "Just to hear the four of us sing about the P word?"

"Look, TV crews, too! I heard there's going to be a photographer from *Life* magazine!" Muffy Peachwick said, pushing up her bra and pirouetting. "Which is my better side, girls?"

"We're going make a mint for Joanie and Hunch!" Kate Howell said, "and I don't think people are really going to care whether we can carry a tune. I would have never guessed . . ."

"What happens if we're kicked out of the Gee Dee House?" Dandy said, her enthusiasm suddenly waning.

"Fat chance, li'l sis," Muffy said, admiring her chesty profile in a full-length mirror. "With all this publicity, we're big-time celebrities. The Mothers Club wouldn't dare kick us out. Do you think they're really complaining with all those 'tsk's, tsk's?' Hell, no! Those conservative old bats are enjoying the vicarious thrills as much as we!"

"Yes," Kate said. "We've become the fabulous 'Four Gee Dee Sluts.' What is this world coming to?"

The P word song, as it was now called, began as a nervous reaction from the unexpected grimness of their part-time work at Yearning Arms. What began as a vicarious, sexual lark had taken on a tedious, serious edge, as the four learned the details of what Wanda Majic and her assistant, Sasha, referred to as "tricks of the trade."

Where was the Joy? The Excitement? The Ecstasy that was supposed to be a part of the sexual experience?

According to the working girls of Yearning Arms, their customers took sex much too seriously. Sasha observed that men's brains and organs were Siamese Twins conjoined and co-dependent.

The quartet had considered quitting as trainees of Yearning Arms, but they had agreed to stick it out until the end of the semester, early February, 1960; and that date was rapidly approaching.

How ironic that their vicarious sexual adventure had propelled them, nay, catapulted them into the campus spotlight as "sexually experienced girls" whose confidence produced a musical composition that titillated the entire campus!

None had admitted it, but they all yearned for their simpler, even mundane, former lives as Gee Dee sorority girls who knew *"who you are and what you represent."* In this momentary, daring flight from their pre-ordained lives working toward the ultimate goal of an "MRS" degree, each knew this brief escape into unchartered territory would truly define *"who they are and what they represent."*

"So let the show begin," Kate said, with a sly wink. She produced a sterling silver flask of *Glen Livet* Casey Lee had given her for good luck. Each took a healthy swig and winced as the licorice-tasting, single malt scotch burned the esophagus.

"Wow," Joan said, in an exaggerated deep voice, "Now, I can reach those low, bass notes."

Dandy belched, giggling, "I don't know if I can stand. I feel super dizzy.".

"I don't care," Muffy said, slugging down another, "I need more liquid courage."

"Two's the limit, 'Sluts,' " Kate said, capping the flask. "At this rate, we'll have slurred singing. It's important we pronounce each and every syllable of the P word song clearly." She held her breath, suppressing a burp welling up her innards.

7:15 p.m.

The last of the SRO crowd had been shoehorned into the concrete nooks and crannies of the Women's Gymnasium, another neoclassical building designed by Julia Morgan, the architect of Hearst Castle. Temporary bleachers and banks of lighting ringed the outdoor pool that had been enclosed by a huge blue and gold tent. The expanse of the pool had been cleverly covered by a portable floor strong enough to support a make-shift stage

Standing at the center of the stage, KALX disc jockey, All-Pro kicked off the program.

"WELCOME, ladies and gentlemen, to this HISTORIC musical

218

event. For the first time ANYWHERE, our own singing sensations, the Woody Wood Pecker-ettes, will perform ORIGINAL lyrics to the song we've come to know as the P WORD!"

A sustained roar of applause and cheers enveloped All-Pro.

"To get this SWINGING crowd in the mood, we've got the INCREDIBLE Big Berry and the Blackouts performing their campus favorite, *"LOUIE LOUIE"* and as a SURPRISE BONUS, we have the DOOCH DOZEN showing off the new FUN AND SEXY Oakland dance moves all of you will want to learn. Here they are, the incomparable BIG BERRY and THE BLACKOUTS!"

"DUH (pause)
Duh-duh-duh. Duh-duh-duh. Duh-duh-duh

With the distinctive syncopated riff of *"Louie Louie"* in the background, the curtain opened to thunderous screaming. A spotlight circled the quintet of black musicians dressed in suits: Big Berry wearing his signature admiral's cap with scrambled egg insignia; on rhythm guitar, a young drummer; a bass guitarist; an older gentleman on keyboards; and Jonathan's Oakland cousin, MJ Jones, on lead guitar.

Below the stage, writhing to the infectious beat of the band were two lines of dancing Dormies:

Royal, Waz, Lizard, Super Sleuth, Tubbins, Mo
Jonathan, Punch, Organ, Hunch, Ruby Lips, Casey

"DUH (pause)
Duh-duh-duh. Duh-duh-duh. Duh-duh-duh."

"C'MON DOWN, GIRLS!" All Pro shouted. "Time for your rock and roll DANCE LESSONS!"

A wave of females oozed onto the floor engulfing the Dormies, emulating their stomping, undulating, twisting, wiggling, twirling, serpentining gyrations.

Big Berry and the Blackouts played four spirited renditions of *"Louie-Louie,"* the rock and roll song with the indiscernible, X-rated-sounding lyrics. For an encore, Jonathan joined the group, reprising his guitar performance at the Gee Dee Halloween Presents Party.

The charged crowd gave the band a standing, five-minute ovation.

Returning to the microphone, All-Pro said, "now that you're revved up and in the MOOD for something NAUGHTY, it's my EXTREME PLEASURE to introduce the SINGING SENSATIONS of the Cal campus, the LOVELY AND TALENTED group, Woody Wood Pecker-ettes, singing the PROVOCATIVE P WORD SONG, you're all been DYING to hear!"

As the make-shift curtain slowly lifted, Big Berry and the Blackouts laid down a background introduction for the WW Pecker-ettes, gamely smiling, but obviously ill-at ease. Flashes of Brownie Hawkeye cameras created a halo of light around the quartet.

A reverent silence gripped the audience, as Big Berry and the Blackouts segued into a discreet chalypso rhythm and sang backup vocals:

"Oooh, oooh, ooh, oooh.
Oooh, oooh . . . Oooh-oooh-oooh.
Ooooh, oooh, oooh, oooh.
Oooh, oooh . . . Oooh-oooh-oooh."

Emboldened by their swigs of *Glen Livet*, the WW Pecker-ettes began, in perfect harmony, sounding like the popular Lawrence Welk group, the Lemon sisters. But a closer scrutiny would have detected, in the their voices, a mocking undertone of swooning irreverence.

Joan Dildeaux had penned the X-rated lyrics to the Frankie Avalon single, *"Venus,"* the number one song in America. The girls of Yearning Arms knew and appreciated something about men that the Gee Dees had never contemplated: that men were totally controlled by their gonads; and according to Wanda Majic, "the penis always has a mind of its own." As Sascha observed, "when women address the male psyche, the brain is nothing more than an intercom to the male organ.".

In an inspired half-hour of creativity, Joan had created the lyrics she, Kate, Muffy, and Dandy sang whenever they heard "Venus."

The WW Pecker-ettes, in their Yearning Arms persona, sang,

"Oh, Penis! Hey, Penis!"

On hearing the P word, the crowd erupted into cheers.

Muffy, outfitted as Daisy Mae from the popular comic strip, *"L'il Abner,"* was barefoot, wearing a pair of frayed, skin-tight cut-off shorts, a red, short-sleeved blouse with bright yellow polka dots from which her ample bosom overflowed. On her face, she wore a light blue, Lone Ranger mask.

Kneeling, with her hands raised to the heavens, Muffy sang the first verse of Joan's lyrics:

> *"Penis, if you will,*
> *Please let me give you a little thrill,*
> *A little something beyond compare,*
> *A thrill that you and I can share."*

"YES! YES!" members of the Guerillas for Free Speech chanted.

Dressed as B-Movie personum, *"Motorcycle Mama,"* Joan wore a black leather vest, knee-length, black leather boots, and a black, kitty mask. In her hand, she snapped a cat-o-nine tails, as she sang the second verse:

> *"Penis, please be clean.*
> *No wayward squirts or spurts obscene,*
> *No icky drips of semen wane,*
> *No sticky globs of gooey stain."*

Shrieks of "OH, my GOD!" and "she didn't say THAT?" emitted from wide-eyed sorority girls in the crowd.

Dressed as 18th-century French Marie Antoinette, Kate wore a silver wig piled high, a white Venetian mask, a backless, white, long-sleeve blouse with the maroon, sequined inscription, *"Let 'em Eat Cake,"* and a white, hoop skirt with petticoats extending only to the thighs.

Folding her hands in mock prayer, Kate sang the lyrics to the bridge of Joan's send-off of *"Venus:"*

> *"Penis - symbol of Manhood you are,*
> *Rigid and tumescent,*
> *King - whether straight or bent."*

Choruses of playful "boo's" rained down from males of the crowd

Dandy Cane dressed as the rhyme, femme fatale, *"Little Bo Beep,"* her hair in pig tails adorned with pink ribbons, and the top half of her face covered by a pink mask, brandished a long, curved, sheep herder's staff. Fluttering her saucer-shaped eyes innocently, Dandy sang the third and final verse of Joan's musical parody:

> *"Penis, if you come,*
> *I'll always be your little chum,*
> *Helping you spill some stored-up seed.*
> *Friends in need are friends indeed!"*

Gales of laughter buffeted the WW Pecker-ettes locked arm-in-arm, swaying back and forth, singing, in four-part harmony, at the top of their lungs, the closing lyrics:

> *"Oh, Penis! Hey, Penis!*
> *Let me be your friend."*

Shouts of "Again! ENCORE! Again! ONE MORE TIME!" echoed through the Women's Gym. Energized by the enthusiastic response, the WW Pecker-ettes again sang the lyrics of their P word song, amid choruses of reverent "shhhh's!"

As the quartet reached the closing lyrics, Joan Dildeaux, shouted, into the microphone, "now, everybody . . ." and the audience joined in a thunderous chorus of:

> *"Oh, Penis! Hey, Penis!*
> *LET ME . . . BE YOUR FRIEND !"*

40

LET'S MAKE A DEAL

"So, we've got a deal?"

The soft-spoken question came from Tom Hobknob, the ruggedly handsome president of Ep Sig fraternity. Hobknob was of medium build with close-cropped brown hair and a perennially sly, toothy grin.

"Possibly," Casey Lee said, glancing at Royal French.

The two Dormie leaders sat on the cantilevered hearth of the Dooch living room, their backs to a flickering, dying fire. The lights of the rectangular, fish-bowl dorm were dark, and as an additional precaution, the visitors had been admitted through the patio.

Seated next to Hobknob was Stefan Tillich, a hulking giant, who was almost as tall as Royal but a hundred pounds heavier. Tillich had deep-set, dark eyes and a pencil-thin moustache, facial hair that was rare for a fraternity man.

The clandestine meeting had originated from a note passed along to Casey from Kate Howell during one of their secret chats in his eighth floor room high up at the top of Dooch.

The hand-printed message read,

> *"We need to meet. Secretly, of course . . .*
> *The Ep Sig's would like to help Hunch*
> *win the Campus Snow King Contest*
> *For a price, of course . . . If Dirk Krum*
> *or the IFC learns of a meeting, we will*
> *deny it, of course . . ."*

"We're willing to turn over all the money we raise for Tillich's Campus Snow King candidacy, in exchange for an endorsement when we run Tillich for Student Body President next Spring," Hobknob said.

"Wouldn't it be political suicide for a member of the IFC to openly solicit non-org, Dormie support?" Royal asked.

"Of course . . ." Hobknob beamed his toothy grin, "but, if the election were close, non-org votes would make the difference. Dirk Krum intends to run his Neanderthal roommate, Chip First, for Student Body President; so Dirk, through his puppet, would effectively control both the IFC and the ASUC - Associated Students of the University of California.

"Of course . . ." Royal said, echoing Hobknob's response.

"There's a greater reality Dirk and the IFC refuse to recognize," Hobknob said, "that the influx of middle-class students will not go away. Look at the 11 new high rise dorms the Administration is planning to build in 1960 and 1961. You, Dormies, could overrun the campus and change the balance of political power in a few years."

"Scary, isn't it?" Casey said. "Imagine, non-orgs controlling Cal campus life, like Genghis Khan knocking on the gates of Vienna."

"Of course . . ." Hobknob said, "unless enlightened members of the IFC formulate a plan to insure long-term IFC control of the campus."

"What kind of plan?" Royal's military mind was now intrigued. "Simple." Hobknob said, "The IFC siphons off non-org leaders, so the Dormies will never effectively organize its masses."

"How?" Casey asked.

"Simple plan, difficult execution," Tillich chuckled.

"What if the IFC changes its rules to accept members of all races, faiths, and socio-economic backgrounds without discrimination," Hobknob said.

"Fat chance," Casey said, "you'd have to eliminate black-balling. Fraternity chapters in the Deep South would never tolerate the end to black-balling."

Casey was referring to the practice allowing a single "no" vote by one fraternity member to block acceptance of a new member, even if all other members of the fraternity vote "yes."

"Why, you might be stuck with untraditional pledges, guys who aren't cookie-cutter handsome, who don't come from rich, socially prominent backgrounds!" Royal said, tongue-in-cheek. "Horrors, the IFC might be stuck with guys who look like Casey, or worse, guys who look like me, or Hunch Hitowski, or Ollie Punch!"

"Of course . . ." Hobknob said, letting the thought sink in. "But I see this as a matter of economic and social survival. If the IFC doesn't broaden its membership, if it doesn't change its exclusive ways, membership will shrink, houses will close, and its power and influence over campus life will disappear!"

"Then we won't have Dirk Krum and the P U's to kick around anymore," Casey said, inducing a loud chuckle from Tillich.

This was the moment the two Dormies were waiting for.

"We'll need more than your Campus Snow King money for our endorsement of Tillich," Royal said, winking at Casey.

"What more do you want?" Hobknob's toothy grin had vanished.

"We need something tangible, something very symbolic," Casey said.

"Like what?" Tillich asked.

"Having our own tree in Dwinelle Plaza where Dormies can hang out between classes," Royal said.

"Impossible!" Hobknob shouted. "Those trees have been the property of the IFC for decades."

"The Jewish fraternities got their trees as a result of the Peace Pact of 1951." Royal said.

"But that was different," Tillich said. "They loaned the IFC a ton of money to rebuild Christian fraternity houses damaged by the earthquake. We had to make way for them. That was part of the deal. That was all business."

"So, losing membership and closing down fraternities are not business concerns?" Casey asked.

"Of course . . . they are!" Hobknob said, "but . . . but you're asking for way too much. Even if we agreed, we couldn't take a Dwinelle tree away from a fraternity, Christian or Jewish, and just give it to you Dormies!"

"We're not asking you do that ," Royal said. "There's an easier way. You talk the Administration into digging a new planter box in the middle of Dwinelle Plaza, and we'll take care of planting a tree suitable to our taste. That way, you and the Ep Sig's won't be blamed for the integration of Dwinelle Plaza's social life."

Hobknob motioned Tillich over to a darkened corner of the living room where they caucused in whispers.

Returning, Hobknob said, "we'd agree no one would ever tell how a new planter box for a Dormie tree suddenly appeared in Dwinelle Plaza, correct?"

"Of course . . . NOT!" Casey and Royal said in unison, extending their hands to seal the deal.

Thus, a deal was struck that would impact the social and political life of the Cal campus throughout the 1960's.

41

THE TWAIN SHALL NOT MEET

It had taken all the resolve Jonathan could muster to invite Pritti Diva to coffee, the only kind of date his meager budget could afford. For weeks, he had sat like a bowl of mush in English 1A class, next to the beautiful green and orange-eyed girl, building up his courage.

Butch, with his New York swagger, was confident Pritti Diva was dying to go out with Jonathan. When he finally stammered an invite, she winked her orange eye and said sweetly, "love to, Jonathan."

Now, Jonathan was a nervous wreck.

What would he say to this gorgeous creature? How would he avoid acting like a puppy dog drooling for approval?

Butch claimed the sure-fire way to impress any girl was to ask a series of questions intended to create an aura of interest and, at the same time, eliminate the pressure of being suave and "de-boner," Butch's pronunciation of *debonair*.

Thus, with dedicated enthusiasm, Jonathan was ready to bombard Pritti Diva with rehearsed questions to mask his social ineptitude.

The couple was seated at a darkened booth in the rear of the Bear's Lair, the student union cafeteria, enveloped in toasty clouds of burnt grease rising from the busy grill. They nursed coffees that cost fifteen cents each, re-fills included. From the juke box, Johnny Tillotson sang *"Poetry In Motion."* On Jonathan's knee sat a 4 by 6 inch index card with neatly typed questions

"I've been wondering . . ." Jonathan murmured, unable to look Pritti Diva directly in either her green or orange eye.

"*Heterochromia*," she said, "You're probably curious about the colors of my eyes?"

Jonathan felt a pang of guilt. He did want to ask her about her exotic eyes; but had discreetly omitted that question from the index card.

"Thanks for telling me, but that's not the question I had in mind."

Jonathan glanced down at the index card for assurance and said, "Pritti Diva sounds so continental. Is it a Neopolitan name?" This was the question Butch promised Pritti would find "incredibly flattering."

"My friends call me by my nickname," Prima said, leaning forward, holding up a diamond studded charm dangling at the end of a gold chain necklace. "Do you know what this is?"

"A snake?" Jonathan asked. His knees were shaking. He felt the index card slip between his knees and slide to the floor.

"It does resemble a snake" Pritti Diva said, with a smile that melted his heart. "It's an 'S.' S for Sascha."

"Wow! Sascha is a cool nickname," he said, sounding her name, *Sascha*, in his mind. "How did you get it?"

"My mother gave it to me. It's a stage name."

"Is your mother in show business?" Jonathan was intrigued.

"You could say it's a form of entertainment," Sascha said.

"Do you know any actors?" Jonathan said, "My mother always said I look like Tab Hunter."

The cafeteria jukebox warbled Sonny James's - not Tab Hunter's - rendition of *"Young Love."*

"Yes," Sascha said, pouring cream into her coffee, "I know some rather accomplished actresses - and I agree with your mother. You do look like Tab Hunter."

"What's your major, Sascha?" Jonathan asked, remembering the second question on the index card.

"Business administration," Sascha replied. "Mom - she's not my real mother - wants me to take over her business when I graduate."

"Is she also a Diva?" Jonathan asked, recalling questions about family history were high on Butch's list.

"In some ways, she might be considered a diva," Sascha said. "No, she has a different last name, Majic. Mom took me in and raised me when one of her former employees abandoned me as a baby."

"Magic, as in magic show?" Jonathan said. "Is that the kind of entertainment business your mother runs?"

"Some of her happy clients claim Mom does performs magic, but

228

Mom spells her name with a J, not a G."

Emboldened by the ease of their repartee, Jonathan made a wild guess. "Does your mother run a theatrical company?"

"You could call it a theatrical company," Sascha laughed. "We do have an extensive wardrobe for every possible role."

"Enough questions about me, Jonathan," Sascha said, with a wink of her orange eye. "Tell me about yourself."

Jonathan was unprepared for the reversal of roles.

"You might say I'm an orphan, too," Jonathan said.

Like water released from a dam, Jonathan spilled out the details of his life: the simple, happy youth as one of the singing duo, the Amazin' Double A's; his family's secret of how Aldon Farms, the largest hog operation in Iowa, was founded; his Uncle Mike and Aunt Pearl's scandalous, interracial marriage; his disinheritance for failing to keep his Three Promises; his recent adventures as a Dormie; and his academic struggle to stay in school.

Jonathan was exhausted. He looked at the beautiful girl who had patiently listened to him paint his tales of woe and experienced a glowing ethereal feeling something like . . . falling in love.

"Sascha," he blurted, "I feel so close to you. I'd love to see you again, soon?"

"Jonathan," a sadness crept into Sascha's voice. "I'm not the right kind of girl for you."

"But, you're wrong. Look how we easily we can talk to each other," Jonathan said, a sound of desperation creeping into his voice.

Sascha whispered, taking his hands into hers. "There are things you don't know about me, things you wouldn't want to know. We come from different worlds. Trust me, when I say that it wouldn't work."

Sascha gave him a dazzling smile and said, "Despite your problems with your parents, you're still the product of your Iowa values, of your Iowa hopes, of your Iowa fears."

Jonathan felt a knot in his stomach.

Sascha continued, "One day, you'll realize I was right. It's not a question of whether you're handsome, intelligent, or charming. You are! It's just that I know where I have to go with my life; and if I told you the truth about me, you wouldn't want to be a part of it. So, I'd rather leave you with a positive image than risk the consequence of how you'd feel, if you knew my secrets."

Sascha gently kissed the back of his hand, "Thank you for the lovely afternoon, Jonathan. For a couple of hours, you've made me feel like a normal, college girl."

"But, you're anything but normal," Jonathan said, now unafraid to look Pritti "Sascha" Diva directly in her green and orange eyes. "You're the most . . . unusual girl I've ever met."

"Yes," Sascha sighed, "that's part of my problem."

42

BOARDWALK AND MARVIN GARDENS

The crystal paperweight, sculptured in the shape of a dollar sign, shattered the mirror, showering shards of broken glass back toward the jagged image of a scowling William Randolph Chandler. How WRC detested moments like this, when control over his world was wrested away by something unexpected!

Money, the feel of it, the smell of it, had been his lifelong ally. The promise of munificence had always helped him have his way.

It had taken two generations of Chandlers to learn this truism. At the turn of the century, when grandfather George Chandler brought his fortune from cutting and selling Lake Tahoe-Carson Range lumber, Grandpa George naively believed San Francisco society would afford him respect. The Chandlers quickly learned that Old Money was somehow better than New Money. Thus, even if the Chandlers were as wealthy as the Old Rich like the Crockers, the Stanfords, the Hearsts, they were dismissed as inferior, New Rich.

But later in the 20th century, new arrivals to The City did not discriminate between Old and New Money. Money was money. While Old Money lived smugly on (S)Nob Hill, three generations of Chandlers had - to use a football metaphor - made an end run, buying their way into the corridors of influence and power creating what Grandpa George affectionately called the "holy matrimony of N and P," the marriage of news and politics. The Chandlers had muscled into the newspaper business and their paper, the *Gazette,* was one of the most influential in the state.

Now that William Randolph Chandler was his party's candidate for Governor, the San Francisco Establishment was showing a belated sense of deference and respect

WRC had just recovered from the distressing news that his worthless, weak-spined professor son-in-law, Ari Scott, was willing to be divorced by WRC's daughter, Cee Cee, than denouncing his recently discovered illegitimate daughter, that Commie bitch, Anna Cappuccino.

Ari will pay dearly for his misguided sentiment, WRC thought.

He had directed his corporate counsel, Barry Dreyersdorf, to hire bombastic trial attorney Marvin Belly for the divorce trial, with instructions that Belly was to destroy Ari's name and reputation.

Any judge will have to be careful not to alienate the future Governor of California, Chandler thought; and there was no doubt, in WRC's mind, that the gubernatorial election was his.

More important than even money and political power was a driving desire to build a monument symbolizing Chandler power and prestige for generations to come. That self-indulgent Hearst had his little castle at San Simeon, but WRC had designs of a grander scale, something akin to what the Statute of Liberty was to New York City.

The Pyramid, a structure of timeless classical design, would harken echoes of the mystical grandeur of powerful pharaohs who ruled Egypt thousands of years ago. When WRC first saw the Cheops Great Pyramid at Giza, he knew he must build his own version in downtown San Francisco. When completed, the Pyramid would be the tallest building west of Chicago, dominating the San Francisco skyline, casting an omnipotent, pointed shadow over the financial district.

The plan had been simple and discreet. Patrick Hoyl, a high-powered realtor, hired by WRC's corporate counsel, Dreyersdorf, would acquire parcels of tenement property along the border between North Beach and Chinatown, offering unheard of sums of money for slum properties. Hoyl would acquire title to two blocks of property in the name of Grand Designs Inc., the dummy Nevada corporation, run by WRC's secret half-brother, Howard Muse.

The first group of properties had been acquired quickly, as descendants of Italian North Beach immigrants happily unloaded unproductive family property. Now, this unexpected turn of events - the problem of acquiring the remaining parcels owned by Chinese families.

"Double the offer," WRC ordered, but the increased offer had been rebuffed. Worse, Hoyl reported the Chinese families had sold their land for lesser amounts to a Madame Lee whose representative in these transactions was a Calphung Quock.

"Who the hell is Quock?" WRC had demanded. "Triple the offer for those Chinatown dumps. If that doesn't work, hire Quock away from this Madame Lee! Money talks, and we'll talk louder than anyone!"

To WRC's surprise, Quock had spurned sums that would have yielded a quick profit to Madame Lee and further, had refused Hoyl's discreet offer of employment.

"Set up a meeting," WRC said. "Nobody in her right mind's going to turn down real money. This is just a small-time shake down."

What had begun as a show of money to intimidate a recalcitrant little old Chinese lady, was now something totally alien to WRC. It began with Quock's instructions that WRC, Hoyl, and Chandler's Chief Financial Officer, Franklin Majestic, meet on a foggy evening under the *"International Settlement"* sign on Pacific Avenue. It had spun out of control when WRC, Hoyl, and Majestic were blindfolded; driven around aimlessly in a large limousine; then blindfolded, and escorted through the putrid stench of Chinatown by Oriental goons.

How I hate the smell of Chinese food! WRC thought.

As WRC's eyesight became accustomed to the darkened room, he felt an uncharacteristic pang of apprehension. The walls of the room, ringed with indirect light, were a deep red, each wall bearing a strange Chinese symbol, framed in gold. The City's cool, grey fog swirled above the arched glass ceiling.

The trio were seated before a dais where eight people sat in shadows. In the center was an empty gold, throne.

A voice shouted a Chinese command, and the eight rose and bowed to a female assuming the gold throne, her face also hidden in the shadows.

"Welcome, Mr. Chandler, Mr. Majestic, " a voice with a British accent said. "Thank you for coming to discuss this important issue. My name is Calphung Quock, Madame Lee's aide-de-camp."

"Yes, Madame Lee, Mr. Quock," Hoyl began. "As you know, Mr. Chandler desires to purchase the ten parcels of Chinatown property you recently acquired. He is willing to extend a most generous offer."

Calphung Quock rose from his seat beside Madame Lee and said, "I dare say, gentlemen, making a profit is not Madame Lee's most important concern."

"Certainly," Hoyl said, "we are not suggesting Madame Lee should only be concerned with money, but Mr. Chandler is willing to offer Madame Lee $1,000,000 for the ten parcels."

Madame Lee's advisors murmured among themselves.

"This is quite a generous offer," Hoyl continued, "since the City of San Francisco has evaluated these lots at only $10,000 each, $100,000 total. A million dollars is a very fair premium for them."

"Madame Lee does not question the generosity of Mr. Chandler's offer," Quock said. "She is deeply concerned where the displaced people of Chinatown will go. There are at least 100 families living on these parcels and not enough room in Chinatown to absorb them."

"Madame Lee," WRC said, rising to his feet. "You obviously are a sophisticated business woman. For the money I am offering, surely there must be a solution for these people. Conditions have always been crowded in Chinatown. What difference will it make if a hundred more families are stuffed into Grant Avenue? As immigrants, they are fortunate to be in America. Even if they are inconvenienced, they will be happy to pay any price to be part of the American dream."

"Mr. Chandler," Madame Lee interjected, "while there are terribly crowded conditions in Chinatown, you miss the point."

My God, Chandler said to himself, *she speaks perfect English. Must have had Catholic education at the Chinatown St. Mary's.*

Madame Lee continued. "The 40,000 people of Chinatown cannot continue to live between Stockton and Kearny, and California and Broadway. They are hard working, loyal Americans. They deserve the opportunity to live in nicer neighborhoods with better schools. It's fine for the wealthy like you, to look on the people of Chinatown as cute, exotic Celestials. The reality is that Chinatown is a slum where people are born, live, work, and die without any hope of escape.

"You want to buy up land that is dear to Chinatown while immigrants arrive every day from Hong Kong whom we cannot accommodate. We don't need your money so much, as we need additional land to take care of our own people."

"Madame Lee," CFO Majestic said, intrigued by the tenor of the discussion. "If it's not money, what may Mr. Chandler offer that will give him what he wants and provide the people of Chinatown what they need."

Such a bleeding heart liberal, Chandler thought. *Maybe, I can close the deal with less money than I was willing to offer.*

"Calphung has done research for me," Madame Lee said. "The Chandler family owns substantial property along Clement Street. I would be willing to trade you my ten parcels for 30 of yours on Clement."

"That's impossible," Chandler said, "Chinese can't buy property outside of Chinatown. It would be scandalous to have your people moving into Clement Street."

"Ten years ago, the California Supreme Court ruled restrictive covenants in deeds illegal," Quock said. "There's no legal reason why Chinese can't move into Clement Street."

"It's ludicrous," Chandler said. "The neighborhood will be angry. Property values will go down. There will be violence."

"Mr. Chandler," Madame Lee said. "I'm offering you Boardwalk for Marvin Gardens. You may lose some votes on Clement Street, but you can take credit for being enlightened, by showing others how you are moving into the 1960's with the welfare of the less fortunate in mind."

"Boardwalk for Marvin Gardens, Mr. Chandler," Calphung echoed. "We can sign the papers this week."

Madame Lee and Calphung were referring to the capitalistic board game, *Monopoly*, where the properties with the greatest value are Boardwalk and Park Place, while Marvin Gardens is one of low value.

"This is too good a deal to pass up, Mr. Chandler," Majestic whispered. "You get the ten parcels you need to build the Pyramid. Your properties on Clement Street are occupied by white trash, middle-class workers who don't vote anyway."

Hoyl nodded in agreement.

"Madame Lee, you are truly an enlightened business woman," WRC said. "The people of Chinatown are fortunate they have such a skilled advocate. We have a deal, Boardwalk for Marvin Gardens."

Turning to Majestic and Hoyl, WRC whispered, "Let's get the hell out of here before she changes her mind and asks for Park Place instead of Marvin Gardens."

43

PARADE OF HORRIBLES

"Professor Scott, is it true you abandoned your illegitimate daughter when she was a baby?"

Flashing bulbs and TV camera lights - a crush of news reporters - wire services, radio, TV, and local media - jostled for position in the hallway of the San Francisco City Hall Courthouse, as Ari Scott and his attorney scurried out the elevator.

"Keep moving, Ari," Mona Morgan said, using her brief case as a battering ram, "don't talk to anyone."

"Miss Morgan, is it true your client will claim temporary insanity as a defense to child abandonment?"

"No comment!" Mona shouted, "Professor Scott will testify on his own behalf." Mona Morgan was dressed conservatively in a black business suit that hid her voluptuous figure.

No need for superficial distractions for the press, she had reasoned.

The number of the press corps covering the child custody trial of *Scott v. Scott* had tripled since Sam Paean's gossip column hinted Marvin Belly planned a parade of famous, powerful witnesses to testify against Ari Scott.

Mona had warned Ari not to be shocked by the circus atmosphere, as Belly had built his by legal reputation by manipulating the press.

Ari and Mona hurried past the media gauntlet to Courtroom 16 of the Honorable Robie Phillips, Judge of the San Francisco Superior Family Law Court. Outside, a knot of reporters huddled around Belly, hanging on his every word. Nearby, stood Cee Cee's father, William Randolph

Chandler and his aide, Lumken.

Behind, a male voice snarled,"Well, well, if it isn't the Great Scott."

Ari stopped, paralyzed by the chill of recognition. It was the dark voice from his past.

Impossible, Ari thought.

The danger from his old nemesis had evaporated when the House Un-American Committee had left the Bay Area for Hollywood. Turning slowly, Ari was shocked to see his ex-wife, Cee Cee, accompanied by the Chairman of HUAC, Congressman Clayborn Muck.

Cee Cee dabbed her eyes with a silk handkerchief and averted looking at Ari.

"This must be your lovely counsel, Miss Morgan," Muck said, doffing his felt hat. "I hear you're quite charming, young lady; but I think you may be in over your head."

"We shall see," Mona said, without rancor.

"Why are you . . .?" Ari stumbled over his words.

"I'm here to offer moral support for the new lady in my life,"Muck said, with a smirk.

"What?" Ari said.

"The Honorable William Randolph Chandler has decided that, since his daughter was single again, Cee Cee should be squired by someone deserving, someone with compatible values, especially political values."

Leaning forward, Muck hissed, "All's fair in love and politics. You stole Sofia from me. Now, I'm getting even by screwing your wife!"

Ari clenched his fist, his face flushed.

"No, Ari," Mona said, grabbing his arm, pushing him into the courtroom. "It's just what that asshole wants you to do in front of the press. Keep cool. We'll be fine."

The gallery was already filled. Ari waived at Anna seated in the front row with Professors Roderick Seakin, Garrick Nelquist and Jacob Aural and his loyal companion Sandy, at his side.

"Thanks for coming," Ari said, patting the dog. "You, too, Sandy."

The courtroom of Judge Robie Phillips was large and airy, with 20 foot ceilings and broad windows overlooking the City Hall Plaza three stories below. Seating capacity exceeded 200. One side was roped off for the press, the other side partially reserved for family and friends, and the remainder filled on a first-come, first-served basis, to the curious. Today, the line of lookie-lou's numbering over a 100, stretched down the hall.

The court staff was in place. Seated at a small oak desk below the Judge's bench was the clerk, a fair-skinned woman with flecks of salt and pepper scattered through her auburn hair. The name plate read: *Clerk Joanne Ferling.* Beside her, the court reporter, Will Hays, straddled a three-legged, stenography machine with a magazine of paper resembling an Army .50 caliber machine gun loaded at the ready. Standing as sentinel was a tall, muscular, bald-headed bailiff wearing a name tag: *TN Phat.*

Mona motioned Ari to sit next to her at the end of the counsel table, shielding him from Marvin Belly's infamous courtroom antics calculated to unnerve opposing counsel and their clients. Belly's law associate, Jacque Citrine, stacking trial books and notes on Belly's side of the table, looked up to cast a dismissive glance at Belly's next conquest.

In contrast, Mona casually produced a single yellow, legal tablet and a fountain pen from her brief case and placed it on the counsel table.

My God, she's cool, Ari thought.

"All rise," bailiff TN Phat announced in a deep baritone voice, "Department 16 of the Superior Court is now in session. Honorable Robie Phillips presiding."

Judge Phillips glided to the bench from his chambers. He was medium height, silver-haired, with twinkly blue eyes.

"Please be seated," TN Phat said.

"Scott versus Scott," Judge Phillips announced, surveying the packed courtroom. "The last time there were this many observers in my courtroom, a tourist had sued San Francisco's famous transvestite, Paulette DuBois, for fraud, claiming Paulette had no business passing himself off as a beautiful woman."

Chuckles rippled through the crowd.

"Would counsel introduce themselves," Judge Phillips said.

Rising, Belly said, "Marvin Belly for the Petitioner, your Honor." Belly wore a silver, metallic suit and a bright red tie. "May I introduce my client, Cecelia Chandler Scott," Belly gestured to his client seated to his left, then added, "Seated behind my client is gubernatorial candidate, the Honorable William Randolph Chandler."

WRC stood, nodded at Judge Phillips, and waved to the gallery, as if he were on the campaign trail.

"Mr. Belly," Judge Phillips said, "This is the first time I've seen you in Family Law Court. Are you contemplating a career change?"

"No, your Honor," Belly said unctuously, "the opportunity to try a case before this Court, with its esteemed reputation for fairness, was too good to turn down."

"Counsel, you may wish to reserve your judgment until after my decision," Judge Phillips said, with a smile. "Opposing counsel?"

Mona rose slowly, knowing her presence drew scrutiny, as she was not only one of a handful of female attorneys in San Francisco, but also by far, the most attractive.

"Mona Morgan for the Respondent, your Honor," she spoke slowly, evenly. "May I present my client, Professor Aristotle Scott."

"It's a pleasure, counsel. Your reputation for skillful advocacy precedes you." Judge Phillips said.

"Opening statement, Mr. Belly?"

"Your Honor," Belly rose and paced leisurely behind Mona and Ari. "The overwhelming weight of the evidence will show Professor Scott is unfit for child visitation rights. We will introduce unimpeachable testimony that he has demonstrated a lifetime of uncaring, callous, profligate behavior, a repetitive pattern that will only inflict irreparable harm to Mrs. Chandler's children, Marc and Monique."

Ari clasped his hands tightly, trying to control his anger.

Lies, lies, Ari thought.

Belly continued. "Professor Scott has distinguished himself in books and teachings with a philosophical doctrine he calls the Higher Truth. But in the judicial spotlight of truth, the evidence will show Professor Scott has not lived up to his so-called Higher Truth, but instead has been a sleazy hypocrite and an out-and-out fraud. The evidence will clearly show that Professor Scott's left-wing, political beliefs will only poison the impressionable, young minds of the children."

The gallery whispered, smelling blood.

Judge Phillips wrapped his gavel twice. "Order in the Courtroom. Outbursts will be not be tolerated. The bailiff is instructed to remove anyone disrupting the orderly progress of this proceeding. Miss Morgan, your opening statement?"

Mona rose and said in a firm, clear voice, "We waive opening statement, your Honor."

A muted murmur swept the courtroom.

Ari turned toward Mona, a look of shock on his face.

We're not going to challenge those untruths? We're going to roll over and let Marvin Belly stomp on us?

Mona put a forefinger to her lips, *shhh'ing* Ari into silence.

"Very well, Miss Morgan" Judge Phillips said. "Your prerogative. First witness, Mr. Belly?"

"I call Petitioner, Mrs. Cecelia Chandler Scott," Belly said, ushering Cee Cee sniffling and red-eyed to the stand.

As Clerk Joanne Ferling administered the oath, Ari saw before him the slightly older version of the wholesome, striking Gee Dee who had pursued "the Great Scott" during graduate school - a girl born of rank raised in the tradition of the Chandler family who never took "no" for an answer.

Cee Cee was still thin, with honey- colored hair and finely chiseled cheek bones. She was dressed in basic black and pearls accented with black high heels and a wide-brimmed black hat. She was dressed to attend a funeral . . . Ari's funeral.

Cee Cee reeked of privilege, and Ari acknowledged, as he sat in this temple of judicial truth, that a great deal of Cee Cee's appeal had been the power and prestige of the Chandler family.

"Mrs. Scott," Belly intoned mellifluously. "Please tell the Court about the qualities you *thought* your husband stood for when you married him."

"I always thought Ari believed in truth and virtue," Cee Cee said softly, looking downcast. "I thought we were raising our two children with those values, but that was before I learned . . ." She began to weep.

"The Court understands your sadness, Mrs. Scott," Belly said, rising and surveying the gallery with a look of utmost sincerity. "Was there a specific incident that changed your mind about him?"

"Yes," Cee Cee said, raising her head and staring at Ari. "When he told me he had fathered an illegitimate child and wanted ME to accept his BASTARD as a member of OUR family." She dabbed away her tears. "I'm sorry, your Honor, I didn't mean to use street language."

Wonderful, just the way we rehearsed it, Belly thought, glancing at the gallery, surveying the effect of Cee Cee's testimony.

"Why did this suggestion disturb you, Mrs. Scott?" Belly asked.

"That's not the way I was raised, and my husband knew it all the time we were courting." Cee Cee's voice gained strength. "Truth and virtue are the hallmarks of the Chandler family. If I had known he had fathered a child out-of-wedlock, I would have NEVER married him. How can we teach our children truth and virtue, if their father has lived a terrible lie all his adult life. I fear his corrupting influence on the children will lead to dire consequences," she sobbed.

Belly paused, counting five to himself, maximizing the sympathetic impact Cee Cee's outburst had on the crowd.

"No further questions," Belly said. "Your witness, counsel."

Don't come across as a ball-busting bitch. Mona told herself.

"Mrs. Scott," Mona said softly, "I want to make sure I understand the reason you feel your husband has been untruthful and lacking in virtue. As I interpret your testimony, truth and virtue were the central values of your Chandler upbringing?"

"Yes, truth and virtue," Cee Cee said.

"You used the phrase, 'hallmark' values, is that correct, Mrs. Scott," Mona said.

"Yes," Cee Cee sniffled.

Mona asked, raising her voice, "And any words and acts that are anything less than truthful and virtuous have no place in your family, is that true?"

"Yes, that's what I meant."

"No further questions," Mona said.

By clarifying Cee Cee's testimony, my own lawyer has pushed the dagger even deeper, Ari thought. *Maybe, I should have accepted Belly's settlement offer.*

"Next witness, Mr. Belly?" Judge Phillips said.

"Petitioner calls the distinguished Congressman, the Honorable Clayborn Muck!"

"Objection, your Honor!" Mona said, springing to her feet. "This witness cannot offer any expert testimony shedding light on my client's fitness as a parent."

"Congressman Muck is not testifying as an expert witness, your Honor," Belly said smoothly. "He is testifying as a percipient witness."

"Objection overruled. The clerk will swear the witness."

Ari watched Clayborn Muck take the stand. Muck had aged gracefully, befitting someone born and bred a Boston Brahmin. He was short, but had maintained his taut, powerful build. Muck wore an ingrained smile, a perpetual grin that prompted one political pundit to describe him as "the smiling pit bull."

"Congressman Muck," Belly began, hooking his thumbs under his suspenders. "Do you know Professor Scott?"

"Yes," Muck said. "As young men, we were teammates on the US Olympic track and field team of 1936. We both ran the metric mile."

"In your capacity as an Olympian, Congressman," Belly said, "did you personally see Professor Scott in and about the Olympic Village?"

"Yes," Muck said, a look of innocence on his face. "It was difficult not to see Ari Scott around the Olympic Village. He spent all his free time chasing a young, teenage Italian swimmer." Muck's voice hardened. "Her name was Sofia Cappuccino, the most beautiful girl at the Olympics. She was as pure as the driven snow until Ari Scott preyed on her innocence, then seduced and ravaged her!" Muck shouted, burying his face into his hands.

The crowd, waiting for dramatic theater, hissed.

"Objection!" Mona shouted. "Move to strike."

"Order!" Judge Phillips said, pounding his gavel. "Congressman, I will strike that last remark, unless you are willing to testify that you witnessed Professor committing the acts you just described."

"I didn't actually see it," Muck said, "but everyone knew what Ari Scott did."

"You are entitled to your feelings, Congressman," Judge Phillips said, "but, since you didn't witness the acts, I'm going to sustain the objection."

"We will prove that fact through another witness," Belly said, nonchalantly. "Your witness, counsel."

Mona walked a few steps to the right of Ari so Muck would be looking in the direction of the press corps. She had learned Muck had a temper that he could not always control, a habit she now hoped to exploit.

The gallery listened intently, as Mona began her cross- examination of the Chairman of the House Un-American Activities Committee.

"Congressman, isn't it true, you had a personal infatuation with Sofia Cappuccino?" Mona said.

"Well, I imagine every red-blooded young man felt something for this lovely creature," Muck said, squirming noticeably.

"But, Congressman, isn't it true you actively competed for the attention, if not the affection, of Sophia Cappuccino?"

"Well, I did . . .like her. She was captivating." His face reddened.

Mona said in an accusatory tone, "ISN'T IT TRUE, Congressman, you became angry and bitter when Sofia Cappuccino chose Professor Scott, over you, as her boyfriend?"

Muck's face turned beet red, as he said under his breath, "I admit, I was a bit disappointed."

"I didn't hear that response, Congressman. Would you repeat your answer?" Mona said in a loud tone.

Muck glowered at Mona, spitting the words out a second time. "I SAID . . . I was a BIT disappointed."

Mona leaned forward and said, in a sarcastic tone, "a BIT disappointed, Congressman? ISN'T IT TRUE you swore revenge on Ari Scott for winning the heart of Sofia Cappuccino?"

Muck sat for several seconds, seething, before he said, in a controlled tone, "Revenge is not the same as disappointment, counsel. NO! I did not swear revenge on your client."

Mona paused for several seconds, allowing Muck's face to turn from scarlet to ashen, then sat down. "No more questions, your Honor."

Ari leaned over and whispered, "We're getting crucified. Should we throw in the towel before things get worse?"

"Be patient, Ari" Mona whispered . "We'll have our turn."

"Mr. Belly," Judge Phillips said, "may we have your next witness?

"Yes, Petitioner calls Professor Werner Von Seller," Belly said.

The Prussian Penguin, dressed in a black suit, white shirt, and black patten leather shoes, waddled up to the witness stand, bowed to Judge Phillips and was sworn by Clerk Joanne Ferling.

"Professor Von Seller, you were part of the American scientific team that developed the atomic bomb that ended the War, is that not true?" Belly said.

"I would not be truthful if I denied it," Von Seller said, smiling. "I am proud to say I helped develop the atomic bomb."

"Professor, you are the Director of the Cyclotron exploring new ways to protect our national security, are you not?"

"I believe my efforts are contributing to world peace, yes." Von Seller said, now glowing with confidence.

"Our future Governor of California, William Randolph Chandler, has asked you to oversee the new publish or perish program at Cal ?" Belly asked.

"Er," Von Seller coughed, "Counsel, it is the Regents, NOT the

Honorable William Randolph Chandler who has asked me to administer this patriotic program."

"My apologies, Professor," Belly said, recovering from his gaffe. "I mis-spoke."

No one was supposed to know that publish or perish was the brainchild of William Randolph Chandler.

"With your history of patriotic contribution to our country and to your university, have you formed an opinion about the patriotism of Professor Aristotle Scott?" Belly said.

"Objection, not relevant," Mona said, in a shrill voice. "This hearing is not about patriotism, your Honor."

"I agree, Miss Morgan," Judge Phillips said softly, "but I'm going to allow it, reserving your right to move the Court to strike this testimony later. Professor Von Seller, you may answer."

The Prussian Penguin had waited for this moment and intended to savor it. Von Seller squinted his monocle into his eye.

"In my view, Professor Scott has done irreparable damage to the cause of freedom and scientific research with his opposition to such patriotic ideas as loyalty oaths and publish or perish," Von Seller said. "If allowed to poison the minds of his children with such insidious thoughts, they will be brainwashed into thinking JUST LIKE HIM!" Von Seller pointed an accusing finger at Ari Scott.

"Your witness," Belly said, sitting, feeling satisfied with the way the testimony was going.

Mona did not afford Von Seller the respect of standing.

"Professor Von Seller," Mona said cooly, " Isn't it true you have no formal training in child psychology?"

"Yes, but you don't have to . . ."

"And you've never had children of your own," Mona said.

"That's also true, Miss Morgan, but . . ."

"So your so-called expertise on patriotism is limited to your observations and experiences with adults?"

"Objection!" Belly said, rising. "Argumentative, mis-characterizes the witness's testimony. Counsel is badgering the witness."

"Let me ask it this way," Mona said, now standing. "For the sake of discussion, let's assume you are an expert on patriotism. Isn't it true that the totality of your experience has been limited to adults?"

"Well, I would disagree. . ." Von Seller stammered.

"A SIMPLE yes or no?" Mona demanded.

"I'm instructing Professor Von Seller NOT to answer yes or no!" Belly shouted. "The witness may answer any way he desires."

"He's not your client," Mona snapped, glowering at Belly. "You can't instruct him how to answer."

"Enough! " Judge Phillips said, pounding his gavel. "Counsel will both conduct their examinations in a professional, courteous manner or face sanctions. Do you understand?"

Belly and Mona nodded.

"Professor Von Seller, you may answer yes or no and offer an explanation," Judge Phillips said.

"I believe you understand the question," Mona continued.

"The answer is no. What I wanted to say, Miss Morgan, is that I have had years of experience with students, many still in their impressionable youth. I have witnessed student values and ideas corrupted by faculty members with left-wing political views, like Aristotle Scott. These leftists have spent a lifetime manipulating young minds. If this can happen to young adults, it is only logical that it is going to happen to young children."

"Professor Von Seller," Mona paused, then asked in an incredulous tone, "Are you accusing Professor Scott of treason?"

"Treason is an extreme word, Miss Morgan," Von Seller removed his monocle and cleaned it with his tie and said. "I think Professor Scott is less than patriotic."

" 'Less than patriotic?' " Mona asked, moving directly behind Ari "That's an odd term, Professor Von Seller. Would you accuse anyone who disagrees with you of being 'less patriotic'?"

"Of course, it would depend on the issue, Miss Morgan;" Von Seller said, reinserting the monocle. "But, if you're talking about matters of public importance, like loyalty oaths and publish or perish, the answer is YES!"

"Professor Von Seller," Mona said, in a clear voice, "you've formed your opinion about publish or perish based on your INDEPENDENT and UNBIASED analysis?"

"Why, yes." Von Seller said, "I pride myself in making up my own mind, FREE FROM OUTSIDE INFLUENCES, of being OBJECTIVE on all the great issues of the day."

"Thank you, Professor," Mona said, winking at Ari.

What does she have up her sleeve? Ari wondered. *So far every witness has hammered another nail into my coffin!*

"We will reconvene after the afternoon recess," Judge Phillips said, striking his gavel.

Suddenly, the gallery buzzed with recognition of the broad, stocky figure looming just inside the courtroom door. Diminutive, *Sentinel* reporter, Jani Kay Fong, burrowed her way to the front of the crush of reporters engulfing the new arrival.

"Here comes the heavy artillery Sam Paean promised," Mona said, directing Ari's attention toward the door.

Oh, my God, Ari thought, staring at Belly's star witness.

The new arrival had a burly build with dark, slicked-back hair and bushy eyebrows. He wore a white panama hat, a three-piece all-white suit, white shoes, white shirt, and a royal blue tie and matching royal blue kerchief peeking from his jacket, breast pocket. His companion was younger, taller, matinee-idol handsome with slick-backed, dark hair. He too was dressed in an all-white suit contrasted with a red tie and matching red kerchief in his breast pocket.

For years, Belly's star witness's picture had been prominently displayed in magazines and newspapers all over the world. He was more than a celebrity, he was a living legend. He was the Director of the Federal Bureau of Investigation, the FBI, none other than J. Edgar Hoover accompanied by his assistant and constant companion, Clyde Tolson!

* * * *

"Next witness, Mr. Belly," Judge Phillips said, reconvening the hearing after the noon recess.

"Petitioner calls the EMINENT federal law enforcement officer, that PATRIOTIC crime fighter, J. EDGAR HOOVER," Belly said.

Belly sounds like a circus barker, Ari thought. *What could the Director of the FBI add to this hearing?*

Ari stared intently at the legendary G-Man. J. Edgar Hoover was not as tall as he appeared in photographs, but, up close, his scowl was wore frightening, more intimidating.

"Welcome, Mr. Hoover," Judge Phillips said.

"Judge Phillips, it is my pleasure to testify anywhere to keep the streets of America free of Communist scum."

"Objection," Mona shouted, jumping to her feet.

"Sustained," Judge Phillips said. "Mr. Hoover, your reputation as an anti-Communist patriot is renown, but you must confine your remarks to questions asked by counsel."

"Sure, Judge," Hoover said.

Members of the press corps listened intently, poised to record every word of the famous crime fighter.

"Mr. Hoover," Belly began, "does the FBI maintains dossiers or files on all suspicious persons in the world?"

"Yes, we do." Hoover said.

"How long has the FBI maintained such files?" Belly asked.

"I instituted most of the programs since the War," Hoover said proudly, "but we've got OSS records as far back as the early 1930's."

"On behalf of Mrs. Scott, did I ask you to search your files for any information concerning Professor Aristotle Scott?" Belly said, rising.

"Yes, you did," Hoover said, snapping open his worn, leather brief case, producing a crinkled, vanilla file. "I have the file here."

"Would you please describe the contents of that file?" Belly said.

Mona and Belly moved toward the witness stand.

"There are three groups of photos," Hoover said, holding the first. "These are a little faded, but they were taken after the '36 Olympics showing Professor Scott and his Commie girl friend cavorting through Europe."

"Objection," Mona said, viewing the photos.

"Sustained," Judge Phillips said, "Mr. Hoover, I'm instructing you to refrain from volunteering your opinions unless asked to give them."

Mona handed Ari the discolored, ancient photos.

They were black and white photographs, each taken at a different stop in the *toure di amore* Ari had shared with Sofia so long ago . They depicted Ari and Sofia smiling before the Coliseum in Rome; walking a beach on the Italian Riviera; sharing a gondola along the canals of Venice; standing before the Uffizi in Florence; and holding hands at the Duomo in Milan.

"Was there a reason the FBI kept tabs on Professor Scott?" Belly asked.

Hoover turned and spoke directly at Judge Phillips. "Initially, we were suspicious about his girl friend and her family, the Cappuccinos," the FBI Director said, arching his thick eyebrows.

"Why were you concerned about the Cappuccinos?" Belly asked.

"The family had made a fortune from their coffee invention, eh, what do you call it?" Hoover asked.

"The Cappuccino machine?" Belly said.

"Yes," Hoover said. "That's it. The FBI thought this might be a left-wing scheme to siphon money from companies selling good old, All-American cup-a java, right here in the States."

"What is this second group of photos?" Belly said.

"These are a better quality," Hoover explained, "taken after the War. They show Miss Cappuccino and her daughter in the company of a young, Italian Communist, Pablo Zarzana."

"What was your concern about Zarzana, Mr. Hoover?" Belly said.

"That he might foment revolution, that he and his Communist party might take over the government. Italy was very vulnerable after the War," Hoover intoned.

"Finally, what is the third group of photos," Belly said, pointing.

"These are the best quality, taken last year," Hoover said, a hint of smugness in his voice. "These photos show how pervasive Pablo Zarzana's influence has become, even in our country." Holding up an enlarged black and white photograph, Hoover said, "In this shot, he's posing with some United States Senators."

Mona glanced at the last batch of photos. There, standing next to Pablo Zarzana was her secret lover, Fitz!

For a moment, Mona was overwhelmed by a sense of nausea. She and Fitz had gone to great lengths to keep their affair secret.

How shockingly ironic that, in the middle of the most important case of my career, Fitz's handsome image appears as part of a trial exhibit!

Mona looked up at Hoover. The Director was half smiling, half smirking.

Does Hoover know about Fitz and me? The FBI was legendary for their surveillance activities. Had she and Fitz been caught on film?

Don't panic, Mona told herself, reciprocating with a forced smile.

"Why do you still maintain this dossier on Professor Scott," Belly continued.

"In my view, the world-wide Communist conspiracy continues from one generation to another. Along the way, it sucks others into its web.

Many don't even know they're pawns of this vast, diabolical plot to take over the world." Hoover snarled.

"Here, you have the Cappuccinos," Hoover extended his left hand, palm up. "The daughter takes up with Professor Scott, has an illegitimate child by him, then later marries Zarzana," he said holding his right hand, palm up.

"Scott returns to teach at Cal and worms his way into the patriotic family of William Randolph Chandler by marrying his daughter, Cee Cee. Then, lo and behold, Professor Scott's love child by his old girl friend 'happens' to enroll at Cal. At the same time, Scott becomes the ring leader of the faculty opposing loyalty oaths and publish or perish. These events are TOO coincidental to be an accident."

Hoover clapped both his hands together. "This is part of the global Communist conspiracy!" he shouted.

Loud murmurs echoed through the courtroom.

"Order," Judge Phillips said, rapping his gavel. "The bailiff will remove everyone who continues to be disrupt this courtroom, and I shall cite them for contempt."

Buoyed by the FBI Director's testimony, Belly bowed and said, "your witness, counsel."

Don't lose your composure, Mona told herself. *Don't appear weak.*

Mona inhaled deeply and approached the legendary FBI Director, J. Edgar Hoover.

"Director," Mona began quietly, "you testified the Cappuccinos have been under suspicion for years."

Hoover nodded, "Yes."

"Isn't it true that, during the War, Mussolini imprisoned the Cappuccinos for being capitalistic traitors?" Mona said.

"Technically, that's true," Hoover said, squinting at Mona, "but the FBI concluded the only reason the Cappuccinos were locked up was they didn't give Mussolini a big enough cut of the profits from their coffee machine."

"From your experience, Director," Mona said cooly, "if it were just a question of money, wouldn't it have been easier for the Cappuccinos to pay Mussolini more money to avoid spending years in prison?"

"You may have a point, Miss, but I think history has validated our theory," Hoover said, rolling his eyes.

"Director," Mona said, moving directly behind Ari. "You seem to place great importance on the fact that Sofia Cappuccino had two well-known men in her life - Professor Scott and Pablo Zarzana - correct?"

"Yes, Miss," Hoover leaned forward, arching his thick brows. "When a woman takes up with not one, but two important men, I think we have to question her intentions."

"Do you believe in love, Mr. Hoover?'

"I, er, . . . yes, but I've never been married," Hoover said, looking uncomfortable. He glanced at his companion, Clyde Tolson, standing at the rear of the courtroom.

"But would you accept the notion that one woman, especially a beautiful and charismatic woman like Sofia Cappuccino, could have two different loves in her life?"

"I wouldn't know, counsel," Hoover said, regaining his composure, "but, I think the strong, moral fibre of America was built on the idea that there is only one woman for one man. When Sofia Cappuccino took up with one man, had his bastard child, then took up with another man, a Communist who helped raise that child, there is definitely something WRONG!"

"I gather, Mr. Hoover," Mona said, leaning toward the witness, "you feel it is not only wrong, but this is part of the insidious world-wide, Communist conspiracy?"

"I couldn't have said it better myself, Miss." Hoover said, clasping his hands, in victory.

"If Mr. Belly has no other questions or witnesses," Mona said, "I would ask the Court to adjourn these proceedings for the weekend. On Monday, we will present Respondent's case."

"Any objections, Mr. Belly?" Judge Phillips asked.

"None at all, your Honor." Belly said, smiling broadly. "I am sure everyone in this courtroom looks forward, with great anticipation, to whatever evidence and testimony Miss Morgan intends to present."

"The Court will be adjourned until Monday morning at 9 a.m.," Judge Phillips said.

* * * *

Mona Morgan exited the Western Union office, near the City Hall Superior Court. She had sent the telegram in the code she shared with her lover, Fitz.

It read:

> "FITZ: (stop)
> Emergency!   (stop)
> Derailed train! (stop)
> Please call!   (stop)
>
> - M.M."

Fitz, my darling, Mona thought. *You've got to come through for me. Ari's future with his children depend on it.*

44

FAMILY TREE

"Wow, absolutely stunning!" Joan Dildeaux said, "Just as beautiful as Jennifer Jones in *'Love Is A Many Splendored Thing.'* How can Madame Lee not be impressed?"

Kate Howell made a graceful turn in her new outfit, a Chinese *cheong sam,* a form-fitting silk dress with high collar and daring side slits extending well above the knee. The baby-blue color of the full length dress was a perfect match with Kate's eyes, and Joan had rolled Kate's long, blond hair up into a "beehive" accented with two, protruding chopsticks painted a matching blue.

"I hope she'll like me," Kate sighed.

"Don't worry, roomie. She'll love you."

Two weeks ago, Casey mentioned that his grandma, Madame Lee, would like to meet his "dear friend," Kate.

"That would be wonderful, Casey," Kate had cooed, "when?"

"Grandma said, 'as soon as possible,' which usually means yesterday," he winked. "But there's a catch."

"What's the catch?"

"She wants to talk to you alone," Casey said.

"Probably just girl talk," Kate said, with confidence, recalling her pleasant, summer, week-end visits with Crazy Aunt Martha at the Peaceful Valley Old Folks Home.

Kate, Joan, and Muffy had shopped Chinatown's Grant Avenue for something appropriate to wear, deciding the baby blue *cheong sam* not only fit Kate perfectly, but also added a nice, *Chinese touch* to her audience with Madame Lee.

Borrowing Rod Organ's ex-cab, Casey drove Kate across the Bay Bridge and parked the woodie in the Portsmouth Square garage near Kearny. Ironically, this street in Chinatown was named after an Irishman who led violent anti-Chinese riots in the 1800's.

"I'll show you the scenic route," Casey said.

Kate slipped her arm through Casey's as they moved through the throngs of jostling, Saturday Chinatown shoppers.

The air was heavy with the pungent mix of salty, sour, sweet, bitter, and burnt aromas. Along Grant Avenue, two-way traffic was held hostage by a teeming mass of humanity, oblivious to honking car horns. Several men greeted Casey with bows, some shook hands with enthusiasm. Elder women waved at Casey. Others, chattering in the cacophony of Cantonese, pointed and nodded toward the exotic sight of the blond *lo fahn* girl wearing traditional Chinese dress.

"Everyone knows you," Kate smiled.

"Everyone knows Grandma," Casey said. "I'm only Madame Lee's lowly grandson."

The couple passed stacks of cages filled with braying animals and crates of exotic shaped fruits and vegetables lining storefront sidewalks. Tanks of live fish and hooks of freshly cooked poultry filled restaurant windows. They followed the series of alleys above Grant Avenue, each one more narrow than the last; then through a fortune cookie factory; past several courtyards and small walk ways; eventually climbing several flights of stairs at the rear of an unassuming building.

Casey rapped rhythmically on a black, lacquered double door with shiny brass trim. The two were admitted by a stern young Chinese man wearing a shoulder holster and pistol, who nodded deferentially to Casey. Behind was a smiling moon-faced man speaking in a clipped British accent.

"Casey, old chap, so good to see you. And this must be your dear friend, Kate."

Casey introduced Kate to his grandma's aide, Calphung Quock, who bowed and shook her hand formally.

"Right this way, young lady, Madame Lee is waiting."

"Calphung will escort you out," Casey said, backing out the door. "Take your time. I'll be waiting downstairs."

Calphung led Kate through a room with the glass cupola and a raised dais into a smaller living room, with luxurious white carpeting, filled with Chinese teak and burnished antiques. The air was redolent with jasmine.

"Madame Lee, may I present Miss Kate Howell," Calphung said, motioning Kate toward the stylishly coiffed, silver-haired woman whose back was to the arrivals.

As Kate bowed politely, she glimpsed Madame Lee's exquisite blood red *cheong sam* with gold embroidery.

Am I glad I'm wearing something Chinese, Kate thought.

Turning, Madame Lee smiled and extended her hand. She perused Kate's *cheong sam* and said, "What a lovely color, my dear. You look absolutely stunning."

Looking up, Kate was startled. Standing before her was a slender, small boned woman in her mid-sixties, with silver hair, fair skin, high cheek bones, and clear, steely blue eyes.

Casey's grandma, Madame Lee, looked like a typical patrician, Caucasian grandmother from her home town of San Marino.

"But, you don't look . . ." Kate stammered, suddenly at a loss for words.

"My dear," Madame Lee said, with an assuring smile. "I believe you started to say . . . 'you don't look Chinese.' "

"I apologize, Madame Lee." Kate said, recovering her composure, "I didn't mean to be rude."

"I may not *look* Chinese," Madame Lee said, "but I assure you, I *am* Chinese *in heart and soul.*" She ushered Kate to two ebony high-backed chairs with inlaid pearl.

As Madame Lee poured Kate a cup of *oolong* tea, she said, "One of the reasons I wanted to meet you was to tell you about my family and indirectly, about Casey."

Madame Lee told Kate her story.

I was born in The City, the only daughter of a Pacific Heights family. When I arrived, my three brothers were already teenagers, attending private school. Wealthy San Francisco families had Chinese servants living in the basements of their mansions known as "the Chinaman's room." Our servant, Chong Lee, was hired as a young teenager and was treated as part of the family, almost a fourth son. Chong was quite modern thinking, dressing in western fashion, and one of the first servants in San Francisco to give up the traditional pig tail queue.

It was the time of the Chinese Exclusion Act. Chinese women were not permitted to enter the country. Chong had worked for us over ten years and wanted to return to China with his savings and marry. My family didn't want to lose their valued servant, so my father used his influence to allow Chong to bring a "picture bride," an arranged fiancee, to San Francisco. Her name was Ming, a pretty teenager with bound feet. The two were married in our family living room, and Ming became Chong's helper moving into the "Chinaman's room" in the basement.

The Lees had a son, Gim, born the same year as I. My family gave Gim the English name, James; and Jim and I were raised like brother and sister.

The Lees who called me "Missy Ah-Bay," my given name was Abigail, let me help them prepare meals, join them on neighborhood strolls, and accompany them to Chinatown for grocery shopping.

In the late 1800's, girls weren't expected to attend school; but my mother insisted I receive private tutoring, so a retired school marm, Miss Jilly Telfird, came to our house for home schooling. Since the Lees were considered family, Jim was allowed to sit in on my tutoring; and Miss Telfird tutored the two of us between the ages five and 17. I must admit Jim was much better at math, science, and proper English than I.

We had a wonderful, carefree childhood learning and playing. When my parents were away, I would sneak down to the Lees's "Chinaman's room;" and Jim and I would play Chinese games like Mah Jong and Pai Gow. I even learned to speak Cantonese.

When we were young teenagers, Jim told me about his parents' hosting a Chinatown meeting for a very important man from China, a young revolutionary who visited Chinese communities throughout California raising money to overthrow the Manchu Dynasty. His name was Dr. Sun Yat Sen who later became the "George Washington of China."

At 17, something wonderful happened. Jim and I fell in love. It was also something impossible, unfathomable, as California law did not permit marriage between Caucasians and members of "the Mongolian race." When I told my parents, my father was shocked and angry. I recall him shouting, "See what happens when you treat these people as equals?" My mother was more sanguine, assuring me that I would forget my "silly, little infatuation," when I met eligible boys of "my own kind." My parents gave the Lees an ultimatum, choose between their jobs and their son.

The night before Jim was to move to Sacramento to live with a cousin, we decided to elope. Looking back, that was terribly romantic, but totally impractical. We couldn't stay in California. Where could we go?

Intrigued by Madame Lee's story, Kate said, "Let me guess. You went to China?"

"Oh, my dear," Madame Lee said, squeezing Kate's hands. "I see why Casey likes you so. You have such an adventuresome spirit! Yes, we decided to join Sun Yat Sen's revolution against the Manchu Dynasty!"

Madame Lee continued her story.

Miss Telfird helped me withdraw money from my trust fund; and we bribed the purser of China Clipper Lines to take us across the Pacific.

The ocean voyage was incredibly romantic. The Captain of the Clipper was Harry Freelander, a second-generation, China hand who befriended us. At each stop, Harry escorted us ashore and showed us the sites. We visited Old Honolulu before there were any high rises on Waikiki. Harry took us through Kowloon and Hong Kong Island when the British colony was still a sleepy little port. Jim and I spent days at sea, holding hands in the sun of the blue Pacific, talking about our future in China.

When we arrived in Shanghai, we were shocked at how awful women were treated, especially a lo fahn who was the "concubine" of an American-born Chinese. We made our way, by ox-cart and mule, joining Dr. Sun Yat Sen and his ragtag band of revolutionaries who were battling the Manchu army. Dr. Sun Yat Sen remembered Jim, the son of the San Francisco Lees who raised money for his cause. He commissioned Jim as Captain, and I worked with women tending the wounded.

When I learned I was pregnant, Dr. Sun arranged for an American missionary to marry us and, later that year, we were blessed with a son, Ock, whom we gave the English name, Errol.

Dr. Sun's revolution was successful. For the next two decades, Jim and I continued to serve Dr. Sun, helping to establish the Chinese Republic, the first democratic government in the thousands of years of Chinese history. During that time, our son, Errol, fell in love and married a lovely young woman, Low, a niece of Dr. Sun.

When Japan invaded China in the late Thirties, Jim and Errol joined the guerillas helping American General Clare Chennault and his Flying Tigers fight the Japanese. When the Imperial Army committed barbaric atrocities against civilians, especially women, in the Rape of Nanking, Jim and Errol feared for my safety and, with the help of our old China Clipper friend, Captain Harry Freelander, I returned to San Francisco.

It was 1939. I had been gone for almost 30 -years.

I returned to The City exhausted and dirty, dressed like a Chinese peasant woman. My brothers refused to see me. In their eyes, I had renounced my family and my race. I was as good as dead. My father had died after the market crash of 1929; but my mother, who was now gravely ill, had set aside my share of Daddy's inheritance, hoping I would some day return. Before passing away, Mother instructed the family's attorneys - Parent David Saint Christine Powell & Diane - to quietly disburse me my inheritance.

"Even with money, where could you live?" Kate asked, understanding Madame Lee's quandary. "You had married outside your race, against your parents' wishes, and had been gone for most of your life."

"Yes, my child," Madame Lee said. "Having money did not mean I could suddenly start a new life, so I decided to live with the people I felt most comfortable with."

"The Chinese." Kate said, feeling enormous empathy for this incredibly courageous woman.

"Yes, I moved to Chinatown," Madame Lee said. "My in-laws, the Lees, had retired and moved to a flat on Grant Avenue. They helped me find a suitable place for their 'Missy Ah-Bay,' and I have been here ever since. At first, the locals, especially men, were suspicious of me; but over time, my dedication to the welfare of the people of Chinatown has earned begrudging respect. But there is still a strong resentment among some, because of my race."

Madame Lee continued her story.

*Later, I learned my husband, Jim, had died fighting the Japanese.
Our son, Errol, and his wife, Low, had a son born to them in 1940.
They named my grandson, Kai See whom you know as "Casey." After
the War, I desperately wanted the three of them to come to America;
but Errol wrote that he and Low's future lay in China. During the
terrible civil war between the armies of Chairman Mao Tse Tung and
Generalissimo Chiang Kai-Shek, Errol and Low refused to take sides
and were ostracized by both the Nationalists and Communists. With
the help of General Chennault's friends, Errol and Low smuggled
Casey out of China before they were arrested and executed by the
Communists for being "enemies of the People's Republic."*

Kate felt a knot forming in her throat.
Madame Lee has endured so much heartache, in the name of love,
she thought.
Changing the subject, Kate asked, "Why do you keep armed guards?
Are you concerned about your ties to Dr. Sun Yat Sen?"
"It's Calphung's idea. I'm not worried about Communists. Very few
people know my history," Madame Lee said. "But Calphung believes
that my work on behalf of the people of Chinatown is important enough
to merit protection. Chinatown is a very patriarchal society. Some have
not welcomed my efforts to help women, children, and the poor."
Madame Lee refilled their tea cups with fresh *oolong.*
Kate looked at the calm, dignified woman who did not outwardly bear
the scars of her traumatic life. *What would I have done in Madame
Lee's place?* Kate thought.
"Actually," Madame Lee said, with a slight smile. "Members of my
birth family are more distressed about my return than anyone in
Chinatown. If revealed, my identity could be embarrassing."
". . . and your maiden name was . . .?" Kate asked.
"My surname is well known to you, my dear," Madame Lee said,
pausing. "My family name is Krum. I was born Abigail Krum."
"The same family name as Dirk Krum III?" Kate said.
"Dirk's grandfather, Dirk Krum I, was my eldest brother."
"That means," Kate gasped. "Casey and Dirk are cousins!"
Dirk's hatred of Casey was more than racial prejudice, Kate

thought. *No matter how superior Dirk felt, no matter how dismissive he was of Casey, he could not escape the fact Casey Lee, leader of the detested Dormies, traced his bloodline to the same Krum great-grandfather.*

"My dear," Madame Lee said, "The more important reason I wanted to meet you is because I am concerned you and Casey are becoming too serious."

"I think the world of your grandson, Madame Lee."

"I don't question your feelings, Kate; but I must warn you of the hardships you two will face." Madame Lee said.

"But it's been 50-years since you and Casey's grandfather . . ." Kate said. "The 1960's will be a different time and place."

"Your youthful idealism is wonderful," Madame Lee said, "but your romance faces terrible odds. It has only been a few years since California abolished the law prohibiting interracial marriage. Unfortunately, such unions generate hatred and misunderstanding. Society still has problems dealing with matters of race. True, the Sixties are upon us, but people are not accustomed to exotic couplings.

"Marriage will require you to turn your back on everything familiar and comforting. Casey tells me your family is socially prominent in Los Angeles. Will your parents tolerate your dating, much less marrying, someone who resembles their gardener? Will they accept bronze-toned grandchildren who have almond eyes? Are you willing to give up your family's love for my grandson?"

"But you made that same choice, Madame Lee."

"I would not have traded my life for anything else in the world, my dear;" Madame Lee said softly. "But I chose to become Chinese and live in China. You two don't have that same option."

"I can see why Casey is so taken with you," Madame Lee said, "You are lovely, intelligent, and sensitive. He cares a great deal about you, probably more than he has expressed, but I don't want my grandson hurt by someone who may be smitten merely because he is different or exotic."

"When Casey was young," Madame Lee said, "I sent him away to private school in Carmel. I wanted to shield him from problems my husband and I had faced. Casey enjoyed an uncomplicated childhood where race was never an issue. His private education fooled him into believing he was a typical, All-American boy. Until he enrolled at Cal, the so-called bastion of liberality, he was sheltered from the problems of race. How ironic that his first encounter with prejudice would be from his own cousin, Dirk Krum!"

"Looking back, private school was a mistake. Casey would have had a better sense of reality had I sent him to public high school with all the Italian kids from North Beach."

"Do you see why I worry about Casey and you? Should you become serious and marry, life will not be as simple as mine."

"Yes, Madame Lee," Kate said. "but my feelings for Casey are much deeper than infatuation."

"Good, then my conscience is clear," Madame Lee said, rising, signaling an end to their meeting. "I've babbled on much too long."

They embraced, clinging to each other tightly, separated by a half century of experiences but joined by the object of their mutual affection.

"Calphung will escort you to the street," Madame Lee said. "Thank you for coming. It has been a pleasure meeting you."

"The pleasure has been mine, Madame Lee." Kate said. "I'll think about everything you've said."

"I'm sure you will, my dear," Madame Lee said. "Please make the right decision for you . . . and for Casey."

After she left, Kate could not have imagined that Madame Lee had broken into tears, sobbing with an intensity the comforting words of her aide, Calphung Quock, could not staunch.

45

TRUTH AND CONSEQUENCES

"You have nothing to fear, Ari," Mona Morgan had said. "Tell the truth and leave the rest to me."

His attorney's words had been comforting, but Ari had spent a restless weekend apprehensive about his testimony. Both Anna and Garrick had stopped by to offer words of encouragement, and Sam Paean and E Lyn had called to convey their best wishes. But the thought of defending himself against the collective accusations of Cee Cee; his old nemesis, Clayborn Muck; the Prussian Penguin, Werner Von Seller; and G-Man J. Edgar Hoover was overwhelming.

How can I counter the combined testimony of my prominent ex-wife, a United States Congressman, a renown atomic scientist, and the Director of the FBI?

On Monday morning, Mona greeted Ari outside the steps to the Hall of Justice. She was again dressed conservatively, but her suit was more tailored and accent colors matched her auburn hair and emerald eyes.

"It's our turn," Mona said confidently. "We've taken their best shots. Now, we'll counter their arguments, one-by-one, and we'll have a few surprises of our own."

The curious and the press were present in even greater numbers, as Ari and Mona pushed their way through the throngs to the Courtroom of Judge Robie Phillips. The weekend TV news and newspapers, local and national, had devoted substantial space to the proceedings of *Scott v. Scott,* highlighting Marvin Belly's parade of celebrity witnesses. Most court commentators concluded Ari would lose his child visitation rights, but *Sentinel* reporter Jani Kay Fong, the only female covering the trial offered a dissenting opinion that Marvin Belly's presentation was fundamentally flawed.

Win or lose, Ari Scott and Mona Morgan were now media celebrities.

Banks of lights bathed the dark hallway in front of Judge Robie Phillip's courtroom in a blinding spotlight white, as Marvin Belly held court in a sea of jousting microphones.

Passing unnoticed behind the media mob, Ari and Mona heard Belly intone portentously, "I have never had a trial where the weight of the evidence has been so clearly in favor of my client. It is inconceivable that Professor Scott can present any evidence that will sway the decision of Judge Phillips. I feel very sorry for Miss Morgan. She is obviously a talented attorney, but there is an old legal saw that you 'win some, lose some.' However, I am sad to say that representing Professor Scott is the epitome of an exercise in futility which, I hope, will not taint Miss Morgan's legal career."

"Condescending SOB," Mona swore under her breath, as she and Ari entered the courtroom.

Please, hurry, Fitz, she thought.

Once again, Ari's loyal friends and family, Anna, Garrick, Roderick, Jacob and Sandy, were seated in the front row. Nearby, Sam Paean and E Lyn sat with Jani Kay Fong, the only members of the press not a part of the media frenzy in the hallway.

"All rise! Department 16 of the Court will come to order," bailiff, TN Phat announced, "the Honorable Robie Phillips presiding. Please be seated."

Judge Phillips motioned the bailiff to summon Marvin Belly from the hallway.

Belly entered hastily and took his seat at the counsel table.

"My deepest apologies for my tardiness, your Honor, counsel," Belly said."Sometimes, the press is your most difficult opponent."

"Your apologies are accepted by the Court, Mr. Belly," Judge Phillips said, "but I'm not so sure Miss Morgan agrees with your assessment of this case."

"Before we begin Respondent's case, I wish to state that I am flattered by the amount of media attention this hearing has generated," Judge Phillips said, "but I remind counsel that I, and not the press, will make the final decision."

Glancing at each other, the opposing attorneys said in unison,"Yes, your Honor."

"Miss Morgan, your first witness?" Judge Phillips said.

"Aristotle Scott," Mona said, watching Ari nervously step forward to be sworn.

Be strong, Ari, she thought.

After preliminary questions to calm him down, Mona began the heart of Ari's testimony.

"Professor Scott," Mona said, "why didn't you tell your wife about your Italian girl friend, before you married her?"

"Until recently," Ari said, "I believed Sofia had died during the War. I didn't think it was necessary to tell Cee Cee about ancient history, especially about someone who had passed on. It had nothing to do with how I felt about Cee Cee."

"Professor, you don't deny fathering a daughter out of wedlock?" Mona said.

She's leading him right into my trap, Belly thought.

"No, but I didn't learn about Anna's existence until the start of the Fall semester when Sofia wrote me about Anna."

"Had you been a loving and caring father to your children, Marcus and Monique, before you learned about Anna?" Mona said.

"Yes," Ari said. "I don't think Cee Cee will dispute that."

"Did you continue to be a loving and caring father even after you learned of Anna's existence?" Mona said.

"Absolutely," Ari said, looking at Anna seated in the front row. "Nothing changed my relationship with Marc and Monique. After I met Anna, I was so pleased she had turned out to be such a lovely young lady, I wanted my wife and children to know her."

"If you had known that telling your wife would result in a divorce and this custody battle, would you still have told her?" Mona said.

"Objection, your Honor," Belly said. "Calls for speculation, not relevant."

"Overruled,"Judge Phillips said. "You may answer, Professor."

"I agonized over revealing Anna's identity to my wife," Ari said. "I hesitated, afraid of hurting my wife; but I eventually decided to do so."

"Why?" Mona asked.

"It was more important for me to tell the truth and run the risk of alienating Cee Cee, than to live a lie the rest of my life."

"How would you describe your relationship with Sofia Cappuccino, when you returned from the Olympics?" Mona said.

"Objection," Belly said. "The answer is self-serving."

"To an extent, all testimony is self-serving," Judge Phillips said. "Overruled. The witness may answer."

"I had proposed to Sofia during our *toure di amore*," Ari said softly, tears welling in his eyes. "She accepted but needed her father's blessing."

"Did Mr. Cappuccino give his approval?" Mona asked.

"No," Ari said. "He could not bless his daughter's marriage to an unemployed graduate student, but he said he would give his approval when I finished school and obtained a job."

"So, you were engaged to Sofia Cappuccino before your return to California.' Mona said.

"Yes," Ari said. "Our marriage was only a matter of time."

"Between your engagement to Sofia Cappuccino and your marriage to your wife, did you have any other romantic relationships?" Mona asked.

"No. Those were the only two romantic relationships I've ever had," Ari whispered.

One chip at a time, Mona thought, surveying the hushed gallery. "Your witness, Mr. Belly."

Today, Belly wore a metallic colored, three piece suit that had seemed to glow golden in the hot, bright lights of the media. He placed his head in both his hands, pretending to be deep in thought.

"If I understand your testimony, Professor Scott," Belly said, "it was ok for you to father a child out-of-wedlock, because you *THOUGHT* you were engaged to the mother?"

Belly now rose, glaring at Ari. "Is that your excuse for having pre-marital sex?"

Cee Cee began to weep.

"Objection to this line of questioning," Mona said. "Counsel is invading the witness's right of privacy."

"I trust Mr. Belly does not intend to delve into intimate details of the witness's sex life," Judge Phillips said. "Professor you may answer in a general sense."

"I have never condoned sex outside of marriage," Ari said, "but the passion of my youthful romance got the better of me."

"GOT the better of you?" Belly snarled. "Isn't it true that you did everything possible to seduce this young woman?"

"NO!" Ari said, "I loved her very much."

"One man's lust is another man's love, isn't that true, Professor?"

"Objection, your Honor," Mona shouted.

"Sustained," Judge Phillips said.

Belly winked at William Randolph Chandler and said, "Professor Scott, isn't it true your alleged engagement is a total fabrication, offered solely to elicit public sympathy?"

"No!" Ari said, "Sofia and I were engaged."

"Professor, you will agree that there are only two people who can corroborate your claim," Belly said. "One is Mr. Cappuccino who is dead and the other is your 'almost betrothed,' Sofia Cappuccino Zarzana, who lives half-way around the world, isn't THAT true?"

Ari wiped a way a tear.

"You must answer, Professor Scott," Judge Phillips said.

"Yes," Ari said.

"I have no further questions," Belly said, beaming a smile at the press corps.

Returning to his seat, Ari thought, *Belly made me look like a criminal.*

"Respondent calls," Mona paused, "the honorable Chancellor of the Cal campus, Roger Haynes."

"Objection," Belly said, "Chancellor Haynes cannot offer any probative evidence in this child custody proceeding."

"Offer of proof," Mona countered. "Mr. Belly's witnesses have advanced the argument that Professor Scott's supposed 'less than patriotic' views would expose his children to unhealthy, if not dangerous, influences. Chancellor Haynes' testimony will offer an opinion as to whether Professor Scott's views are, in fact, 'less than patriotic' or dangerous."

"Mr. Belly, " Judge Phillips said, "you opened the door on this issue. It's too late for you to close that door. The witness may testify."

Chancellor Haynes, a distinguished looking academician, with thick, wavy, white hair and wearing glasses, was sworn.

"Chancellor Haynes," Mona said, "does the University of California recognize a specific definition of 'patriotism?' "

"We do not." Chancellor Haynes said, "The Cal campus has always been a place of divergent views, some popular, others unpopular. Times and issues change from year- to- year, but we always believe the campus should be a marketplace of ideas, where students and faculty can test the strength and validity of views by open and unfettered debate. Some call this Free Speech."

"Would you tell us the reasoning of this attitude?" Mona said.

"Certainly." Haynes said, "Our student body represents the best and brightest from all over the world. We trust our students' ability to analyze and test ideas presented and to decide what is right for them. In terms of your specific question, students are expected to question the notion of patriotism."

"Are you saying, Chancellor Haynes, that anyone, is free to say whatever he wishes?" Mona said.

"There's no such thing as total free speech," Haynes said. "Courts have ruled you can't yell 'fire' in a crowded theater, when there is no fire. You can't incite people to violence. You can't slander someone's reputation. But, short of these exceptions, anyone on campus is free to say whatever he or she believes, without fear of censorship."

"For the sake of discussion," Mona said, "what if someone, like Professor Scott, were to advocate certain views and students following those views make stupid, if not horrible, decisions?"

"That's possible," Haynes said. "Professors have been known to offer views that are considered stupid by the general public."

Muted laughter filled the courtroom.

Haynes continued. "One of the flaws, yet the beauty of a democracy, is that the majority rules, so long as certain basic rights of the minority are protected. Sometimes, the majority is wrong, but it's better that the majority make mistakes, than permit the few to control the opinions of the many."

Mona paused to allow Chancellor Haynes's statement to sink in. "Your witness," she said, sitting.

Belly walked leisurely to the witness stand and said, "Isn't it true, Chancellor, that you agree more with Professor's Scott's views on patriotism than those of Professor Von Seller's?"

"That's true, Mr. Belly, but it's not important whether I agree or disagree with any professor. The important thing is that all professors exercise the right to express themselves."

"Even, if you personally disagree with someone's views?" Belly said, a tone of disbelief in his voice.

"Absolutely, Mr. Belly. During speeches by Professor Von Seller, I admonished an unruly crowd at the Greek Theater. Recently, at Dwinelle Plaza, I reminded the crowd that whether one agrees with Professor Von Seller, Cal students owe a duty to listen to his opinion."

"But wouldn't you agree, Chancellor, that by allowing what you call Free Speech, you may incite unruly behavior."

"That's possible, Mr. Belly, but it is only through the open airing of opposite views that any democratic society may make intelligent decisions."

Belly rolled his eyes in mock disbelief. "No further questions."

"Now, we're going to have some fun," Mona whispered

There's nothing fun about this ordeal, Ari thought.

"Respondent calls Professor Roderick Seakin," Mona said.

Belly glanced at the tall lanky, professor, carrying a large brown paper bag, taking the stand.

Belly looked at William Randolph Chandler quizzically.

What could this professor possibly testify to?

"Professor Seakin," Mona said, "have you ever had a discussion with Professor Von Seller about his role in the publish or perish program?"

"Yes, I have," Seakin said.

"What did Professor Von Seller tell you?" Mona said.

"He told me it was William Randolph Chandler's idea to have the Regents' pass the publish or perish program."

"What else did Professor Von Seller tell you?"

"That publish or perish was the best way to punish the Cal faculty, especially Ari Scott."

The audience erupted in murmuring.

"Order!" Judge Phillips said, banging his gavel.

"Did Professor Von Seller tell you anything else?"

"That William Randolph Chandler had ordered him to hire Teaching Assistants from USC with the marching order to make Cal students undertake irrelevant and unreasonable class room assignments, while Cal professors are busy trying to complete their publish or perish requirements," Seakin said.

"Did Professor Von Seller ask for anything in return?" Mona said.

"Yes, Professor Von Seller wanted William Randolph Chandler to appoint him Chancellor of the Cal campus," Seakin said.

Gasps, then angry muttering erupted among the audience, as all eyes turned toward the crimson face of William Randolph Chandler.

"Objection!" Belly shouted, jumping to his feet. "Irrelevant! Move to strike! Lack of foundation! Motivated by partisan politics! This testimony is intended to inflame the passions of the audience!"

"Order! Order! Judge Phillips shouted, pounding his gavel. "I will clear this courtroom if the audience cannot control itself."

"Mr. Belly," Judge Phillips said, "I agree that Professor Seakin's assertion that gubernatorial candidate, William Randolph Chandler, conspired with Professor Von Seller to initiate the publish or perish program to punish the Cal faculty is inflammatory, and, if spoken outside this courtroom, may be slanderous. However, the accusation is subject to cross-examination and its weight, if any, is still subject to proof. I'm going to allow it."

"But your Honor," Belly bellowed. "What does this testimony have to do with child custody?"

"May I address that issue, your Honor?" Mona said.

"Very well, Miss Morgan," Judge Phillips said.

"As I recall," Mona said, "Mr. Belly called Professor Von Seller to buttress the argument that my client's opposition to loyalty oaths and his stand against publish or perish is, in Professor Von Seller's words, 'less than patriotic' and would, therefore, poison the minds of Professor Scott's children."

"On cross-examination, I specifically asked Professor Von Seller if his support for publish or perish were based on his unbiased and independent analysis."

"I recall that line of questioning," Judge Phillips said.

"Professor Von Seller's answer and I quote from the reporter's transcript," Mona said, reading from a copy of the transcript she had ordered from court reporter, Hays:

"QUESTION: 'And, Professor Von Seller, you've formed your opinion about publish or perish based on your INDEPENDENT and UNBIASED analysis?' "

"ANSWER: 'Why yes. I pride myself in making up my own mind, FREE FROM OUTSIDE INFLUENCES, of being OBJECTIVE on all the great issues of the day.' "

Mona continued, "If Professor Seakin's testimony is credible, it tends to discredit the truth and veracity of Professor Von Seller's testimony."

"That is an absurd stretch of relevance," Belly said.

"Counsel, Judge Phillips said, "if you had not introduced Professor Von Seller's testimony on this subject, I would sustain your objection. However, since you elicited it as part of Petitioner's case, Miss Morgan has the right to rebut it. Do you wish to cross-exam Professor Seakin?"

Rising, Belly glanced at William Randolph Chandler whose face was now purple with rage.

"Professor Seakin, isn't it true that you disagree with Professor Von Seller's position on publish or perish?"

"Yes, totally," Seakin said.

"When and where did this alleged conversation with Professor Von Seller take place?"

"About two weeks ago, on campus."

"Were there any witnesses to this purported conversation?"

"Yes, Professor Nelquist was present," Seakin said, pointing at Garrick Nelquist.

Belly held his arms up in feigned shock. "Professor Garrick Nelquist was a witness to this alleged conversation?"

"Yes," Seakin said.

"The same Professor Garrick Nelquist who has written newspaper articles AGAINST HUAC, the committee Professor Von Seller avidly supports?" Belly asked.

"Yes, the very same person," Seakin said.

"Pray tell, Professor Seakin," Belly said with a snarl, "can you explain why Professor Von Seller would tell you and Professor Garrick, two faculty members who vehemently disagree with him, enemies so to speak, something so outrageously inflammatory and politically damaging as you've related?"

"I'd be happy to," Seakin said.

"We're all dying to hear the reason, Professor Seakin," Belly said sarcastically.

"It's simple," Seakin said, "Professor Von Seller thought he was talking to William Randolph Chandler and his male secretary, Lumken, instead of Nelquist and me."

"Oh, a simple case of mistaken identity? Is that your explanation?" Belly said.

"Absolutely," Seakin said.

"With leave of the Court," Belly said, "I ask William Randolph Chandler and his secretary, Lumken, to rise and be formally identified."

"Granted," Judge Phillips said, "please stand, Mr. Chandler. If your secretary, Lumken, is present, may he also stand."

Both WRC and Lumken rose and stood side-by-side, in the front row of the gallery.

"The record will note that William Randolph Chandler was present, along with his secretary; Lumken," Judge Phillips said, "and the Court took judicial notice of both their physical appearances. Thank you, gentlemen."

"Mr. Chandler's famous face speaks volumes to the lack of credibility of Professor Seakin's claim," Belly said, sitting down. "No further questions, your Honor.

Muted laughter rippled across the audience.

"Professor Seakin," Mona began her redirect, "would you tell the Court why Professor Von Seller believed you and Professor Nelquist were William Randolph Chandler and his secretary, Lumken?"

"Yes, in fact, I'll demonstrate," Seakin said, reaching into the paper bag and producing a makeup kit.

"First, I change my hairstyle to resemble Mr. Chandler's by combing it this way," Seakin said, slicking his hair back. "Then, I darken my face by using pancake makeup. Most importantly, I add false eyebrows to make mine look as thick as Mr. Chandler's."

"Describe the lighting conditions when this conversation with Professor Von Seller took place?" Mona asked.

"It was late at night," Seakin said. "and we spoke in dim candle light. Professor Nelquist was standing in a darkened corner where only his silhouette could be seen."

"Describe your position relative to Professor Von Seller during this conversation," Mona said.

"Yes, Miss Morgan, if I turn my profile toward you and place my chin on my fist, posing like the statue of Rodin's *Thinker,* then ask the drapes of the windows be drawn, and further ask Professor Nelquist to stand in the corner behind me."

"The bailiff will please draw the drapes," Judge Phillips said."If Professor Nelquist is present, he will come forward and stand in the corner behind the witness."

"Your Honor," Mona said, "may we ask William Randolph Chandler to come forward and stand next to Professor Seakin with his profile facing the same direction as Professor Seakin's and ask Mr. Chandler's secretary, Lumken, to stand next to Professor Nelquist."

"Ridiculous," Belly shouted, "cheap courtroom theatrics."

"Mr. Belly, if that is an objection, I'll overrule it. I believe you are known to be an expert in courtroom theatrics. Mr. Chandler will come forward and pose next to Professor Seakin and his secretary, Lumken, will stand next to Professor Nelquist, in the manner requested by Miss Morgan."

The courtroom took on an eerie silence, as William Randolph Chandler, his face etched in anger, walked slowly to the witness stand and turned his profile in the same direction as Professor Seakin's. A grinning Garrick Nelquist assumed a standing position in the corner behind Seakin, next to WRC's secretary, Lumken.

Gasps greeted the comparison. In the dimmed light of the courtroom, the profiles of Professor Seakin and gubernatorial candidate, William Randolph Chandler, bore an uncanny resemblance, and the silhouettes of Professor Nelquist and Lumken were of similar height and shape!

Polite, then loud applause broke out among the audience.

Judge Phillips loudly gaveled order back into the courtroom, as the witness and the human exhibits, William Randolph Chandler, Lumken, and Garrick Nelquist, returned to their seats and the drapes were re-opened.

"Your Honor," Mona said, "our final witness has transportation difficulties. I respectfully request a recess until tomorrow morning to accommodate the witness."

"Objection," Belly shouted. "The witness had all weekend to arrange transportation to this Court. Petitioner desires the matter be submitted, for decision, NOW!"

Please hurry, Mona said to herself.

"I'm inclined to agree with Mr. Belly," Judge Phillips said, "the weekend recess should have been more than enough time for your witness to reach the courthouse. I'm going to . . ."

On hearing the courtroom door open, all eyes turned to the person entering Courtroom 16.

"Oh, my God . . ." Ari said, jumping to his feet.

Anna's mouth was agape with surprise. Cee Cee began to sob on recognizing the new arrival.

"Your Honor, our witness has arrived," Mona said, "Respondent calls . . . SOFIA CAPPUCCINO ZARZANA."

Fitz, my darling, you came through with flying colors.

Loud whispers swept the press corps.

Judge Phillips gaveled the gallery silent. "Mrs. Zarzana, you may take the witness stand."

The soft click of Italian high heels echoed through the hushed courtroom, as Sofia approached the witness stand.

In spite of the long journey, she looks absolutely fabulous, Ari thought, noting Sofia's perfectly coifed hair and her designer Italian suit that appeared to be wrinkle free.

"Mrs. Zarzana, have you or any member of the Cappuccino family ever been a member of the Socialist or Communist parties?" Mona asked.

"Never," Sofia said emphatically. "Before the War, my family were wealthy industrialists. Mussolini imprisoned us for being bourgeois capitalists."

"Would you describe your relationship with Professor Scott after the 1936 Olympics?" Mona said.

"We were madly in love," Sofia said, "Ari proposed to me during our *toure di amore*."

"What was your response, Mrs. Zarzana?" Mona said.

"I accepted; but my father was old fashioned. He would not give his consent to someone who was unemployed. He told us we could not marry until Ari finished school and had a teaching job."

"Mrs. Zarzana, did you have a child with Professor Scott?" Mona said.

"Yes," Sofia said proudly. "We have a beautiful daughter," Sofia pointed at Anna, "who spent her first years of life with me in Palermo Prison."

"Did you tell Professor Scott about the Anna?" Mona said.

"I did not tell Ari about Anna until last year, when she enrolled at the University of California."

"How did you meet your husband, Pablo Zarzana?" Mona asked.

Sofia retraced her past.

"After the War, my Mama, Anna, and I moved back to Milan and lived with my Aunt Marguerite who had a second floor apartment overlooking the large square, Piazza del Duomo and the Cathedral. Mama helped Aunt Marguerite wash restaurant linen to pay the rent.

Although I was young and single, my illegitimate child made me an undesirable among the bachelors of Milan.

I worked part-time at a coffee house on the Via Manzoni, near the1867 Galleria where the coffee drink Papa invented was popular. Serving cappuccino was a bitter reminder of what our family had lost. I escaped my misery by volunteering as an usher at the La Scala Opera House. Whenever Puccini's Madama Butterfly was performed, I cried my eyes out, as the story reminded me so much of my love affair with Ari.

In the mornings, I would walk Anna to the Piazza and listen to speakers voicing their post-War views. One was a young, firebrand who advocated overthrowing the rich. His name was Pablo Zarzana. He had charisma that held crowds spellbound. Pablo was arrested several times but always returned to speak to adoring crowds.

One day, he introduced himself. "You are the brave mother who brings her beautiful little girl to hear speeches that could get you arrested, eh?" Pablo teased. "Would you allow me to buy you a cappuccino and your daughter a soda?" he asked.

"You may not want to be seen with a mother whose child has no legitimate father," I said.

"That makes both of us undesirable," Pablo said. "My opponents call me a bastard, so I will take my chances."

"How do you feel about your husband's politics?" Mona said.

"I don't care about politics," Sofia said, "his or anyone else's, but politics is a part of who Pablo Zarzana is. My husband's love of politics is as strong as his love for his family. I have often joked that politics is our son."

"How would you compare your feelings about Professor Scott and those for your husband," Mona said.

"Objection," Belly said. "Mrs. Zarzana's feelings are irrelevant to this proceeding, your Honor."

"You may be correct, Mr. Belly," Judge Phillips said, "but since this witness has come half-way around the world to testify, I want to hear what she has to say. Objection overruled. Mrs. Zarzana, you may answer."

"My love for Ari Scott was the romantic love of youth. Sometimes, I wonder how things might have turned out if the War had never come between us. But we had our daughter, Anna, who represents the best of both of us, and I am thankful that she has had the opportunity to know her birth father.

"My love for Pablo Zarzana is different. It is the kind of love that comes with maturity and perspective. He welcomed Anna as his own and helped me raise her. In my country, not many men, especially political men, would have done so. They would have wanted me only as a mistress, for fear of what marrying a woman with an illegitimate child might do to their careers. For his courageous decision, I am forever grateful to Pablo Zarzana."

Ari felt tears steaming down his face. He saw Cee Cee dabbing her eyes. He heard sniffles among the audience.

"Mr. Belly," Judge Phillips said, "any cross-examination?"

Belly stood and surveyed the sea of sympathetic faces.

Better leave well enough alone. Belly thought. *Cut losses, by not compounding the effect of her testimony.*

"No, your Honor, we'll submit the matter."

"Thank you counsel. I am ready to rule," Judge Phillips said. "This has been a most unusual hearing. Press coverage has been unprecedented. The Court has never had such distinguished witnesses. What began as a child custody hearing became a public forum debating such lofty issues as the nature of patriotism, the notion of free speech, the definition of love, and a suggestion of partisan intrigue and political manipulation.

"What I, as the trier-of-fact, must never lose sight of is that the welfare of the two minor children, Marc and Monique Scott, are of paramount importance.

"What are the best interests of the children? It is a difficult decision in any divorce; and the public nature of this custody proceeding makes the Court's decision even more difficult. But it is the Court's duty to exercise its best judgment and render a decision based on the evidence presented and the laws of the State of California.

"As the Petitioner seeking to deny her husband's visitation rights, Mrs. Scott has the burden of proving that substantial harm would occur from the exercise of Professor Scott's visitation rights. The eminent Marvin Belly, Esquire, has produced an impressive list of witnesses to bolster his client's case. If this were a Congressional hearing, many of his arguments might well be persuasive.

"But this is not a Congressional hearing. This is a judicial determination as to what are in the best interests of the minor children.

"The law recognizes that parents, be they an ex-husband or ex-wife, have a fundamental right of child visitation. This right is not conditioned on money, social standing, politics, or even citizenship.

"There must be persuasive evidence presented to the Court that Professor Scott is unfit to exercise his basic child visitation rights.

"Being controversial does not make Professor Scott unfit. Nor does being unpopular make him unfit. Espousing political views that are bitterly opposed by others does not make him unfit. Having well-intentioned friends who impersonate famous public figures does not make him unfit.

"Accordingly, I find Professor Scott's parenting of a child out-of-wedlock, by itself, although unacceptable by most of American society, does not make him unfit.

"I find Petitioner has not sustained her burden of proof. Applying California law, I have no alternative but to deny her petition to prevent Respondent from exercising his child visitation rights.

"Respondent Aristotle Scott shall have the usual rights of visitation of every other weekend, every other major holiday, and one month during the summer, subject to the mutual convenience of the parties.

"This Court is adjourned!"

The gallery broke out in applause. Ari was mobbed by well-wishers. An enraged William Randolph Chandler and angry Clayborn Muck ushered Cee Cee quickly from the courtroom.

Jani Kay Fong was the first reporter to reach Mona Morgan's side.

"How did you get Sofia Zarzana here from Italy, on such short notice?" Jani asked.

"I, too, have influential friends," Mona said, wondering when she would see Fitz next.

"But those propeller-powered Constellations flown by commercial airlines aren't fast enough to get Sofia Cappuccino from Italy to San Francisco . . ." Jani began.

"I said, I have influential friends," Mona said, leaning forward, whispering in Jani 's ear. "We borrowed the President's jet airplane - *Air Force One* - to fly Sofia Zarzana here from Italy, in time to testify. That's your news scoop."

"But why would . . .?" Jani stopped, suddenly remembering the

President and J. Edgar Hoover had publicly clashed over the FBI's clandestine surveillance of U.S. citizens.

"Let's say the President of the United States has made an indirect political statement," Mona said, winking.

Packing up his books and papers, Marvin Belly turned to Mona and said, "Nice job, counsel. Thanks for the lesson in courtroom theatrics. If you ever change your practice from family law to suing insurance companies, there'll be room for you in my firm."

"Thanks, Marvin," Mona said, extending her hand that Belly gripped firmly. "If you ever need a divorce attorney, you know where to find me," she smiled.

"Tough case, Mr. Belly," bailiff TN Phat offered, as the famous trial lawyer exited Department 16.

"Yeah," Marvin Belly Esquire sighed. "Win some, lose some."

46

THE BIG SNOW SHOW

The banner of the *Daily Californian* trumpeted:

"HOLLYWOOD INVADES CAL CAMPUS
Movie Sex Symbols Vie For Dollars

The two leaders for Campus Snow
King and Queen pull out all the stops
today at Harmon. Gym. Handsome,
leading man, Rock Hudson, will sell
autographs for the first place team,
P U-Kappa's, while Dooch-Gee Dees
counter with sexy, blond bombshell,
Suzette Mew Mew. $100 separate
the two teams."

The Art Deco facade of Harmon Gym was hidden behind tons of fresh Sierra snow hauled in by the IFC, creating a hill four stories tall. A twisting slide, three feet wide, had been sculptured into the slope of the man-made "Bear Mountain" allowing students to body slide from open windows near the roof.

Television stations, drawn by the appearance of the two movie stars, recorded the faux winter scene. The Cal Band wearing reindeer antlers, performed winter tunes. Oski dressed in Eskimo gear and snow shoes, padded through the drifts, inhaling Kerrs beer through a piece of plastic tubing inserted into his eye hole. Crunchy Munchy - impervious to the winter scene - sold Eskimo Pies at the edge of a temporary ice-skating rink, while Jericho Slabio and Guerillas for Free Speech protested the spoilation of nature with signs urging:

"Leave Mother Nature Alone!"
"Snow Must Go!"
"No Snow Jobs On Campus!"

Inside, long lines of students waited patiently to pay a dollar for a Hollywood star's autograph. Under one basket, at the P U table, Chauncey Remington kept a watchful eye on the rugged actor dressed in a dark suit and thin tie, scribbling *"Love, Rock,"* for screaming coeds. Under the opposite basket, Ollie Punch - his wandering eye spinning furiously - stood as a salivating guard over the sexy blonde, in a skin-tight, gold lame dress, scrolling, *"Love & Kisses, Suzette,* for a line of over-sexed college boys moaning at the Dooch table.

Along one side of the basketball court, competing food stalls hawked college favorites: greasy corn dogs, butter popcorn, sticky cotton candy, and gooey pizza slices.

Across the way, booths hosted games of eye-hand co-ordination: dunking machine, horse shoe pit, dart board, basketball free throw, and coin-toss. There, two duels reprised last Fall's Big C Sirkus among shouting throngs. At the horse shoe pit, Casey Lee squared off against TA Brewster whom the Dormie leader had upset in the Frisbee toss at the Mining Circle. Nearby, IFC members and non-orgs wagered bets as Monty Maitland, the tart-tongued, penny pitching ace, tried to avenge his Big C Sirkus loss to Jonathan Aldon. This time, Montgomery, grim and tight-lipped, was the object of relentless abuse from Ollie Punch who showered Maitland with barbs: ""Don't choke, Maitland!" and "Gonna let a Dormie frosh embarrass you again?"

At mid-court, oblivious to the bedlam, All Pro sat cooly, on a raised platform, broadcasting his KALX radio show. Dropping head phones over his ears, All Pro set the diamond stylus on Barrett Strong's, *"Money"* and cued up Lee Dorsey's, *"Ya Ya."*

All Pro's given name was Garth Uvula. His mother claimed Garth emerged from the womb, wailing in deep, resonant tones. During her son's childhood, Mrs. Uvula taught young Garth to emulate the rich

278

speaking voice of her favorite crooner, Bing Crosby. She was convinced a mellifluous voice would compensate for Garth's plain looks. What Mrs. Uvula had not anticipated was Garth becoming a popular high school disc jockey, the "Undulating Uvula," and now, Cal radio station, KALX's All Pro, "the man with gonads in his Adam's apple."

The Dormies had donated the $500 reward for retrieving Oski's head and the $750 Calphung Quock collected from the casino winnings. Almost $600 was raised by the WW Pecker-ettes at the P Word concert An additional $300 had been raised from raffles, car washes, and spaghetti feeds. Despite these efforts, the P U-Kappa team was leading.

The score board totals read:

Penny-a-vote
| P U-Kappa: | 234,913 |
| Dooch-Gee Dee: | 219,411 |

Further down the list of contestants:
Ep Sig & Little Sisters: 61,776

"Hope the Ep Sig money puts us on top," Royal said, eyeing the score board.

"If we stay close, the Ep Sig's contribution should be enough," Casey said, giving Tom Hobknob a discreet thumbs up.

The Dormies and Gee Dees huddled in a tight circle, in front of the official counting table, soliciting donations for Joan Dildeaux and Hunch Hitowski. For the first time, since high school graduation, Hunch was dressed in a suit and tie. Joan was radiant, in the dress she had worn at Gee Dee Presents three years ago.

"THIRTY MINUTES before the EXCITING close of the Annual Campus Snow KING and QUEEN contest," All Pro boomed into the PA system.

"WHO WILL WIN? Will it be the MIGHTY P U-Kappa team? OR will it be those DARLING UNDERDOGS, Dooch-Gee Dee? Round up those LAST MINUTE pennies, boys and girls. We're going RIGHT DOWN the wire in A PHOTO FINISH!

"For those out in radio-land, here are the Ventures with their instrumental hit, *'WALK, DON'T RUN.'* "

"Looks like a toss-up, Dirk," Jefferson Warring said, pushing through the crowd. "I've been comparing Rock's line and Mew-Mew's. It's pretty even. If it weren't for her big boobs, we'd be winning in a landslide."

"How did the Dormies find out about Rock?" Dirk said, scowling.

"Got me," Chip said, "I thought only the four of us knew."

"If it's close, I'll use our emergency fund," Dirk said, fingering the wad of $100 bills in his pocket. He had borrowed $1,500 from his father with the understanding that if the loan were used, the P U's would owe Dad, Dirk Krum II, a weekend of shagging balls at the Pebble Beach Country Club driving range.

"Let's put a little damper on Dormie enthusiasm," Dirk said, eyeing Casey and Kate in animated discussion. "Add these to our total," he said, handing five $100 bills to Warring.

That fucking Chinaman and his Dormies are not going to embarrass us again, Dirk thought, recalling the shame when Dooch had edged the P U's for second place in the Big C Sirkus. *When it comes to money, there's no way the Dormies can compete with the P U's.*

Overflow crowds now filled the first ten rows of the gym, as the Cal Band, Oski, Crunchy Munchy, cheer leaders, pom-pom girls, and revelers swarmed into Harmon Gym.

"NEW TOTALS," All-Pro said, as crowd noise subsided. "With ONLY TWENTY MINUTES left, the Ep Sig's and their Little Sisters HAVE WITHDRAWN and donated their ENTIRE TOTAL to the Dooch-Gee Dee team!"

Gasps and boo's emitted from members of the IFC. Cheers and applause broke out among Dormies and non-orgs.

Hobknob, you two-timing traitor, Dirk thought.

"WAIT! Here's another FIVE HUNDRED dollars to the P U-Kappa cause. LATEST COUNT:

	Penny-a-vote
P U-Kappa:	*338,413*
Dooch-Gee Dee:	*301,597*

"Damn," Butch said, "Ep Sig money's not enough. We're doomed!"

"Let's not give up yet," Casey said, watching the crowd part, admitting a trio of Negro boys, one dressed in a suit, a second in a high school letterman's sweater, the third sporting a black beret and bandoleer. A buzz of recognition, then polite applause, as students recognized MJ of Big Berry and the Blackouts, and his two brothers.

Jonathan pressed forward to greet his Oakland relatives.

"Cousin Jonathan," MJ said, "this is from Reverend Ike and the congregation, a humble donation to your cause. It's not much, little more than a $100."

"We couldn't," Casey said, "this is only a college contest. Your church needs this more than. . ."

"Hush, Brother Casey," MJ said. "You, cousin Jonathan, and the Gee Dees gave Big Berry and the Blackouts their first big break. With our recent success, the band is donating ten percent of its income to the church, so please accept this contribution as a token of the band's and the church's appreciation."

"We'd like to make a donation too," a voice shouted. Behind the Jones brothers stood Professors Scott, Nelquist, Seakin, Aural, and Sandy.

"We passed the hat at the Faculty Club," Ari said.

"Damn near 100% participation," Nelquist said. "Didn't think a bunch of old faculty farts were still interested in young babes like Suzette Mew Mew."

"They all want separate autographs," Aural said. "Sandy and I want one too."

"Here's $200 for the cause," Seakin said, handing Casey an envelope bulging with bills.

"Wait," Kate Howell said, pushing her way through the group. "I have another $100 from an anonymous source." Jonathan noticed a smiling Pritti Diva slipping Kate a wad of bills.

"And $25 bucks from the non-orgs on the football team," star quarterback, Joe L. Capp said, handing Mo McCart a fistful of ones.

"NEW TOTALS! A quick response from Dooch-Gee Dees," All Pro intoned."WHAT A COMPETITION! With ONLY FIFTEEN MINUTES left, it's a HORSE RACE!"

Penny-a-vote

P U-Kappa:	*360,127*
Dooch-Gee Dees:	*346,559*

"They can't keep this up," Dirk said, a sneer creeping across his face.

"They've got to be tapped out. Jefferson, add this to our total." Dirk peeled off the remaining ten $100 bills and handed them to the P U frosh president.

"A $1,000 bucks should put our total out of reach," Chip said, snapping his fingers in approval.

Both applause and groans greeted the new totals.

"With ONLY TEN MINUTES left, the P U-Kappa team has opened AN INSURMOUNTABLE LEAD," All Pro said:

Penny-a-vote

P U -Kappa:	*485,016*
Dooch-Gee Dee:	*355,875*

"It's hopeless," Waz said, "we're more than a grand behind."

Destiny, Living Buddha thought. *You cannot alter destiny.*

A ripple of recognition greeted the balding man and his entourage elbowing through the crowd. The arrivals included an older man in a white, cowboy hat and a middle-aged man in a nautical cap.

"In the nick of time," Sam Paean said. "You all know E Lyn. Some of you know these distinguished gentlemen."

Jonathan gulped.

"Holy shit," Butch said.

"I can't believe this," Waz said, shaking his head.

"Bad karma, " Living Buddha whispered.

Standing beside Paean were Zephyr Cove Sheriff Will Bartone and Tahoe casino owner, Billy Hurry!

"Don't worry boys," Sheriff Bartone said, tilting his cowboy hat. "I can't arrest you outside my jurisdiction."

"E Lyn and I are here to help broker a deal,"Paean said.

"A deal?" Waz said. "The last time we saw the Sheriff, the deal was jail time unless we ponied up a $100 bucks a piece!"

"Boys, let by-gones be by-gones," Sheriff Bartone said. "Your jail break was the best thing that happened. Douglas County built me a brand new hoosegow! You guys aren't the first under-age boys to gamble at Hurry's and you, sure as hell won't be the last. In fact, technically, there's no crime when the victim decides not to press charges, right Billy?"

"Absolutely," Hurry said. "When Sam and E Lyn explained that the Beatniks I posed with on New Year's eve were the same boys who had the big craps run, I had to track you down. Thanks to them, I'm here to make a financial proposal."

"Can't give you back the money we won at your casino," Butch said.

"We've already donated it to the Campus Santa King and Queen Contest," Jonathan said, pointing to the score board.

"I don't want the money back," Billy Hurry said, chuckling. "Hurry's Casino can afford to lose a few hundred bucks. This is strictly business. You have something I want, and I'm willing to pay for it."

The Dormies exchanged puzzled looks.

"I want to buy back the pair of dice you used during those 52-straight passes. My pit bosses told me they were missing after your arrest."

"If . . . we have them, what will you do with them?" Waz said, remembering he had given them to Jonathan as souvenirs.

"I'm going to display them in a place of honor," Hurry said. "How does $500 sound?"

"I'll throw in these as part of the deal,"Sheriff Bartone said, pulling a pair of black hornrim glasses from his jacket. "One of you left them behind. I don't need these beat up specs."

Oh, my God, Jonathan thought. *Buddy Holly's glasses!*

"$500 is not enough," Casey said, calmly. "$2,000."

There was a collective gasp, then silence.

Hope Casey's not overplaying his hand, Royal French thought

"You drive a hard bargain, son" Hurry said. "How about a $1,000?"

Royal looked at the gym clock. There were less than three minutes left. Money raised from the dueling autograph signing tables of Rock Hudson and Suzette Mew Mew had already been tallied.

Casey glanced at the current totals on the tally board:

	Penny-a-vote
P U-Kappa:	*519,431*
Dooch-Gee Dee:	*399,586*

"Split the difference," Casey said, extending his hand. "$1,500."

"Now, let's be reasonable, boys," Sheriff Bartone said.

Billy Hurry turned and looked at the "Beatniks" who had posed with him on New Year's Eve, each now perfectly clean-shaven: Jonathan,

Butch, Living Buddha, Waz, and Casey.

"Blown more money than that on parts for the ghost of the SS Tahoe," Hurry said, gripping Casey's hand firmly. "It's a deal."

Amid whoops and shouts, Billy Hurry peeled fifteen $100 bills from a rubber-banded wad.

"Go!" Casey shouted, handing the money to Jonathan.

With Royal, Butch, and Mo forming wedge through the crowd, Jonathan scampered up to the counting table and slapped the bills down, with authority, as All Pro began the count down, "TEN, nine, eight . . ."

The total was quickly tallied, as the crowd joined the count, "THREE, TWO, ONE!"

"Time is UP! All Pro announced.

A buzz of anticipation spread through the crowd as last minute donations were verified.

"Ladies and gentlemen," All Pro announced. "THANKS to all of our contestants. A NEW RECORD for money raised for underprivileged children . . . OVER SIXTEEN THOUSAND dollars!"

Cheers and applause swept Harmon Gym.

"Now, it is my PLEASURE to present the 1960 CAMPUS SNOW KING AND QUEEN. WINNERS, at a penny-a-vote, by the slender MARGIN of LESS than TWENTY DOLLARS."

All Pro paused, ". . . JOANIE DILDEAUX AND HUNCH HITOWSKI!"

Sheer bedlam broke out on the floor, as Dormies and Gee Dees jumped for joy. Kate and Casey hugged. Joanie and Hunch, once denigrated as Dildeaux and the Dwarf, were paraded, in make-shift sedan chairs before the standing, cheering crowd. The Cal Band played *Pomp and Circumstance.* Crunchy Munchy tossed Eskimo Pies to the new royalty. Oski cracked open two Kerrs to toast the Royal Couple.

On the floor, side conversations bloomed. Paean and E Lyn congratulated Billy Hurry on the return of the now legendary, pair of dice. The four Cal professors examined the ancient Colt 45 of the Nevada lawman. Prima Diva tried on Buddy Holly's glasses. MJ signed autographs. Joel L Capp chatted up AJ, hoping to recruit the high school football star to Cal. Guerillas for Free Speech peppered RJ with questions about the philosophy of the Black Panther Party.

284

The final totals:

Penny-a-vote

Dooch-Gee Dee:	*549,521*
P U-Kappa:	*547,829*

"Without the reward for Oski's head, the Tahoe gambling winnings, and Billy Hurry's purchase of Waz's hot dice, we would have been goners," Casey said.

"Destiny," Living Buddha muttered, shaking his head in disbelief.

Royal French, a dazed grin on his face, nodded in agreement.

"Don't forget the Ep Sig money, Casey," Royal said. "In the end, it did make a difference, so we'll have to round up votes for Tillich when Hobknob runs him for ASUC President in the Spring."

"Let's get the hell out of here," Krum said, leading a dejected group of P U's out of Harmon Gym.

As the P U's passed the Ep Sig contingent, Tom Hobknob saluted Krum with a forefinger to the eyebrow, while Stefan Tillich waved an exaggerated farewell.

"A new day has dawned for campus politics," Tillich said, watching Chancellor Haynes and last year's Campus Snow King and Queen, ASUC President Ralph Van de Kamp and pretty A Chi O Kathy Mellory, crown Hunch Hitowski and Joanie Dildeaux as 1960 Campus Snow King and Queen.

"Of course . . . " Hobknob replied with a toothy grin.

47

DEAD WEEK

"P-E-D-R-O!   P-E-D-R-O!   P-E-D-R-O!"

The plaintive cry of students studying for exams echoed through the eastern foothills. The period between the end of classes and the start of finals was known as Dead Week, a week of all-day, all-night frenzy and hysteria.

There were several theories about the origins of the tradition The most popular is that Pedro was the lost dog of the University President who promised to cancel exams if the dog were found. Another was that Pedro was the handsome lover of the daughter of Don Jose Domingo Peralta, an early Spanish settler, who owned all the land that is now Berkeley. When Pedro disappeared, the young woman wandered the ranch lands broken-hearted, calling out his name in vain. On moonlit nights during exams, her ghost returns and, with the help of students, resumes the search. A third was that Pedro is the name of a student who dropped dead from shock on receiving all A's in his exams. In desperation, students call "P-E-D-R-O!" for "H-E-L-P!"

The body fell silently from the Campanile but landed with a thunderous *plop*. The impact ripped the belt from the victim's tan khaki's and somersaulted his Bass Weegun loafers along the brick esplanade. Campus police found the crystal of the victim's Rolex watch unscathed, at the base of a English plane tree 25-yards away. The tragic death brought a new, somber unintended meaning to Dead Week.

The banner of the *Daily Californian* screamed:

"CAMPUS SUICIDE!
Despondent Student Jumps From Campanile

Cristopher Papis, a member of Phi Chi fraternity, leapt to his death from the belfry of the Campanile at noon yesterday.

According to carillonneur, Hunch Hitowski, Papis peered over each of the four sides of the bell tower before vaulting onto a ledge and jumping off the west face.

Phi Chi fraternity members said Papis had been depressed about "mediocre" grades. Several horrified students studying inside the Main Reading Room of nearby Doe Memorial Library witnessed Papis's jump.

Papis was the son of David Prestone Papis, Class of 1934."

The Main Reading Room of the Doe Memorial Library - a cavernous enclosure Butch estimated was as large as the Main Reading Room of the New York Public Library - is 210-feet long, rising 45-feet to a curved, coffered, vaulted ceiling with three elongated, rectangular skylights. A large, Roman-arched window at each end dominates the Main Reading Room, especially the eastern exposure framing a panoramic view of the eastern foothills and the nearby Campanile.

Jonathan sat, elbow-to-elbow, with students in curved, oak seats jammed into long, blond oak tables lit by inverted troughs of light. Tension in the Main Reading Room was palpable, a cloud of anxiety hovering over the 400 students hunched over stacks of books and notes. The only sounds: turning pages and scratching pencils.

Preparing for finals, Living Buddha had extended Jonathan's nightly hypnotic, tutoring sessions from two to four hours during which a stream of Dormie upperclass men imparted whispered pearls of wisdom and tips on taking exams.

Living Buddha, Royal French, and Casey Lee were confident the intensive tutoring, along with moral support from Butch, Tommy Tubbins, and other freshmen, would earn Jonathan the necessary 27 units above a C average: in Poli Sci 1A, Chem 1A. Rhetoric 10, and compulsory ROT-C.

The consensus was that Jonathan's academic survival would turn on how well he did in Professor Aural's English 1A exam. Achieving a B would earn him the three additional units necessary to salvage the semester. A C grade or worse, and Jonathan would be another academic casualty of Cal's fierce undergraduate competition. The problem posed by Professor Aural's exam was that it had nothing to do with facts, figures, or phrases.

Jonathan recalled Professor Aural's comments at his final lecture.

"No matter how difficult the exam questions may appear, the most important thing is to THINK creatively. I will give special consideration to imaginative responses. If you've learned nothing else from my class, you should understand I do not want rote answers. My goal has been to make you appreciate the fact that problem solving requires critical thinking and human perspective. Our class discussions and your reading assignments were examples of this goal.

The liberties I have taken with some of you, especially, Mr. Aldon, were done, in good humor; and men wiser than I, have suggested that humor may be one of the highest forms of human perspective.

Sandy and I have enjoyed your participation and wish you Good Luck in your quest for critical thinking and human perspective."

Jonathan's reverie was interrupted by the fleeting sight of a an object falling from the Campanile. Others saw it and issued screams that echoed throughout the Main Reading Room.

Pandemonium! Eye-witnesses shared their horror. Some released pent-up anxiety by crying. Others screamed, "Oh, my God!" "Another suicide!" Several dashed to the base of the Campanile in disbelief that another tragic Dead Week suicide had occurred.

Jonathan felt oddly detached from the hundreds chattering aloud in the Main Reading Room. He had felt the heat and fire of Buddy Holly's plane crash. He had smelled death at close range. The glimpse of the suicide jumper had been disturbing, but not as shocking as bearing witness to the death of his rock and roll hero.

Despite the uproar swirling through the Main Reading Room, Jonathan sat motionless, grappling with disquieting thoughts. With all his heart, he desperately wanted to make his grades and continue as a

Cal student. To this end, he would consider making a pact with the Devil. And yet, if he failed, what would he do?

His options were limited. He could not return to Clear Lake, as his parents had disowned him. He might join the Navy and see the world like Uncle Mike had done in his youth. He could enroll at a Junior College for two years and transfer to a four year university that would accept a former Cal flunk-out. As a last resort, he could work a couple of years while deciding what he wanted to do with his life.

But who would hire him?

His work experiences had been limited to being an amateur rock and roll singer with the Amazing Double A's; a fortune teller's assistant;, a belfry window cleaner; and an assistant ID forger, none of which he could list, with any pride, on a job resume.

Were attaining good grades a matter of life and death? Would he follow in the steps of the pair who jumped off the Campanile?

Professor Aural's words echoed in his mind, *"problem solving requires critical thinking and human perspective."*

In his mind, Jonathan screamed for help:

"P-E-D-R-O!   P-E-D-R-O!   P-E-D-R-O!"

48

BEGINNING OF THE ENDING

"San Francisco will never be the same," Paean said, watching an army of construction workers swarming over the doomed real estate in the chilly, foggy mist of a February morning. The deafening vibration of pile drivers shook the earth, underscoring Paean's personal loss. He felt utter defeat, a failure in galvanizing public opinion to halt the monstrosity that signaled the death knell of his 25-year love affair with The City That Knows How, the San Francisco of his youth.

Across the street, a tall cyclone fence surrounded the mammoth project with billboards proclaiming,

*"Future Home of The Chandler Pyramid
Largest Skyscraper West of Chicago"*

"You did your best, darling," E Lyn said, kissing Paean lightly on the cheek. "Too many political and financial obstacles to overcome." She added cheerily, "but you did help some people escape Chinatown."

E Lyn had been thrilled by the recent front page headline of the *Sentinel:*

*"CHINESE INVADE CLEMENT
Exodus from Chinatown*

By Jani Kay Fong - Staff Reporter"

The newspaper had promoted her former Cal roommate from "Cub" to "Staff" status in recognition of Jani Kaye Fong's coverage of the Scott custody battle. The racial barrier at the *Sentinel* had been broken!

"At what price?" Paean said, stamping out a smoldering Lucky Strike. "Soon, San Francisco's skyline will look like Manhattan with sterile skyscrapers sprouting like weeds." He sighed, "From my flat, I won't be able to see the Campanile in the morning sun."

"Nothing is forever, Sam" E Lyn said, slipping her arm through his. "You've said it many times. It's impossible to stop the advance of the Sixties, the good or the bad."

Paean kissed E Lyn on the forehead. "You're right. I've spent a lifetime creating the myth of San Francisco Past with no room for The City of the Future. I've failed to consider where the fickle finger of fate is taking us. I should look myself in the mirror and admit I've become San Francisco's oldest dinosaur waiting for pickling and mounting in the San Francisco History Museum."

"Stop feeling sorry for yourself, Sam." E Lyn said, elbowing Paean in the ribs. "As long as you're breathing, you'll always be the social conscience of The City, pricking the public conscious with your wit and wisdom. You may lose a few, but you'll win most of your crusades. I can envision your epitaph:

"Here Lies One Loveable Paean in the Ass"

"That's why you're so enchanting," Paean said, hugging E Lyn.

"I thought it was my great legs."

"Yes," Paean said, "and the fact you know how to put my maudlin sentiment in its place."

"Let's celebrate a wake with some Bloody Marys," E Lyn said.

"Sure," Paean said. "Bloody Marys for a bloody mess."

Turning, they walked, arm-in-arm, away from the symbol of San Francisco's future and disappeared into the cool, gray mist of . . .

The City That - Once Upon A Time - Knew How.

* * * *

Kate Howell, Joan Dildeaux, Muffy Peachwick, and Dandy Cane, in bathrobes, with no makeup, and hair gathered up in towels, huddled around the package, wrapped in gold foil, sitting on the bridge table of the Pink Palace. From under the curled, royal blue ribbon, a red envelope with ornate script bore the salutation,

"Kate, Joan, Muffy, & Dandy
Happy Valentine's Day"

"Wanda Majic gave this to us on our last day at Yearning Arms," Kate said. "She said it'd be ok to open it before Valentine's.

"Open it now," Joan said, "I'm not getting anything for Valentine's anyway."

"Yes," Dandy said, "I love presents. Open it now."

"Business first, girls," Muffy said, reminding them of the reason for the meeting.

"I'll be chair," Kate said, surveying the serious faces of the other three. "In November, we all agreed to go on The Pill until the end of the semester and compare notes on how Enovid has affected us. Exams are over, and Spring semester will begin next week," Kate paused. "This, ladies, is our day of reckoning."

"We've been through so much together," Joan said, "so let's be brutally honest . . . Who got laid?"

"Dil-dee, please," Muffy said. "Can't you put it in more romantic terms? It's much more than squirming and humping."

"I'll take your word for it, Muffy-kins; because I didn't get one taker," Joan said, "even when I asked for it, begged for it is more accurate. All I got were chuckles!"

"Men are such asses," Kate said, her profanity shocking her sorority sisters. "I offered Casey my virginity, and he was more concerned about my 'saving it' for my husband! What's all the BS about nice girls being raised that way?"

"In your heart, you know it's true," Dandy whispered. "I'm not sure if I actually did it or not. Every time I got the nerve to try, I'd drink too much and fall asleep." She smiled brightly. " The good news is I'd wake up with my panties on. I'm really glad my dates thought enough of me not to take advantage of the situation." A sly smile crept across Dandy's face. "But one time, I did find a squirt of sticky stuff on my sweater."

"Spare me your freshman innocence, Dandy," Joan said. "Ok, who's going to fess up."

"If you insist," Muffy said. "It wasn't from the lack of desire . . ."

"C'mon, get on with it, Muffy-kins."Joan said, "what happened?"

"I got drunk at the P U exchange and wound up on Chip Fist's bed." Muffy said.

"In 'Mr. Neanderthal's boudoir?' " Joan said.

"There are days of the month, when I get VERY horny," Muffy said. "If there happens to be a guy handy, I have to satisfy my needs."

"But, Chip?" Kate said, envisioning suffocating under the weight of the fat P U, football player.

"I'll be honest," Muffy sighed. "Nothing really happened. I got on top; and between his Mt. Everest stomach and his teensy dick . . . it was not meant to be!"

"How teensy?" Joan asked, suppressing a giggle.

"I think I hurt his feelings by calling it, a 'peck-ette,' " Muffy said.

"Oh, poor little big boy," Kate cooed.

"I wasn't being mean," Muffy explained. "I was frustrated trying to move his quivering belly out of the way of the action."

"Three 'no's' and one 'almost,' " Joan said. "There's no way anyone's going to brand us the sex kittens of the Sixties."

"We haven't counted our handy encounters at Yearning Arms," Kate said. "That was quasi-sex, wasn't it."

"Pulling puds was disgusting," Joan said.

"Wanda Majic didn't make false promises." Kate said. "She told us what we could do without compromising our virginity, remember?"

"It was disgusting, stupid, boring, like milking cows," Muffy said, "but we had some laughs with the girls of Yearning Arms."

"So, what did this all mean?" Joan sighed.

"Taking The Pill put too much pressure on us," Dandy said.

"From the mouths of babes . . . ." Muffy said.

"Maybe Casey was right," Kate said. "As much I wanted to go to bed with him, I might have regretted it. It could have ruined our relationship. Taboo things are absolutely irresistible."

"The Pill hasn't made me any hornier than I am," Muffy said. "I've always had a healthy appetite, and nothing we've done the past two months has changed me."

"Muffy-kins," Joan said. "It's easy for you to poo-poo this experiment. You've always had a line of guys waiting to jump your bones. What about us?"

"Dil-dee, baby," Muffy said, "what I said is I'm liberated without it. The Pill's real benefit will be to straight-arrow types, like you."

"Muffy's got a point," Kate said. "Imagine what Phoebe Apperson would have preached had The Pill been around in her day. She was way ahead of her time."

"So, who's going to continue with The Pill?" Joan asked.

No one raised a hand.

"I guess we'll save The Pill, like we'll save our virginity . . . for marriage," Kate said.

"I've given little v's away so many times, I guess I can save the Big V for my wedding night," Muffy winked.

"Open the package!" Dandy squealed.

"Why not," Kate said. "The Campus Snow Queen should have the honors."

Joan carefully ran a finger nail file under the seal of the red envelope, plucked out a pink card, and handed it to Muffy. "I don't have my glasses on, Muffy-kins."

Muffy read the message out loud:

> *"To our sweet, Gee Dee Virgins,*
> *Thanks for your great work at*
> *Yearning Arms. You wanted to*
> *broaden your experiences, but*
> *you may have gotten more than*
> *you bargained for. Tokens of*
> *appreciation while you await*
> *your honeymoon night !*
>
> *Fondest regards,*
> *Wanda and Sascha.*
>
> *PS Virginity is <u>not</u> a four-letter word"*

As the note was passed around the table, Joan untied the royal blue ribbon and carefully removed the gold foil wrapping.

"Oh, my," Joan said, handing each of the four an identical, shiny pink, plastic object. "Vibrators!"

"How do they work" Dandy said, turning one over in her hands.

"Flip the switch on the bottom, li'l sis," Muffy said.

"Might give good facials," Joan said, placing the buzzing sex aid against her cheek.

"To V and V! Virginity and Vibrators!" Kate said, raising her Yearning Arms, projectile-shaped souvenir.

"VIRGINITY AND VIBRATORS!" the other three shouted, saluting Kate with their humming sex toys.

Downstairs, housemother Miss Willa Havisham, drank deeply from the silver chalice of *Jack Daniels* and toasted her silver-haired image in the mirror. *Remember who you are and what you represent,* she said to herself, as the stereo played Little Brenda Lee singing *"All Alone Am I."*

* * * *

In the patio of the P U house, the hulk of the Seeburg KD-200 Select-O-Matic sat splattered and forlorn, awaiting pickup from the Salvation Army, its electrical system damaged beyond repair by the tidal wave of sludge that had engulfed it.

In the dank darkness of the P U living room, Chip Fist, Chauncey Remington, and Jefferson Warring tried valiantly, without success, to console their despondent, drunken President.

"Guys, where did I go wrong with Kate?" Dirk Krum III whispered.

* * * *

The Pilgrimage is a campus tradition in which graduating seniors take a final stroll about campus, reviewing with nostalgia the familiar sights of their days at Cal. It had been Casey's idea for Jonathan to celebrate a freshman Pilgrimage before facing the Angel of Death.

The pair left Dooch, hiking up Channing, passing the P U house where during dorm registration, Jonathan and Butch had joined Casey's commandos in a retaliatory stink bomb attack on their rivals. Turning north on College, they crossed Bancroft, retracing the route past the bronze Pelican, through the peaceful hillside lawn of Faculty Glade, and over gurgling Strawberry Creek to the base of the Campanile where Mo McCart had distributed fake computer cards that helped Dooch freshmen secure classes in the stampeding madness of Class Registration.

The two rode the Campanile elevator past the neatly stacked rows of dinosaur bones, stopping at the bell tower office where Miss Burdick offered freshly baked cookies and her well-wishes. At the belfry they inhaled the sweeping panorama: of the Golden Gate Bridge and the Pacific beyond; of Memorial Stadium where the Dormies had carted off the goal posts; of the classic design of the Greek Theater, site of the Pajamarino- Bon Fire Rally; of the Beaux Arts jewel box, the Mining Building, where Jonathan had competed with the Dormies in the Big C Sirkus.

Ignoring the chilling reminder of the student suicides, the two peered down the face of the Campanile where Jonathan, Butch, Tubbins, and Fart-ing had implemented Royal French's RF in protesting HUAC's call for loyalty oaths.

Exiting the Campanile, the pair walked downhill passing venerable South Hall, where Jonathan had suffered repeated embarrassment from Professor Aural. They made their way through the throngs in front of Wheeler Aud and Dwinelle Plaza, passing the ringed trees surrounded by fraternity and sorority members and the newly-installed planter box, the future site of the Dooch palm tree.

Approaching Sather Gate, Jonathan stopped, surprised by the sight of an aisle formed by the people who had been so much a part of his semester at Cal. Each shook his hand, bear-hugged him, and offered a hearty "good luck."

Fellow freshmen: Butch Tanenbloom, Tommy Tubbins, even Jerry Fart-ing.

The duo dabbling in aerial dynamics: Ollie Punch and Campus Snow King-Campanile carillonneur, Hunch Hitowski.

His mentors in fortune-telling and academics: Ruby Lips and Living Buddha.

Crunchy Munchy offered a free Eskimo Pie.

Tears streamed from Jonathan's eyes.

Comrades from the Stan-furd Axe RF: Mo McCart and Rod Organ.

Dooch's resident experts in beauty, art, and culture: Super Sleuth, Waz, Lizard, and All Pro.

Seventh floor Eng-ineers wearing their slide rules like swords: Dick Phuncque and Hormone Lennings.

Surprise! Gee Dees: Kate, Joan, Muffy, and Dandy, giving him sweet pecks on his cheek.

More Surprise! Big Berry and the Blackouts. MJ and AJ, even RJ.

Still More Surprise! Orange and green-eyed female fatale, Pritti "Sascha" Diva! Amid a chorus of hoots, Sascha gave Jonathan a long, wet kiss . . . .*right on the lips!*

Even More Surprise! Calphung Quock handing him a frosty can of Kerrs, with a hearty, "cheerio pip-pip, sport!"

A curious Ludwig Von Schwaren ambled over from his fountain, intrigued by the gathering.

"I'll . . . I'll," Jonathan tried to speak.

"Will you hurry up and spit it out, Aldon," Ollie Punch barked. "Don't bore us with your sentiment."

"No matter what happens," Jonathan croaked. "I'll never forget you . . . all of you."

Hoots and applause mingled with the gurgling of Strawberry Creek.

Casey Lee placed a firm hand on Jonathan's shoulder, nodding at the figure walking slowly down the Sproul Hall steps.

"Time to cheat the Angel of Death, Jonathan," Casey said.

"Go Bears!" the well wishers shouted, as Jonathan emerged from beneath Sather Gate.

Jonathan wiped away the tears and walked purposely toward the bulletin board where the Angel of Death was posting lists of students who had failed. The Angel of Death was a small, thin, middle-aged man with a large Adams apple who wore small spectacles perched on his hook nose. He wore a dark suit, starched white shirt, and a thin black tie. The Angel of Death turned, as if expecting Jonathan's arrival, and grinned from ear-to-ear.

Jonathan stopped, turned, and gave a sweeping wave toward the crowd at Sather Gate.

Today was February 3, 1960, the one year anniversary of the day he retrieved Buddy Holly's glasses from the fiery site of the deadly plane crash near Aldon Farms and exactly five months since his arrival on campus from Clear Lake, Iowa.

Jonathan was floating, buoyed by a feeling of contentment, no longer afraid of his fate. He had been blessed by the wonders of friendship and suffused with lessons from the University of Life.

As he marched confidently to meet his destiny, Jonathan thought, *The Angel of Death be damned! Go Bears!*

* * * *

"All of you gentlemen are so wonderful! Charming and handsome too!" Anna Cappuccino said, with an earthy laugh that evoked in Ari Scott warm memories of her mother, Sofia.

"You Italian ladies have a way of making a man feel so damned special," Garrick Nelquist said, tamping a wad of tobacco into his meerschaum.

"I second that observation," Jacob Aural said, patting the head of his loyal companion. "Sandy does too."

"So does Alexander Graham Bell," Roderick Seakin said, dressed as the famous inventor.

Anna was seated before the warmth of the Great Fireplace of the Men's Faculty Club, commanding the undivided attention of Professors Scott, Nelquist, Aural, and Seakin.

"I apologize for being such a suffocating, hovering father," Ari said, taking a large sip of brandy, "but I can't tell you how happy I am that Jericho Slabio is out of your life."

"Papa, I was such a fool, a silly girl whose mind was twisted by the sound of pretty, empty words," Anna said, placing her arms around Ari's shoulder. She shuddered at the mistake she had almost made.

"Speaking of twisted," Garrick said, "Super Sleuth's photos of Jericho Slabio and Lotta Ackshon imitating human pretzels should be donated to The Contortionist Hall of Fame."

"They looked like a DNA double helix," Seakin said.

"Let's speak of something pleasant," Anna said, blushing. "Professor Aural, tell us an amusing story, something that will cheer our spirits."

"Yes," Nelquist said, "like whether any of your freshmen students earned an A in your hard-ass exam?"

"Ah," Aural said, "like Ari's Higher Truth, earning an A in English 1A is reserved for only the few who dig through the intellectual obtuseness of my lectures and get down to what Garrick calls the 'nitty-gritty.' "

"You're not admitting to the dissemination of academic BS, are you, Professor Aural?" the Alexander Graham Bell look-alike said.

"You might say that is the Highest form of Truth," Ari said, wading into the irreverent discourse.

"Gentlemen, we have a lady present, and I would not want her ears turning red from our base feelings about academia," Aural said.

"But," Nelquist persisted, "did anyone hit the academic jackpot?"

" I gave only two A's," Aural said, "one to the most brilliant student, Roz Tess, but let me share the other one with you. Using Garrick's expression, 'lighten up,' I posed the following problem:

"Write a CONCISE essay containing the themes:
RELIGION, ROYALTY, SEX, and MYSTERY."

"Unfair," Nelquist chuckled, "religion, royalty, sex, and mystery?"

"Concise?" Ari added. "That's impossible. Students love to disgorge as much useless data as possible."

"That's the point," Aural said. "I wanted them to think, not parrot information. Critical thinking and human perspective should be the most important factors in problem solving."

"Lofty goals," Jacob," Seakin said, "but asking students to write a short essay on religion, royalty, sex, and mystery is worse than making my students sit through my impression of Madam Curie."

"To prove that it can be done," Aural said, breaking into a broad grin. "I gave an A to the following concise, imaginative response:

"My God," the Queen said. "I'm
pregnant! Who did it?"

"Wonderful," Ari said, wiping away tears of laughter.

"Who was the ballsy, imaginative student who gave you the retort you so aptly deserved, Jacob?" Nelquist asked.

"He's a foreign student," Aural said, stroking Sandy's head.

"Good for him," Anna said. "Foreign students are just as smart as American students.

"How foreign?" Ari asked.

"From an exotic, far away land?" Nelquist asked.

"Must be an English-speaking land, judging from the sophistication of the response," Seakin said.

"Correct on all accounts," Professor Aural said. "I gave one of only two A's to a foreign student - one from that exotic, English-speaking exotic land ... far, far away ... Clear Lake, Iowa."

49

EPILOGUE REDUX
(*denotes subjects not featured in *A Golden State of Mind*)

The P U-Dormie rivalry raged for two more years until Dirk Krum, Casey, and Kate Howell graduated with the Cal Class of 1961.The struggle between the two living groups became a footnote to the dramatic changes in the campus demographics.

In the early1960's, the California legislature approved millions of dollars for the construction of new student housing to accommodate the anticipated influx of Baby Boomers. A dozen high-rise dorms sprouted up on the Cal campus, all identical to the prototype, Dooch Hall.

By 1980, the ratio of men to women equalized, forcing the campus administration to convert all high-rise Cal dorms which had been previously segregated by gender into coeducational living groups with communal bathrooms.

By the year 2000, Dirk Krum's worst fears had been realized, as the influx of middle-class Baby Boomers reached epic numbers. In 1959, the student population was 65% male - 35% female; and ethnically: 93% White - 7% "Other." By the new millennium, the student makeup was 48% male-52% female; and by ethnicity: 38% Asian; 35% White; 10%; African-American; 5% Hispanic; 12% "None of Your Business."

Spurred by Civil Rights legislation and the need for survival in the face of dwindling membership, the Greek system at Cal abandoned its policy and practice of discrimination based on race or religion.

For Jonathan Aldon and his clan, life made a serendipitous circle. Under the mentorship of Living Buddha, Jonathan survived his freshman year. Graduating with the Class of 1963, Jonathan followed JFK's advice and joined the Peace Corps. On some enchanted evening, in the Fiji Islands, he fell in love with Peng Kai, "Pinky" Hwang, a graduate student at the University of the South Pacific. The two were married in Hong Kong, on Living Buddha's estate, high on the wind-swept slopes of Victoria Peak. Ziggy, on leave from Viet Nam, served as best man. Mike and Pearl were the only Aldons in attendance. .

After service in the Peace Corps, Jonathan remained in Asia for 20-years as a U.S. State Department farming advisor. A daughter, Kelly Ming Aldon, was born in Singapore and educated in American schools, including Cal. The highlight of Jonathan's Far Eastern career was appearing, with Pinky and a group of Chinese hog farmers on the cover of *National Geographic*.

When Murle Aldon died of cancer in 1975, Mike, Pearl, and their son, Francisco (Frisco) moved from Minneapolis to manage Aldon Farms. For the rest of her widowed life, Gertrude Aldon dedicated her life to martyrdom. In 1980, Gertrude suffered a fatal heart attack after seeing Jonathan and "that Oriental woman" on the cover of *National Geographic*. She was laid to rest beside Murle in the ornate Aldon mausoleum at the God Be With You Sanctuary, once an empty field where Buddy Holly's plane crashed in February 1959.

In 1988, Mike and Pearl retired from hog farming to spend more time with their son, Frisco, now a Minneapolis judge, and their grandchildren. On Mike and Pearl's urging, Jonathan returned to Clear Lake for the first time in 28-years. He and Pinky moved into the family Tudor along the whale-shaped shores of Clear Lake to manage Aldon Farms.

After a 30-year hiatus, the Amazin' Double A's resumed their musical career on Oldies Night at Buddy's Place (formerly the Blue Horizon Inn) now owned by Ziggy and his wife, Zelda. The middle-aged rock and roll duo's signature song remains *"That'll Be The Day."*

Jonathan's Oakland cousins, the Jones's, answered Destiny's call. Reverend Ike and Doris retired from their radio ministry after the City of Oakland claimed their home on Heavenly Court through eminent domain to construct a football coliseum for the new NFL team, the Oakland Raiders.

After starring as a Cal football player, AJ graduated with a degree in Political Science and served consecutive terms in the California state legislature. MJ pursued a music career, producing 12-Grammy winning albums. In 1968, RJ died in a shootout between the Black Panthers and the Oakland police.

From his *"Louie, Louie"* royalties, Alfonso (Big) Berry acquired controlling interest of a corporation developing cemeteries in upscale communities. One of the company's most profitable units is the God Be With You Sanctuary in Clear Lake, Iowa.

For many of the Dooch Dormies, their Cal education paved the way to life-long adventures.

Bernard (Butch) Tanenbloom married a Jewish American Princess, a five star-general and enjoyed a successful career as a prosecuting DA in Manhattan before running for public office. Tanenbloom is serving his third term as Mayor of New York City.

Ruppert (Ruby) Lips founded the San Francisco Gay Men's Opera Company that has performed to enthusiastic audiences throughout the world. Ruby and his partner of 30 years live in a stately mansion along embassy row, overlooking the Golden Gate.

Royal French formed a security service for celebrities and married noted contemporary artist, Marilyn Anglais. The couple raised their children Mitch, Charles, and Julie at *Pickfair*, the former Hollywood home of silent film actors Douglas Fairbanks and Mary Pickford.

Julio (Hunch) Hitowski became a millionaire from his invention, a musical dial tone for telephones, and settled in Malibu with his wife, Lynda Svelter, a former Miss California.

Homer (Waz) Wazlewski is the New Jersey Director of Lottery.

Michael Hu (Living Buddha) manages the many dot.com ventures of his worldwide conglomerate, Living Buddha HK Ltd.

Cable television's most popular show, *Wide World of Wrestling,* is owned by Oliver (Ollie) Punch dba HA! HA! HA! Productions.

Marty (Super Sleuth) Silverstein served as Director of the Secret Service under three U.S. presidents. Retired, Super Sleuth resides in Palm Springs where he enjoys daily strolls along El Paseo, ogling the parade of stylish, women shoppers.

Garth Uvula (All Pro) received a PhD in Speech and established the Cal Department of Media Studies. The former Rooster Face is the International President of the Eddie Fisher Fan Club.

*Rod Organ and his heiress wife, Careen, founded an international airport shuttle service, "The Faster Organ."

After earning an MBA degree, Mortimer (Mo) McCart became a sports agent. In 1990, Mo was elected Commissioner of the NFL.

* Harry (Hormone) Lennings is Chief of Sanitation for the City of Mill Valley. He and his wife, Lonnie, have two children, both noted endocrinologists.

A few Dormie lives took curious turns.

Robert B. Jean (Lizard) gave up a promising art career and returned to the family business. Lizard is Chairman of the Board of Le Bleu Jean Co., the world's largest manufacturer of denim clothes.

After retiring as Chief Eng-ineer of the Kennedy Space Center, Dick Phuncque opened a popular fast food chain, Wienies 'R Us.

Tommy Tubbins dropped out of Cal in his junior year to travel Nepal and Kathmandu before settling in Marin County where he and his wife, Keckee, breed pet llamas.

Some Cal traditions survived the new millennium, others have fallen by the wayside.

Oski, the Cal Bear mascot, still prowls mischievously about campus, inhaling beer through plastic tubing inserted in his eye hole. The synchronized Cal band, now 50% female, marches to the delight of generations of long suffering Cal football fans who bear witness to the Cal tradition of gridiron futility.

The cannon, above Memorial Stadium, still fires, during football games, commemorating the occasional Cal score, while a new generation of young Cal freeloaders on Tightwad Hill, wear T-shirts bearing the genealogical message:

"I was conceived on Tightwad Hill
during a boring Cal football game"

The Campanile's 61-carillons, 49 acquired during the long tenure of chime mistress, Betty Burdick, continue to serenade the campus daily. At Ms. Burdick's memorial service, her ashes were scattered from the bell tower, while her favorite protégé, Hunch Hitowski, chimed *"Nearer My God To Thee."*

*After the rash of student suicides of 1960, the Campanile belfry was enclosed with protective glass, preventing further aerial deaths.

*Defying mathematical probabilities, Cal lost six football games, in a row, to Stan-furd, from 1961 to 1966, prompting the Dooch Sexy Six to honor their vow to return the Axe from its tomb beneath South Hall. The Axe is now awarded to the winner of the annual Big Game.

*Protests led Leland Stanford Junior University to change its mascot from the Indian to The Cardinal which apparently is a tree. In the campus vote, the actual winning name, Robber Baron , was invalidated by a red-faced Stan-furd University President. Robber Baron would have been not only politically correct, but also historically accurate.

The insanity and hysteria of mass Reg Lines have been replaced by electronic enrollment by phone and computer.

There is still a Dead Week before final exams, during which frantic, forlorn cries of

"P-E-D-R-O! P-E-D-R-O!"

echo throughout Berkeley's eastern foothills.

Frozen Gremlins were banned at Cal football games after an incident of mass ptomaine poisoning overtaxed the campus sewer system, the day after the all-men's rooting section was formally integrated by angry females demanding equal seating along the Bear 50-yard line.

The Reserve Officers Training Corps, ROT-C, was eliminated as a mandatory class for frosh and sophomore males after student demonstrations against the Vietnam War raged through America's college campuses in the late Sixties. Now voluntary, ROT-C offers co-ed membership for future military officers.

Dwinelle Plaza is no longer the private preserve of fraternities and sororities. Today, Greeks and non-orgs mingle freely at the ancient Wheeler Oak and the other concrete-ringed trees, including the Dooch palm tree, but smoking has been banned on campus.

International House (I House) maintains its tradition of nurturing future world leaders, infusing foreign students with the spirit of the Cal experience. Like Anna Cappuccino, visiting students have met and mingled at I-House, sharing the youthful vision of goodwill and optimism for a lasting world peace.

Telegraph Avenue continues to be the central nervous system of activity near campus. Telly teems with tourists taking photos of bearded and silver-haired, aging vendors peddling beads and trinkets left over from the psychedelic Sixties when these same merchants were protesting America's "bourgeois, capitalist society." Many of today's Telly entrepreneurs are college dropouts from USC and Stanford.

On the wall of a small smoke shop on the corner of Bancroft and Telly, a small weather-beaten plaque commemorates the 500,000-Eskimo Pie ice cream bars Crunchy Munchy sold from 1946 until his death in 1981.

The uproar over loyalty oaths and publish or perish foreshadowed the unrest that would sweep the Cal campus in the turbulent decades to follow: the Free Speech Movement, anti-Viet Nam War sit-ins, People's Park riots, and affirmative action demonstrations.

In the aftermath of HUAC and publish or perish, Cal professors had varied careers.

Werner Von Seller (Prussian Penguin) served as Chairman of the Atomic Energy Commission under Lyndon B. Johnson. In 1974, the Prussian Penguin died in a freak accident when he waddled, stumbled, and fell into Cal's atom smasher, at the Cyclotron. His monocle and sterling silver cigarette holder were retrieved and are on display at the Visitor's Center of the Cyclotron.

Governor Ronald Reagan appointed Garrick Nelquist State Boxing Commissioner. Later, Nelquist returned to Cal before retiring to a small Cotswold cottage near London.

*After winning a Nobel Prize in 1970, Roderick Seakin retired to La Jolla, an upscale enclave north of San Diego, where he acted in regional theater until his death in 1992.

Jacob Aural declined a cabinet position with John F. Kennedy and continued to teach at Cal. Both he and his loyal seeing-eye dog, Sandy, passed away in 1985. The pair are buried on the hillside above the Big C. The inscription on their gravestone reads:

Hallmarks of creative thinking and perspective:
Excellence, Humor, Tradition, Diversity

The Gamma Delta (Gee Dee) sorority motto, *Remember Who You Are and What You Represent,* took on new meanings for members of the House of Beauty.

Joan Dildeaux married a Swedish doctor who pioneered a plastic surgery technique that transformed her into a stunning beauty. The ex-homely legacy enjoyed a brief modeling career and is manager of her husband's Beverly Hills Before & After Body Sculpturing Clinic.

After five failed marriages, Mergetroid (Muffy) Peachwick returned to Cal and earned a PhD in Human Sexuality. Today, Muffy is a recognized sex therapist and hosts a nationally syndicated radio talk show, *Sex and Stuff With Dr. Muff.*

Gee Dee housemother Miss Willa Havisham retired and moved to the Peaceful Valley Old Folks Home where she was the bridge partner of Crazy Martha Howell. When Crazy Martha passed away, Ms. Havisham buried her friend with a box of rum-soaked cigars.

Dandy Cane flunked out of Cal in her sophomore year and joined her sister, Candy, as a stewardess for CAT Airlines. Dandy married an older, wealthy USC alum - President of Stretch-em Condoms, Inc. The couple settled in Newport Beach where they raised their ten children.

Among the P U's, Chip Fist tied his career to a conventional product, as owner of Bitchin' Beer Co, the largest distributor of Kerrs.

*Jefferson Warring produces premium wine in the Napa Valley, sold under the popular label, Thunder Burp. Every year, Warring dutifully visits Dirk Krum III on Krum's birthday.

Gerald Farthing, formerly Dormie Jerry Fart-ing, served 12-years as an Air Force pilot and married a belly dancer. The couple own Fart-ing Enterprises, a sales outlet for tofu products.

Other campus notables had divergent careers that spanned a spectrum of endeavors.

*Wanda Majic sold Yearning Arms in the mid-Sixties, when tear gas from the Free Speech demonstrations put a damper on business. Wanda moved to Nevada where she opened a popular brothel named Back In The Saddle. Retiring in 1981, Wanda was elected Nevada Congresswoman, running on a pro-business platform.

*Pritti (Sascha) Diva attended medical school after Wanda Majic closed Yearning Arms. Dr. Diva is a successful eye surgeon in the Contra Costa bedroom community of Lafayette.

*Jericho Slabio gave up public speaking after he failed to earn his PhD within 15-years. Slabio is a prosperous Amway salesman.

After leading the Bears to an upset victory over Ohio State in the Rose Bowl - the last time Cal went to Pasadena - Joe L. Capp became Cal's football coach, then Athletic Director for 25 frustrating years.

*Tom Hobknob replaced Dirk Krum as IFC President in 1960. Hobknob is serving his 17th term as Congressman from Santa Barbara.

Student body president, Ralph Van de Kamp, made and lost several fortunes in junk bonds. In early retirement, Van de Kamp participated in a landmark medical study for a revolutionary new drug for male erectile dysfunction.

*Stefan Tillich - backed by Dormie and non-org support - succeeded Van de Kamp as ASUC Student Body President. Tillich owns a string of upscale lap dance clubs in The City frequented by foreign tourists, especially dictators from emerging countries, newly recognized by the United Nations.

*Pete Mewell coached "Mewell's Mules" to an NCAA basketball championship and the USA Olympic team to a gold medal. Still active in his 90's, Mewell runs an annual camp for point guards in Kauai.

T A Brewster, Casey's competitor in Frisbee at the Big C Sirkus, became a popular folks singer, then a respected movie actor, under the stage name, Geoff Geoffstopherson.

Monty Maitland, the penny-pitching hustler, played minor league baseball before turning to sports officiating. Maitland is Executive Director of the Major League Umpires Association.

*Disgusted by the crowds and the National Guard generated by the Free Speech Movement, Ludwig Von Schwaren moved to Sonoma County where he died peacefully in 1972. Ludwig's Fountain, in Sproul Plaza, still bears his name.

*Lotta Ackshon dropped out of school after her twisted affair with Jericho Slabio and became a Carmelite nun.

Portions of the campus forest were bulldozed in the 60's and 70's, making way for the construction of sterile, blocky edifices to accommodate the influx of Baby-Boomers.

A charmless, modern monolith now towers over the Mining Circle where the Big C Sirkus competition once raged. An annex to Doe Memorial Library replaced the wooden T-Buildings after 50-years as "temporary" offices.

Cal's bucolic charm and architectural gems have, for the most part, endured the onslaught of modern progress.

Strawberry Creek continues to swirl and gurgle beneath Memorial Stadium, through Faculty Glade, and past the eucalyptus grove.

Descendants of Brutus, the chirpy squirrel, still inhabit the family estate in the Old Buckeye tree, in Faculty Glade.

*Camphor-scented Eucalyptus Grove is still a barrier against prevailing Bay winds. On his retirement, Professor Ari Scott donated a permanent wooden bench where, once-a-day, the singular shaft of sunlight pierces the thick canopy of blue gum eucalyptus, highlighting the site of his former, temple of camphor.

South Hall was spared from the wrecking ball; and, with its bulky neighbors, Wheeler and Dwinelle, remains the central axis of the Cal campus. The nude panels Mary Sather once had removed as an affront to the memory to her husband, Peter, are now a part of Sather Gate.

*Senior Men's Hall was renamed Senior Hall when the Order of the Golden Bear Honor Society accepted female members. The OGB still meets in the "secret" back room behind the stone fireplace.

The stately, clubby comfort of Morrison Library reading room remains an island of quiet civility, while the Mining Building is still a symbol of the timeless beauty of Beaux Arts architecture.

*Anthony Hall - with its bronze Pelican statue - now houses the Cal Institute of Humor. The fireplace mantle still bears the inscription:

"Be Good - If you can't Be Good - Be Careful"

*Sproul Hall, the site of the Free Speech Movement, became a backdrop for scenes from the 1967 movie, *"The Graduate."*

*Under the guidance of Werner Von Seller, the Cyclotron tripled in size. On a clear night, approaching jets can see the Cyclotron glowing blue and gold as it smashes atoms.

*Women's Gym has been converted to academic studies and houses the Graduate Center for Junk Food Nutrition.

*Doe Memorial Library houses the second largest university book collection in the country, trailing only Yale.

*Dooch Dorm, now co-educational, displays the goalposts toppled by Dormies after the historic upset of USC in 1959.

*Berkeley's Women's Club, blessed with its Beaux Arts architecture, is headquarters for the World Peace and Freedom Movement to Legalize Marijuana.

*Harmon Gym's classic Art-Deco facade was preserved in 2000 by a magnificent renovation and expansion creating the multi-purpose Walter A. Haas Jr. Pavilion, housing the Mewell Basketball Court.

*The vacant hole where Phoebe Appleton Hall for the Advancement of Female Studies once stood was turned into a tree-lined, Koi fish pond, an area of peaceful solitude, in the middle of the bustling campus

History has not always been kind to public figures of the late 1950's and early 1960's.

After Congress dismantled HUAC, Clayborn Muck remained active in national politics for three decades. Between 1964 and 1996, Muck was the presidential candidate of the Christian Anti-Communist Party, finishing a dismal last in each of his nine runs for the White House, breaking Harold Stassen's record for futility.

William Randolph Chandler took an opposite tack. The revelations of the *Scott v. Scott* child custody trial derailed his political ambitions. After losing his gubernatorial bid, the embittered WRC became a recluse, at the family estate, Xanadu, until his death in 1981.

Cee Cee Chandler Scott was appointed by her father WRC, Society Editor of *The Gazette*. Later, Cee Cee became a born-again Christian and married television evangelist Jimmy Faretheewell.

Muck's henchman, Seymour Graft, reinvented himself and started a new career in show business as Willie D. Wadd, producer of infamous porno movies. Since 1980, Wadd has lived as a retiree and registered sex offender in the Mojave Desert community of Blythe.

*In 1968, Colonel McReynolds Jones was awarded a posthumous, Congressional Medal of Honor for "courage above and beyond the call of duty" when he fearlessly drew enemy machine gun fire, allowing a platoon of young recruits to escape a Viet Cong ambush.

For decades, San Francisco wrestled with its civic schizophrenia. Proud of the Manhattanization of its skyline, Ess Eff remained narcissistically deluded in its self-image as romantic Baghdad-by-the-Bay perpetuated by Sam's *Paean to the City*.

In a moment of illogical weakness, Sam and E Lyn Chamberlin married in 1960 and divorced a year later, both realizing that Paean's true love and mistress was The Column. E Lyn continued as Sam's trusty assistant for five years after the divorce.

Sam continued to write *Sam's Paean to The City* until his death in 1998. At his memorial service, the University of California awarded Paean an honorary degree in Journalism.

E Lyn later married a wealthy widower who was elected Mayor of The City for most of the 1970's. Because of her second husband's long tenure in office, E Lyn became known as "Mrs. San Francisco."

San Francisco's institutions and citizens chronicled in Paean's column, as "notables and quotables" flourished.

In retirement, famed transvestite, Paulette DuBois, entertained at senior citizen communities.

*Jani Kay Fong spent ten years as a staff reporter for the *Sentinel* until her hire by the *New York Times* where she won a Pulitzer Prize for investigative journalism.

*Madame Lee (Abigail Krum Lee) remained a dominant social force in Chinatown until her death in 1982. The *Sentinel* reported her funeral procession, over three miles long, was the largest in San Francisco history. She is buried at the St. Mary's Chinese Cemetery.

*Calphung Quock was elected CEO of the Chinatown Chamber of Commerce. He married a former Miss San Francisco Chinatown, and their five children attended schools and universities in England.

*Mona Morgan was the first woman appointed to the San Francisco Superior Court. As a single working mother, Mona raised two Viet Nam orphans whose adoption was facilitated by lifetime lover, "Fitz."

*Marvin Belly made a career of suing insurance companies. After losing the custody battle in *Scott v. Scott*, Belly refused to accept any other divorce cases. Marvin was married and divorced eight times.

*Judge Robie Phillips was elevated to the California Supreme Court and served until his death in 1993.

*Dawna Plumber earned a PhD from Stanford in Hindu Studies. After teaching throughout the sub-continent, she returned to Palo Alto and formed a radical feminist group.

*Barnaby Person closed El Toro to protest The Pyramid. Person moved to the south of France where he writes travel books and runs a bistro for ex-patriots.

*In the 1980's, The Pyramid was sold to a Japanese conglomerate and still commands The City's skyline. Its new owners renamed it The Mount Fuji West Building.

*Clement Street is now called the "new Chinatown" with over 100-Chinese restaurants packed into six square blocks.

*At the Tahitian Room of the Hotel Mark Fairmont, the tropical rainstorm still rages at the end of each musical set.

*At Lake Tahoe, life continued on a predictable course.

*Will Bartone retired as Sheriff of Zephyr Cove in 1965 and hired on as a part-time greeter for Hurry's Casino until his death in 1975.

*Ted Grebits provided guided, moonlight tours of Lake Tahoe from Homewood until his death in 1984.

*Howard Muse took Kerrs beer through a profitable Initial Public

Offering (IPO) and retired after the death of his mother. Muse established the non-profit Preserve Lake Tahoe Foundation before his death in 1981. He was buried next to his mother, Miss Kerrs.

*Billy Hurry built three high-rise hotel casinos and became the largest employer in the State of Nevada. He married beautiful, blackjack dealer, Kandace Kaltwell, and continued to restore antique cars and boats until his death in 1979.

*The Tahoe Tavern served its last meal on September 5, 1964. Her furnishings were sold at auction, and the complex was demolished, making way for a condominium complex.

*The wreckage of the *SS Tahoe* was located at the bottom of Lake Tahoe. Private funds are being solicited by *National Geographic* to raise the steamer from her watery grave.

*Despite the use of mini-submarines, the site of the rumored, underwater cemetery of perfectly preserved corpses in the deepest part of Lake Tahoe has yet to be located.

True Love Ways had many twists and turns.

Anna Cappuccino married a Cal graduate student and returned to Italy to teach at Milan University and raise her two children. After the assassination of Pablo Zarzana, Anna entered politics and enjoyed a brilliant political career, culminating in her election in 1998 as the first female Prime Minister of Italy.

Ari Scott taught Medieval Philosophy and coached the Bear track team until 1974, when he retired to marry Anna's mother, Sofia Cappuccino, widow of Pablo Zarzana. Now in their 80's, Ari and Sofia share their golden years along the shores of Lake Como, enjoying visits from their Italian and American grandchildren.

Dirk Krum III was admitted to the Napa Valley Institution for the Incurably Insane in 1965, after Kate Howell spurned his repeated marriage proposals. Krum spends his days watching a video of *"High Society,"* in which Grace Kelly and Bing Crosby singing *"True Love."*

*The Kate Howell-Casey Lee romance became a casualty of the traumatic upheaval of the '60's - Civil Rights, Viet Nam, Kennedy-King assassinations, drugs and rock & roll - although both realized in retrospect: no love is as pure and perfect as First Love.

Casey Lee became a professional song writer. His musical *Dormie* displaced *Grease* as the longest running show on Broadway. He married country-western singer, Em Hanna, and the couple live with their adopted daughter, Katie, along the waters of Long Island.

Kate Howell never married.

During the '67 Summer of Love, the Golden Goddess had a brief romance with the son of an oil sheik. The affair produced twin boys who were kidnaped by their father and spirited to the Middle East. A year later, the children were rescued in a daring paramilitary operation by a squad of former Green Berets led by Royal French. With her inheritance from her aunt, Crazy Martha's estate, Kate Howell moved to Big Sur where she raised her twins, Casey and Lee.

Silver-haired and still stunning, Kate Howell lives alone in a glass aerie on a rocky outcrop high above the pounding surf of the Pacific Ocean. Occasionally, during the burnished glow of sunset, the former Golden Goddess sips *Glen Livet* and meanders through the recesses of her memory, calling up echoes of that soothing voice, envisioning the indelible image of those exotic eyes, recalling her halcyon days as a member of the House of Beauty . . . and Cal.

Mementos of this by-gone era took on unexpected prominence.

*The picture of JFK, RFK, and Miss Burdick, snapped by Jonathan, is part of the Campanile's celebrity visitors photo wall.

*Rod Organ's yellow and chrome woodie taxi is displayed at San Francisco's Museum of Modern Art as "classic art in action."

*The P U's Seeburg KD200 Select-O-Matic found its way to Seattle's EMP (Experience Music Project) where it is displayed as an antique of the golden age of 45 rpm singles. Frozen in time, in the Select-O-Matic, is the last selection before the sewer flood of '59 shorted out the juke box: Connie Francis's, *"Among My Souvenirs."*

*Lizard's nude mural that adorned the fence surrounding the former site of Phoebe Appleton Hall became a famous poster in the Haight-Ashbury of San Francisco in 1967, the Summer of Love. First edition copies can be purchased on an Internet auction site for $1,000.

*The pair of dice Waz rolled during the Dormies' Beatnik gambling RF is on display at the Gambling Museum of Hurry's Hotel-Casino, South Lake Tahoe, Nevada.

An engraved, brass plaque commemorates the event:

> *"On New Year's Eve, 1959, a young*
> *craps player used this pair of dice*
> *to roll a record 52-straight passes*

At the end of the hour-long roll,
the shooter had won only several
hundred dollars, to the relief of.
Hurry's nervous Pit Bosses."

At the Rock and Roll Museum, in Cleveland, in a darkened corner of a floor dedicated to the pioneers of rock and roll, a single beam of light illuminates a glass case sitting on a black marble pedestal.

Visitors, studying the exhibit, wear headphones attached to CD's playing Buddy Holly's hit recordings: *"That'll Be The Day," "True Love Ways," "Maybe Baby," "Peggy Sue," and "Every Day."*

Affixed to the display is a small mounted, sterling silver plaque:

"Buddy Holly Died In A Small Plane Crash
February 3, 1959 - His Glasses
Recovered & Donated By Fan,
Jonathan Aldon

Within the case, a pair of black hornrim glasses rest on a scarlet cushion turning slowly on a golden, lazy susan.

As the hornrims rotate, visitors scrutinize the scuff marks on the frames, squint at the minute bubbling of the skull temples, and stare at the clear, unblemished lenses.

Unnoticed is a single thread that begins as a knot at the bridge, follows a crease, then curls out of sight beneath the cushion. Unseen at the end of the tether is the remnant of an ancient ice cream stick.

On the frayed shard of wood, in a faint, childlike scrawl, are the penciled words,

. . . Not Fade Away - Crunchy Munchy . . .

BIBLIOGRAPHY

Bell, Jim. *Tahoe's Gilded Age* 2000

Campus Planning Study Group. *Campus Historic Resources Survey*: University of California 1978

Fong-Torres, Ben. *Louie On Parade*: SF Chronicle May 1988

Garchick, Leah. *For Whom The Bells Toll? A Carillon Call Around The World:* SF Examiner August 1978

Gentry, Curt. *J. Edgar Hoover - The Man and The Secrets* 1992

Helfand, Harvey. *Campus Guide - University of California, Berkeley* 2002

Kantor, James. (Ed) *Centennial Records of the University of California:* University of California 1974

Matteucci, David. *College Pranks of The Sixties* 2002

Paltridge, James Gilbert. *A History of the Faculty Club at Berkeley* 1992

Peri, Camille. *Ivory Tower*: SF Examiner Showcase March 1986

Pfaff, Timothy. *Leaves Of Class*: California Monthly May 1982

Scott, E. B. *The Saga of Lake Tahoe Vol. II* 1985

ISBN 141200124-2

9 781412 001243